are systematically interrelated, it is argued, they turn into their opposites. The system is thereby shown to be internally consistent and inclusive. The final section of the book deals in fresh and searching ways with such basic questions as the One and the Many and the nature of knowledge, both in general and as having a bearing on the philosophic system.

In tone and content *Modes of Being* is decidedly speculative. A pioneer work, it is nevertheless the result of thirty years of strenuous and sincere reflection inspired by the determination to do justice to all the principal aspects of knowledge and being.

A new, creative enterprise, *Modes of Being* challenges in a radical way both the analytic approach now dominant in Anglo-American thought and the existentialist trends so characteristic of the continent today. In this respect, especially, the book will be of interest to students of art, history, and literature, as well as to philosophers and theologians.

PAUL WEISS is the founder and editor of the *Review of Metaphysics* and the founder and first president of the Metaphysical Society of America. He is a former Guggenheim Fellow. In 1954 he was the Orde Wingate Lecturer at the Hebrew University in Jerusalem. He is also a consultant for the Great Books Foundation and for the Institute of Philosophical Research and a member of the board of *Philosophy of Science* and of *Science and Culture*. His previous works include *Nature of Systems* (1929), *Reality* (1938), *Nature and Man* (1947), and *Man's Freedom* (1950). Since 1946 he has been a professor of philosophy at Yale University.

D1233070

Modes of Being

Other Publications of Paul Weiss

By Paul Weiss

MODES
OF BEING

SOUTHERN ILLINOIS UNIVERSITY PRESS

CARBONDALE, 1958

© 1958 BY SOUTHERN ILLINOIS UNIVERSITY PRESS
LIBRARY OF CONGRESS CATALOG CARD NO. 57-11877

PRINTED IN THE UNITED STATES OF AMERICA BY
VAIL-BALLOU PRESS, INC., BINGHAMTON, NEW YORK

AB

TO MY CHILDREN

A WHILE BACK I completed a manuscript for a book about this size. I showed it to Richard Sewall, a most perceptive friend. He said it was hard to know what the work was about; it seemed to have no focus, no thesis, and to offer very few clues as to where it was going and how. When, because of his reaction, I once again reread what I had written, I thought his criticisms quite just. Throwing away some of the manuscript, treating other parts as material for articles, and putting the rest aside, I thereupon sat down to state as clearly as I could the pivotal points around which my discussion had ranged. The result was a new book, the heart of which was contained in some four hundred brief propositions, divided into four chapters. Those propositions, somewhat modified, are the theses of Chapters 1 to 4. Despite a most enthusiastic response which this new work elicited from such perceptive philosophers as Jacob Taubes, Irwin C. Lieb, Ellen Haring, and W. H. Sheldon, and despite the endorsement of a number of publishers' readers, I could not interest reputable publishers in the work. It seemed to them that the propositions were not self-explanatory, that they often sounded dogmatic and sometimes even wilfully paradoxical. I thought it wise, therefore, to try to clarify and justify the propositions, and I consequently set about to provide commentaries for each of them, in the guise of essential distinctions and proofs and necessary analyses. The shape of most of the commentaries was determined in good part by my need to make the propositions clear and plausible to a very able and highly critical group of graduate students, and to take care of searching criticisms made by Ellen Haring, Nathan Rotenstreich, and W. H. Sheldon. Each proposition could use much more explication than it now receives. But mindful of my experience with the original manuscript, I have thought it most desirable to keep the commentaries brief. To make them longer would be to risk once more losing the opportunity to see the system and thus presumably the universe as a whole.

Preceding the four chapters of pivotal propositions and commentaries is an introductory essay which places the work in relation to what is being done in philosophy today, and offers a kind of autobiographical account of the way in which the four crucial ideas of the book developed. These chapters are followed by a section offering a brief formulation of some of the denials that could be made to what is here said. These denials, it is contended, mute one another, and taken together add up to what has been affirmed. The next section deals with the nature of the system as a whole. In addition to summarizing and interrelating some of the major points made earlier, it discusses the basic problems which any system acknowledging a plurality of realities must face. At the very end, all the pivotal propositions are re-presented without comment, in order to provide an easy means of reference and to make it possible for the reader readily to envisage the intent of the entire work.

The above paragraphs were written as the preface of a multilithed edition of this book. I used that edition in my graduate classes last year, and distributed it privately to various philosophers who were interested in the work. I also subjected it to a rather close rereading and took account of the criticisms made by my colleagues, students, and friends—particularly those made by Charles Hendel, Robert Brumbaugh, and Vere Chappell. As a consequence I found it necessary to rewrite a good deal of it. Many of the changes are in the form of rephrasings and shifts in nuance, but I did find it occasionally necessary to make some radical restatements, deletions, and additions. It is now at the stage where I, at least, can make no further appreciable improvements; it must at last be allowed to be free of me, and I perhaps of it.

It would be wrong to let the work appear without notice being taken of the signal sensitivity, interest, and judgment shown by Mr. Vernon Sternberg and his excellent staff of Southern Illinois University Press. I have been indeed fortunate to have had the benefit of their thoughtfulness, wisdom, and help.

P.W.

December, 1956

CONTENTS

Part III. THE MODES TOGETHER

Modes of Being

THIS IS a book in philosophy. As a philosophic work should, it attempts to articulate a vision of the whole of things. This means that it must run counter to the temper not only of critics of philosophy but of many contemporary philosophers as well. Every one of us, in these last decades, has often heard the complaint that the world of knowledge has grown enormously and that it is now too big for anyone to envisage. Too many of us have too quickly said that it is futile to hope that the meaning of the whole, or even of man's place within it, can be grasped by anyone. A man must be content, it has been supposed, to master limited branches of knowledge, to try to learn exactly what is the case here or there; he should give up the attempt to say something more. No one seemed to have a real fear that such self-restraint might turn him into a partial man. Encyclopedias and staff conferences, surveys and texts, it was felt, could bring him and all the rest together and in harmony. Co-operation, interchange, and communication would produce well-made parts, and interrelate them, to give a clearer, more lasting, a better articulated account of whatever fraction of the totality of things was available for knowledge. As a consequence, many today are somewhat content to be community thinkers, union men, who know how to work together.

It seems safe to say that the intellectual advances made in recent years over a wide range of disciplines are in good part traceable to the fact that we have specialized together. But it is equally safe to say that these achievements depended in part on our refusal to use our rational powers to the full. A world of experts, each concerned with asserting only what he himself really knows, is a world of men who must accept without cavil what the other experts offer to them as data, method, and outcome—or it is a world of separated items, cut off from all else. Such experts practice what none is willing to preach. On the one side they accept nothing but what they can themselves certify, and on the other they embrace with equal confidence that which they confessedly could not possibly certify.

He who simply accepts whatever others affirm unwarrantedly supposes that those others are right in result, method, and value. He does not really know whether or not their frames are wide enough, their methods sound enough, their values rich enough for the world in which we all live. By putting the actual failure or inadequacy of other disciplines outside the reach of real questioning he denies himself the opportunity of knowing whether or not they are really sound, and whether or not they will ever betray him. To know how reliable other disciplines are, he must know something more than what they report of themselves.

It is fairly safe to say that the successes of our modern ways of thought depend in good part on the chance that the methods and outcomes of our different specialized inquiries happen for the time to fit together. When parts are dealt with in independence of one another, discords almost inevitably arise among them. Even now different disciplines are sometimes found to conflict. The realms of specialized knowledge are not yet integrated. There are methods and results in almost every vigorous science which no one has made cohere with the rest. Nor has anyone ever related the achievements and methods of all the sciences to one another, or brought the natural sciences into harmony with history, law, and anthropology. And what has been discerned by the poets, the mystics, the philosophers is still far from being united with what has been learned elsewhere.

But, it will perhaps be said, this is as it should be. Every living enterprise is incomplete; its problems are its nerve ends, its growth tips. It would be foolhardy to force the different disciplines into harmony now, to try to get rid of the gaps in and between them at once. The critical powers, it can justly be urged, should not be suspended, nor should they be allowed to destroy the tolerance on which co-operative inquiry depends. We should be patient. The occasional breaks and discords in and between the different disciplines will soon and surely must eventually be overcome. Knowledge is accumulative and grows in cohesiveness as it grows in magnitude. Ignorance, and ignorance alone, is what keeps honest inquiring men apart.

There is force in this reply. We have a right to expect, as we progress in our mastery of the world and of ourselves, that what we know will form a more solid block than it now does. Yet, what might at the end of an inquiry have the status of knowledge in that inquiry may not have had that status when outside it or when it is made part of a different inquiry. There are certainties in some disciplines and only probabilities in others; some prefer local truths while others specialize in cosmic ones. Their different claims must be assigned different weights; account must be taken of their different methods and ranges. What we call knowledge in physics is not exactly what we call knowledge in history or philosophy or perhaps even biology. The items in one discipline are obtained along a different route and must meet criteria and be certified in ways not relevant to the items in other disciplines. It makes no difference whether or not we take one of the disciplines as the model for the others, or whether or not we look outside them all for some standard in terms of which we can determine what is and what is not knowledge. In either case we are forced to evaluate and perhaps modify or qualify the claims which each, even at the end of its road, takes to be reliable and true. Some, and perhaps even all of a given discipline's certified truths might have to be altered if they are to be brought into accord with the certified truths of other inquiries. Unless we can somehow stand outside all disciplines, unless we can somehow use common principles, categories, values, we cannot hope to adjudicate authoritatively the claims which each discipline makes even within its own framework; we can therefore have no surety that its results will ever form part of a single harmonious body of knowledge.

It seemed for a time as if this challenge would be accepted in a most promising way. A group of well-trained, meticulous, energetic "analytic" philosophers seemed willing to take as their task the discovery of criteria and principles by means of which the efforts and outcomes of the different disciplines could be evaluated and organized. Through a fresh union of modern logic, linguistics, and methodology, they produced a new discipline, and used this to promote and clarify other subjects. The gathering of data they left to others; it was not their task, they thought, to try to add more facts to those which the empirical sciences provided. They sought only to occupy themselves with a study of the structures, procedures, implications,

grammar that are inevitably exhibited in every sound scientific inquiry; nothing was sensible or legitimate, they claimed, unless it was
certifiable by the methods which such inquiries endorsed.

Bold, perhaps even a little arrogant and contemptuous of older
ways, these thinkers were nevertheless at once modest and cautious.
They said of themselves that they were just inquirers, without set
dogmas or pre-established goals. They sought only to be clear, precise, rigorous, and thorough. But very soon, and perhaps inevitably,
they turned themselves into another race of specialists, alongside the
others, concentrating on the quite restricted task of clarifying the
intent, language, usage, or practice of scientific men. They were
forced to take for granted the suppositions, methods, claims, tests,
and outcomes of fields which, by the very nature of the case, they
could not know firsthand or really master. As a consequence, while
presenting themselves as at once careful and open-minded, they rather
uncritically and dogmatically adopted views which should have been
examined, criticized, and perhaps discarded. The irony of history was
once more manifest: those who set themselves to be merely critical,
sceptical, hesitant, modest, often become great dogmatists.

These analysts have accomplished much. But they could not do all
that needs be done if knowledge is to make—at least in principle—
one exhaustive, coherent whole. For that, their specialty would have
to become all-encompassing. Not only the methods, assertions, structures, but the values and results of the various disciplines need evaluation. Ends as well as means must be critically examined. We must
know not only how sound the various procedures are but what place
the different results of the different disciplines can have within a
comprehensive account. But then something must be known of the
whole. We ought not be content to be solely one among many inquirers; we must also be a one for them, a one over against them,
including them and much else besides.

No one of course knows everything. No one even knows one limited field exhaustively. Yet if we did not somehow grasp the nature
of all there is, we would not be able to have specialties, nor could we
deal adequately with their different claims and contributions. Only if
we know what it is to be a man can we engage in co-ordinate investi-
gations into his nature; only if we know what it is to be a man can
we estimate the rival contentions of doctors, biologists, psychologists,

anthropologists, and the rest. Only if we know what it is to be, to inquire, to understand, can we recognize that we are all dealing with different phases of the same subject, and can know how to bring together the different results that were obtained along different routes of investigation. Before, while, and after we specialize, we have and must have a grasp of the whole, vague, blurred, and even incoherent though this may be. To ignore that whole is to ignore our roots, to misunderstand our aims, to lose our basic tests. It is to forget that we engaged in limited inquiries in order to understand what is real from many independent and, we hoped, convergent sides. It is to adopt the prejudice that only the limited and piecemeal is significant and intelligible, and that without any guidance each bit will inevitably form one seamless unity with all the rest. It is to be so impatient to get down to work that no time is left to ask what it is that is being sought, and why. If we are to engage in limited enterprises, if we are to know what they diversely seek and express, if we are to understand what contribution they can make to the enterprise of life and learning, we must somehow take account of all there is and can be known. Whether we wish it or not, we must, we do think cosmically. Our choice is only to do it uncritically, precipitately moving to the body of some limited enterprise and vainly trying to remain there always, or critically, by taking some thought of where we start and ought to end, and in a sense always are.

No matter how much this last observation be softened, it can, I fear, never be entirely freed from the smell of paradox and dogmatism, presumption and foolhardiness—and of decayed and discarded systems of the past. There is something repugnant in the temper of the grand philosophers, the system builders, the wholesale thinkers. They sound like gods and yet are only men. Even the best of them contradict themselves and one another, omit much that should have been included, and at crucial points are most unclear and unreliable. Their errors are fabulous. But then so is their vision. They leave us with no alternative but to try for ourselves to understand the real world in a way they could not. And this is possible, for they taught us through their achievements and by their failures something of what we ought to say and what we ought to avoid. And we also have at our disposal, as they unfortunately did not, such excellent guides and instruments as the history of later thought, modern science, modern poetry, modern music, modern painting, recent analysis, and symbolic logic.

There are today, I think, signs of a renewed interest in fundamental questions on the part of many thinkers. There is a new spirit just beginning to stir, transforming the world of ideas. Occupied primarily in getting a firm grip on reality, it has so far ignored the question of how to judge and adjudicate the various specialized inquiries. These must eventually look to it, and it to them. But first it must come to clearer and more systematic expression. What now seems likely is that a re-examination of fundamentals will force us to entertain a view of ourselves and of the world which is quite different from that entertained in the past.

We must become at once more bold and humble, more catholic and cautious, freer and more disciplined than before. For too long a time prejudice has been allowed to narrow our perspectives; for too long a time impatience has made us receptive to ideals and values not adequate to our full being and the world. We need a new viable systematic philosophy which is alert to the basic questions raised by the various sciences, by metaphysics and theology, by history and the arts, if we are to remain intellectually abreast of the world in which we live.

One of the objectives of the present work is to outline the nature of this new philosophy. Its main features were unknown to me until after I had struggled through the writing of three books. Reflections on the implications of the first of these drove me on to the second, and this in turn led to the third. The present book in a way continues the progress. An independent venture, it systematizes while it purges, moves beyond while it takes advantage of the previous works.

The first of the books, *Reality*, presented a systematic account of what I took to be the essential features of both knowledge and nature. It maintained that knowledge and nature presupposed one another, making the philosophic enterprise a circle, but one large enough to encompass all forms of thought and reality. Every item of knowledge and being was seen to be incomplete since there was something beyond it, real and obstinate, which it needed and sought. The book made an effort also to work, not as Russell does with a minimum vocabulary, or as others do with a minimum number of acceptable ideas or beliefs, but with a minimum number of presuppositions. It tried in fact to avoid taking for granted anything outside the system, except of course the world which that system portrayed. The world it knew was not philosophy; but philosophy, it also knew, had to omit nothing of the essence of the world.

It is sound, I still think, to hold that philosophy is a circle, that every item in thought and in being is incomplete, and that what a good philosophic account presupposes is not beyond its capacity to encompass conceptually. It is sound too, I think, to maintain as was done in *Reality*, that each thing necessarily points to all the others, as the object of its needs, what it must take account of in order to be complete. The rest of the world must be considered, if we are to understand a thing's nature and why it acts as it does. But the point needs supplementation. Alone it cannot stand, since it fails to do justice to what now seems to me to be a rather obvious truth.

If, as *Reality* maintains, each thing is directed towards and acts in terms of all the rest, no two things would have exactly the same objectives. No two would point in exactly the same direction. Each would act to realize a partly different objective, and thus a different prospective future from that which concerns others. Since the existence of each would be spent in the area defined by its distinct objective, there would be no assurance that any of them, contemporaries at one moment, will be contemporaries at the next. Each would confront the world from an independent standpoint; there would be no necessary connection between the various standpoints. Each being would have its own private time, and this would have its own characteristic rhythm, divisions, pace, not necessarily shared by other times. But then, what reason would there be for supposing that the private time of one would intermesh with the times characteristic of others; how could there be a single time and thus a single cosmos in which all things dwell together?

If each being is occupied with a future proper to it, it will endeavor to make it present in its own way and at its own pace. The different futures would of course share a number of features, making it possible to treat the things as members of various classes. But the things would not act in terms of those common features. The features, because abstractions from, derivatives of a set of disconnected singular objectives, could not possibly keep contemporary beings in temporal accord.

This is a serious difficulty, and not peculiar to the system explored in *Reality*. It faces Aristotle's philosophy, and Whitehead's too. Aristotle's contemporaneous objects move together in time, not on their own account, but because they are confined within a single spatial whole whose rhythms and pace limit the rhythms and pace of the subordinate realities within it. Whitehead's contemporaneous objects keep abreast in time, not because they must intrinsically do so but because the diverse final causes which govern them are under the supervision of an interested God. Whitehead here reminds one of Leibniz with his doctrine of a divinely pre-established harmony which guarantees that the independent adventures of things are in accord with one another. Aristotle here reminds one of Kant and his attempt to treat time as having two sides, the one private or ideal, the other public or actual, which, though quite different in purport and in experienced content, are thought somehow to have the same divisions and rate of passage. Aristotle and Kant overcame the difficulty, of showing how distinct beings can be persistently contemporary, by means of special cosmological assumptions; Whitehead and Leibniz did it by introducing a special theological twist. But these are exteriorly imposed devices. In principle these thinkers allow that things may move in time independently of one another and therefore may, if contemporary today, not be contemporary tomorrow. Yet no matter whether beings are sluggish or quick, asleep or awake, lost in privacies or engaged in public work, all, while living at their own pace, live together in a common time.

There are contemporary beings. Otherwise there would be nothing to interact with us, nothing with which we could be together, nothing which could limit us and thus define us as incomplete. And some beings, contemporary now, are contemporary later. All move into the next moment together, some altering in nature or position, others remaining unchanged or unmoved. One can imagine all of them in the grip of some single cosmic being, some dialectical force, or some all-encompassing power which both drives them forward and keeps them concordant. But this idea compromises the basic fact that it is individuals who act, and act in their own ways and at their own rates. The time through which I live is my own; if there be another time or temporal power keeping me abreast of others, it is more powerful than I and they, and wise beyond belief. There must of course be something common to us all, which limits and even controls us somewhat, so as to enable us, despite our independent existence and adventures in time, to be co-ordinate now and later. But if we suppose it to be something like a cosmic agent running alongside or overhead, keeping us adjusted one to the other, or some all-embracing time or being out of which the individual times are conjointly precipitated, we reverse an obvious state of affairs, since we then overlook the irreducible ultimacy of individuals, and the fact that it is they who spend energy and dictate what the common pattern of the world will be. Things are members of various groups, not because they happen to share some character but because they all have the same objective. Despite their individuality, spatiotemporal beings form a single contemporaneous set of actualities, because each inevitably points towards the very same prospect pointed towards by the rest. A number of them may further specify that common prospect in common ways, and thereby reveal themselves to be members of some more limited group as well. But whether they do this or not, each and every one of them acts as a distinct being, and thus brings the common objective to realization in an individual way.

It is desirable to show that there is and must be one objective, subtending whatever limited objectives individuals or groups of them may be directed towards. And it is important to know the nature of that common objective. *Nature and Man*, my next book, was written in part to satisfy these reasonable and therefore imperious demands. The book stresses the fact that the common objective is essential, that it is inseparable from the very being of individual things. Nothing existed, it saw, solely in the present; each being was partly in the future and was governed in part by that common objective in which it essentially terminated. This defined its direction, and, when specialized as a limited objective, defined the range of things the being could do.

The discovery that all beings inevitably point to the same common future objective made it possible to show how they could exist together in time even though they acted independently, and sometimes even came into conflict. And an awareness that the common objective was itself somewhat indeterminate in nature made it possible to understand why it needed realization and could be realized—questions which were unanswerable by Plato and others who, like him, recognize that there is a common objective to which all beings are directed, but who mistakenly suppose that it is itself perfect, complete, wholly determinate.

If one avoids the Platonic supposition that the idea of perfection is itself perfect, that the idea of the good is itself the best of beings, one could safely agree with Plato to call the common inescapable objective of all beings by that grandest of titles, The Good. A recognition of the nature and needs of that Good makes it possible to offer new ways of understanding the nature of causation, inference, action—all change in fact. Every occurrence, it could then be shown, is at once limited and free, occurring in the present but within bounds determined by what is still future. The separation of theories of artistic creation and logical deduction, of history and physics, which had ruined so many philosophies, could at last be avoided. Every act and thought, *Nature and Man* saw, was present, concrete, transitory. It recognized that they were unpredictable in their full concreteness, because produced only then and there, and thus were incapable of being known in advance. Every act and thought it also saw was, while still future, indeterminate and fixed but yet predictable because entailed by present actualities. Art and history, logic and physics have both an unpredictable and a predictable side, the first two stressing the one, the second two the other. Although they have different starting points, media, objectives, and go through different processes, they exhibit the same fundamental laws and principles.

Nature and Man affirmed, even more vigorously than did *Reality*, that man was not only an integral part of nature, but also a product of evolution. It tried to show that the advance which began with the inanimate, moved through the animate, and ended with man was the consequence of an occasional successful strategy on the part of frustrated beings. These, to overcome grave obstacles, to avoid defeat and annihilation, changed their directions, pointed to new relevant objectives, thereby becoming transformed in nature and in promise.

The book concluded that man, while distinct in kind and not merely in degree from all other beings, alone possessed a persistent self. That self stood out over against the body and the rest of the world because it alone was persistently occupied with the realization of that single, all-inclusive objective, The Good. And because he had a self, it said, man had self-identity, and was capable of self-discipline and self-criticism, privileges which were outside the reach of any other being in nature.

The position explored in *Nature and Man* does not I think have to be changed in any fundamental respect. But it has important implications which it did not pursue. It was one of the tasks of *Man's Freedom* to note these implications and to complete the account. The book stressed the fact that the Good was focused on and striven for by man, for the most part without consciousness but with a freedom peculiar to him. This freedom was exhibited primarily in three more and more effective and inclusive forms, as preference, choice, and will. They were man's primary agencies by which he freely adopted and tried to realize the all-inclusive Good.

Man does and man ought to try to bring the Good to its most complete realization. It is his task to do good, and nothing but good, to every being whatsoever. But he is finite, feeble, ignorant; he must inevitably fail to do what he ought. Man is the guilty animal. But this is paradox. That paradox cannot be overcome by narrowing the range of man's obligations. No area of responsibility is so small as to be within the power of man to fill completely. No one ever does all that ought to be done even to only one other being. No one does or can do all he ought, even to himself. A man has too little knowledge, too little strength, too unstable a constitution to be able to do full justice to the rights of any being. Nor can his knowledge, strength, and constitution be so improved that he will eventually do all he ought. Finite always, he will always fall short of his full obligations.

I find this paradox intolerable. My struggle with it led me to see my previous speculations as part of a much wider four-dimensional whole. Suggestions of the nature of those four dimensions can be found in *Reality* and in other places, but they became clear to me only when I turned to the study of ethics and saw the full force of the paradox that a man had obligations which he could not himself fulfill. As long as I worked with anything less than a four-pronged view I found that the paradox could not be resolved. One had, I became convinced, to distinguish and assume in turn the perspectives of four distinct realities—Actuality, Ideality, Existence, and God. All four, one had to affirm, are final, irreducible modes of being with their own integrity and careers. The universe they together exhaust requires for its understanding a system in which each is recognized to be as basic, as explanatory, and as incomplete as the others.

It is the task of this work to lay bare the nature of these four beings and to grasp something of the way they affect one another. Before engaging in it, it is desirable, I think, to know why it is necessary for any one—not only the author—to consider these four. It may be worth while too to have some preliminary idea of their diverse natures and roles.

Actualities are finite beings in space and time. To complete themselves they strive to realize relevant, essential objectives which, in different ways, they specify out of a single common future Good. Since man is the only Actuality who can focus on the Good in its full universal form, only he can seek to realize that Good in himself and in others. He cannot, as an individual, do full justice to that Good. That can be done only through the conjoint effort of all that there is. A man can hope to do all he ought only if he can accept as his own all the work done, on behalf of the Good, by all the rest. We would, with this observation, reach an end to our system were it not that we had presupposed Existence as an energizing field in which Actualities act. This terminates in the Good, and endows the divine with a temporal dignity. We also presupposed God as a unity in which all Actualities and the Good can be together, and in which Existence finds the unitary essence it needs in order to be intelligible. Both Existence and God are of course also presupposed by the Good; these sustain it in different but necessary ways.

And we ought to make a beginning with Good—or rather with the Ideal, which is the Good when this has been freed from an exclusive reference to realizing Actualities. It has a nature of its own, as is evident from the fact that it is striven for. Indeed it has power enough to attract a man and to make him concerned with its fulfillment. The Good is a correlate of Actualities, a possibility which acts to master Actualities by turning them into types, meanings, representatives of itself. From the standpoint of the Good all that ought to be done is done if whatever there be is idealized, turned into an instance of the Good. This action of the Good on Actualities is the reciprocal of action by those Actualities on it. And, like those Actualities, the Good presupposes material to work upon. Just as Actuality presupposes the Good, the Good presupposes Actuality, and both of them presuppose Existence and God as regions in which they can be together.

The Good is incomplete, indeterminate. It needs completeness, and achieves this only so far as it is fractionated into more determinate and limited forms of itself. It demands not specific activities by Actualities but the provision of opportunities so that it can transform those Actualities from what is external to it into what is subordinate. By offering the Actualities attractive objectives, desirable goals, commanding choices, obligating goods, restraining laws, and finally a luring destiny, it turns the Actualities into purposive, preferring, choosing, willing kinds of beings, into citizens of a state, and finally into beings who could fulfill themselves while enabling all other Actualities to be similarly idealized.

From the perspective of the Good men are required to adopt roles, to become public and representative beings. So far as they achieve this status the Good becomes determinate, not by virtue of the introduction of alien material, but by the Good's adoption of what for it are nothing more than diverse, fragmentary, and harmonious parts of itself. Man's task from the standpoint of the Good is the making of this fractionization easy, complete, and concordant, just as it is the task of the Good, from the standpoint of man, to be receptive of his efforts to make it concrete. The Good ennobles, universalizes Actualities when and as they sustain it, just as Actualities enrich the Good, make it concrete when and as it lures and guides them.

Actualities and the Ideal, even when made one by mastery or fractionization, have an integrity of their own, continue to enjoy an independent status. An examination of them separately and in relation to one another enables us to encompass much of what is—but not all. God and Existence are also essential realities, inescapable dimensions of the universe, illuminating what is left dark by the joint use of the perspectives of Actuality and Ideality.

God is that being who, among other things, makes a unity of what otherwise would be a detached set of occurrences. He sees to it that the Ideal is realized, and that Actualities are perfected. This means that men should recognize that they inevitably submit themselves and their acts to God, as the being who alone can make them adequate to the demands of the Ideal. Since men, their acts, and their

aspirations are part of a realm of Existence, where alone they can
be vital and present, no account of God can be complete which forgets that Existence is his counterweight, the locus of the data he
supports and interrelates.

Existence is a restless force at once ingredient in and overflowing
the borders of Actualities, connecting each with every other and
coming to a focus in the Ideal. Actuality and Ideality are consequently
subject to a single, cosmic flux. But any study which begins with
Existence should be supplemented with accounts where God, the
Ideal, and the Actual are recognized to have independent natures
and functions. Without them there would be no unified world of
values, no focused and uniting futures, and no distinct loci of action.

Actuality, the Ideal, Existence, and God are data for one another.
Each has a role to play in relation to the others, and requires the
others to assume a role for it. In addition, all merge with and qualify
one another. They can have these different functions only because
each has an irreducible, final being of its own, outside of which and
over against which the others are. Each stands out against the rest
as possessing a distinctive career and a characteristic way of dealing
with the others. Actualities strive to be completely adjusted to all
there is; the Ideal strives to encompass everything; Existence is engaged
in a perpetual effort to separate itself off from all else; God strives
to make unity present everywhere. Each helps and restrains the
others, making it possible for them to attain a greater success than
they otherwise could, and preventing them from ever achieving perfect success. No one of them can ever advance beyond the stage
where it is but one of a number of beings. Being is diversely and exhaustively exhibited in four interlocked, irreducible modes.

This swift survey through which I have just gone will arouse
rather than quiet a number of persistent questions and doubts: Is
there a real need to acknowledge as many as four fundamental, irreducible realities? Are just the items here isolated *the* modes of
being? Is there not a need to acknowledge five or six or perhaps
even a greater number, as basic and as essential as any of these? The
work as a whole, and particularly the last chapters offer answers to
these questions. But it may help now to remark that no one can
avoid acknowledging something Actual, for that is what each one of

us is, and what each one of us daily confronts. But Actuality can be made intelligible, we will find, only if account is taken of the other three modes as well. Each of these three in turn demands the acknowledgment of Actuality and two other modes. Each mode requires at least three others. We cannot acknowledge any less than four modes without being confronted with insoluble problems, and without making something in the nature or function of the universe unnecessarily mysterious or unintelligible. But there is no need to acknowledge more than four, until and unless there are difficulties which cannot be resolved except by taking this further step. One ought not to multiply entities beyond necessity.

Each mode stands apart from the rest, and is also a component in them. Each offers evidence regarding the nature and reality of the others. But so long as we remain with any one of them, those others will seem to be nothing more than attenuations of it, imagined or fanciful objects, or the termini of hazardous inferences. One must get over to where those others are. Nothing less than an adequate grasp of the other modes in their own terms will enable us to have the data in terms of which an initially accepted mode can be fully understood. There are many ways in which this result can be achieved. Dialectic is a primary way, but there is also sympathy and imagination, direct encounter and a use of abstractions. All will be acknowledged in their appropriate places.

Each mode of being needs the others to enable it to be itself. The universe is an interlocked whole of four modes of being, no one of which can be unless the others also are effective in it, and effective apart from it. The names that have here been assigned to them may occasionally prove misleading, for while the ideas are somewhat new the language is rather old. Some of the functions of the modes have perhaps even been misconstrued, for not all parts of the cosmos come equally well into the focus of one endeavor. In view of the manner in which the view gradually unfolded, and in the light of our western tradition's emphasis on things and men, and its readiness to look with suspicion at anything which is not directly known, there may be an undue stress here on Actuality. The greatest obstacle in the way of understanding what is here intended is, more likely than not, the author's and perhaps the reader's tendency to minimize the reality or the function of the Ideal, Existence, or God. Completeness and impartiality require that all four modes be dealt with as equally basic, equally real, equally indispensable.

We are confronted, evidently, with a vast and complex set of ideas. It is desirable to bring them within a small compass, so that they can be readily grasped in themselves and in their bearing on one another. The warming flesh of rhetoric must be cut away, and the somewhat ugly naked musculature of a systematic account exposed. In the following four chapters I have tried to make evident the pivotal ideas which the foregoing sketch hints at and demands. I have tried to state with stark simplicity those truths which seem to me to be important either by virtue of the facts which support them, the arguments on which they rest, or the light they throw on what else there is. There are definitions here and there, but for the most part, the distinguished numbered assertions are conclusions rooted in observation and sustained by dialectic. The accompanying commentary usually provides the evidence, argument, or explanation.

The various theses which are here isolated are all on a level, offered as equally basic and true. Those that are presented later should however help to articulate or develop those presented earlier, at the same time that they fixate some new facet of reality. Ideally it should be possible to make a start with any one of them and to utilize the others so as to articulate or develop it, at the same time that these others are used to focus on and to explain some further phenomenon. Strictly speaking, the four chapters that follow, and the theses in them as well, are all co-ordinate. They could have been presented in a different order. For convenience's sake I have tried so far as possible to avoid making forward references.

PART I

The Four Modes

CHAPTER I

Actuality

I THE IMPERFECTION OF ACTUALITIES

1.01 An Actuality is a being in space.

(See 4.62)

WHATEVER we empirically encounter is spatial. What is not spatial may be experienced, imagined, expected, remembered, lived through. It may be an idea, a mathematical entity, and even space itself. Though these have some reality, and even somewhat independent careers of their own, they are derivatives from, dependent on, or parts of what is empirically encountered.

Some Actualities are more than physical or chemical entities; they are quickened by a life or sustained by a unitary self. But this means only that Actualities are of various kinds. Actualities are any beings that have or are bodies.

Actualities are spatial, and they are in space. This space in which they are is a domain of symmetrical, extended relations. There are no relations, however, without terms, and spatial relations are no exception. The being of space is inseparable from the Actualities which are related in and by means of space.

Space is not a form or matrix which men impose on what otherwise would be nonspatial. Not only are things in space even when no one attends to them, but the imposition of a spatial frame on nonspatial beings will not make them spatial. A nonextended entity remains nonextended even when looked at through spatial spectacles. Nor is space a concept. As Kant observed, a concept is unextended and has subordinate members or constituent parts; but space is extended, single, and its parts are only delimited portions of it. Nor is space a substance, a concrete entity; it lacks finality, individuality, and the capacity to act. But it has a status apart from the objects in it, for all of them can be replaced by others. In fact it has properties and a structure, an extensive geometry of its own.

Possessed of some reality and with an independent nature, space is nevertheless dependent on Actualities to provide it with terms, while it in turn offers them a place in which to be contemporary and in which they can move, be in contact, and be over against one another.

1.02   Some Actualities are active.
(See 1.44)

TO ACT is to produce, to make something come about. It is to cause. The causation may involve the use of bodies, or it may occur solely in the mind. There is activity when one thinks and when one communicates, as well as when one pushes or resists or merely maintains one's ground.

What is normally termed an activity is a series or combination of unit activities, each of which begins at one moment, at a "cause," and ends at another, an "effect." Just how long a unit activity lasts is a difficult matter to determine, but for the present purpose it is sufficient to note that every activity, a unit or larger, links a cause with a subsequent effect. An activity takes time; it is temporal, a process of causation which together with the cause issues in the effect. This does not mean that only the nature of antecedent causes and the process of causation need be known in order to understand what the effect will be. In some cases activity is guided by the prospect of the effect that is to ensue, in which case an understanding of the effect will require a reference not only to the antecedent or efficient cause and the process of causation or activity, but to a final cause as well.

1.03   "Some Actualities are active" is necessarily true.
(See 1.02)

IN 1.02 the fact of activity was affirmed. The present proposition maintains that the denial of that affirmation is absurd, for the denial of it would require activity on the part of an actual man. The denial of "Some Actualities are active" therefore necessarily presupposes its truth. That denial is of course not self-contradictory, internally at odds with itself, known to be absurd because of what it says by itself. It is not, in short, logically absurd. But it is existentially absurd, absurd in the sense that what it says is at odds with its own occurrence. This absurdity is significant, so that what it opposes must be not only necessary but significant as well. "Some Actualities are active" is a synthetic though unavoidable truth, presupposed both by its affirmation and its denial.

1.04 Some Actualities cannot act.
(See 1.02)

THERE ARE Actualities which have neither aims nor energy of their own. Their characteristic careers are the resultants of the activities of their parts. Such Actualities are compounds. These are of two types, aggregates or wholes. An aggregate, e.g., 'this table and that shoe,' has no other nature but that which results from the mere conjunction of its components. A whole, such as a stone or a piece of paper, has a nature of its own. Unlike an aggregate, it has a career, though like an aggregate, it has no power of its own. Wholes are not true substances, with individuality, interiority, and aim. But they have a kind of logos, a rationale, limiting the kind of things which their active constituents together can bring about.

1.05 There are two types of primary, or active, Actuality: simple and complex.
(See 1.01, 1.03)

SIMPLE primary Actualities are spatial beings. They have a magnitude. Mathematically they can be divided further, but ontologically, in fact, they are ultimate units, quanta beings. One of the persistent searches of science is for such primary Actualities, in terms of which all others are to be understood as the outcome of some mode of aggregation or compounding. There are, however, complex primary Actualities as well. Organisms are complex, but unlike compounds they have careers whose natures are not wholly determined by the actions of their constituents. They have a power of action all their own; they can, in fact, so act as to limit the actions and thereby dictate to the natures and careers of their constituents. Although a man is a complex Actuality, he is capable of actions by which he expresses himself as a single being and in which he dictates—as when he moves about—just when the primary Actualities in him are to move across space, and where.

It is a hard question to determine whether or not trees, sponges, etc. are genuine complex but primary Actualities, since they seem to lack the individuality and unity characteristic of such Actualities. But there seems to be no doubt but that all animals, birds, and fish are Actualities of this type.

Atomists tend to deny that there can be any complex primary Actualities. Humanists tend to deny that there can be any simple primary Actualities. The former hold that any complexity is but a confused or blurred external conjunction of simple Actualities; the latter hold that any simple Actuality is but an abstract and fictional derivative from such a complex primary Actuality as man. Both evidently affirm correctly but deny wrongly.

1.06 Actualities are temporal beings.
(See 1.05)

THE INITIAL presentation of Actualities as beings in space in 1.01 made it necessary for us to take for granted only a spatial world. Time was evidently presupposed in the discussion from 1.02 on. What is now being stressed is that even a stable world of Actualities is temporal. Such a world is the product of activity, but one which reinstates the nature or situation that had been before.

It is hard to see how Aristotle could do justice to the idea of rest. For him rest is the opposite state from motion, related to it as zero is to some quantity. When he comes to discuss the vacuum he finds grave difficulty in any attempted passage from a density of any degree to a density of zero degree. A similar difficulty should have been noted by him in connection with rest; a moving thing which comes to rest must pass from some finite quantity to zero. Aristotle also thought that if no things changed there would be no time; yet it seems true that a universe could conceivably remain unchanged for a long or for a short time.

Newton viewed rest as occurring in time, but thought of it as a state which need not be achieved. He set it over against accelerated motion as that which required no explanation. For him only the coming to rest or the coming out of rest had to be explained. But there is no such state as mere self-maintenance, without effort, sheer unaffected existence over which an indifferent time perpetually flows.

Each primary Actuality is always in the process of losing and recovering its equilibrium; if it recovers it persistently, the Actuality is at rest. Even as resting, then, it is actively in time. And compounds, though not necessarily active, also are necessarily in time; their parts and the action of others make them into temporal beings.

1.07 Actualities have characteristic natures which enable them to be known and distinguished.
(*See 1.01*)

THERE ARE apples and men, horses and teapots. These Actualities have characteristic natures. Otherwise they would be differentiable by something irrational or external. Their difference would then not be known or could be eliminated; they would differ in an incomprehensible way, or would be identical in fact.

If it be affirmed that there are natures but denied that the natures are integral to the things, the things as outside those natures will be unintelligible, and we would have no reason for saying that those things existed at all. Nor can integral natures be rightly said to be adventitious; otherwise we could separate those natures off to give us irrational surd things all over again.

1.08 Primary Actualities are distinctive, persistent, resistant, insistent beings in space and time.
(*See 1.01, 1.04, 1.06*)

PRIMARY ACTUALITIES are final, irreducible, active substances which persist over a period of time. They are not momentary Cartesian or Humean atoms passing away in the very moment they appear. Each resists pressure by virtue of its irreducible reality; each urges itself on the others, maintaining itself for a while so far as it can fend off or master that which intrudes on it. Compound Actualities are also distinctive, resistant, and insistent, and occasionally might be said to be persistent, with longer time spans than those possessed by some primary Actualities. But they exert no power, even when they influence and compel. Their natures do not permeate them in their entirety, affecting and delimiting the activity of their parts. They frame or condition those parts rather than control them. But there would perhaps be no great harm in speaking of them too as substances.

1.09 There are primary beings which are not Actualities.
(See 1.05)

A PRIMARY being which is not an Actuality is one of three kinds. It may not be in space, though spatializable. A possibility is such a being. It may not be in time, though dynamic. An existent field is such a being. It may not be in space or time, but be capable of entering both. Such a being is divine.

Possibilities do not have extensionality but can acquire it by being realized in Actualities. They are not in time, of course, in the way in which Actualities are; but they are time-toned realities in the sense that they are at the limits of present time, constituting the Future. A field is spread out, and is like space, except that it has a being all its own, pulsating, rushing forward, self-divisive, serving as the locus of relations of comparison as well as of relations of distance. Space is in fact a delimited version of an existent field, the field frozen and conditioned in nature, and bounded by Actualities. Conversely, a field is space made substantial, transitory; it stands outside and over against and yet infects and is infected by Actualities as these seek to maintain themselves in existence. God is nonextended both spatially and temporally; he begins outside these altogether. He is thus to be distinguished from a possibility, for this begins where the present ends, and is to be distinguished from a field, for this is divisible and is partly expressed in the guise of space.

1.10 There are derivative modes of being.
(See 1.01, 1.08, 1.09)

WHAT IS NOT an Actuality, a possibility, an existent field, or an eternal being is a derivative. The past is a derivative; so are space, colors, sizes, shapes; so are compounds of all sorts.

There are at least three kinds of derivatives to be obtained from Actualities: the *analytic*, the *produced*, and the *residual*. An *analytic* derivative is a feature—such as shape, color, size—which has no being of its own but which can be prescinded or abstracted from Actualities. A *produced* derivative is the product of the interplay or inter-relationship of Actualities. Space is the most obtrusive case. Since compounds and other secondary Actualities are essentially modes of spatial togetherness, they are evidently all produced derivatives, though they do not necessarily occur later in time than the primary. A *residual* derivative is an Actuality deprived of some vital feature. A fact, or an Actuality as past, is a residual derivative.

Other modes of being allow for similar derivatives: limited logical possibilities, specific essences and real possibilities are derivatives from Possibility; spatial regions, time and flux are derivatives from Existence; divine attributes, an eternal evaluation and an eternal unity are derivatives from God.

1.11 There must be possibilities.
(*See 1.09*)

AN ACTUALITY must either continue to be or pass away at every moment. This means it is faced with the possibility, "to-be-or-to-pass-away." The acknowledgment of this truth is not tantamount to an acknowledgment that the possibility has a being of its own, on a footing with the Actuality. What is now being asserted is only that a "can be," a possibility, is presupposed by every Actuality at every moment. The possibility could conceivably be resident in some other being, such as God—a supposition which, however, will subsequently be shown to be untenable (see 2.100). In any case, possibilities must be over against Actualities, since Actualities are temporal beings which *can* do the things they in fact do. For an Actuality to pass away or to continue to be for a while, it must first have before it the possibility of such a condition. Were there no such possible condition confronting the Actuality the condition could never be realized; the Actuality would not be able either to pass away or to continue.

1.12 There must be a field.
(*See 1.01, 1.09*)

TWO BODIES distant from one another in space are then and there in a relation of bigger and smaller, darker and lighter. They do not acquire these correlative characteristics only when brought together in one place or one mind. If they did, they would have to be amorphous before they were so related, and would have to move concordantly from a position of nonrelation to a position in which they could be related, or they would be definite entities in a common universe and yet be in no relation of comparison. In the latter case, bigger and smaller, darker and lighter, and so on, would be irrelevant features of these things and could conceivably be interchanged. But the smaller is in one-to-one relation with a part of the bigger; to interchange these denominations in given things would be to treat the part as though it were bigger than the whole. Co-presence is a precondition for action, and not conversely, as some Einsteineans seem to hold.

Co-presence could be a static condition; it could require, if the relations between co-present items were extensive, nothing more than space. But Actualities remain co-present; they are concordant in time. As maintaining this concordance, as having spatial relations to one another for a period of time, they are in a field. This has a dynamics and being over against them; it is not an irreducible mode of being, and it could conceivably be nothing more than an expression of some such mode of being as God. All that it is now necessary to acknowledge is that there is an extensive domain in which Actualities can be, and can move, and across which they can be extensively related and in which they can be kept abreast in time.

1.13   There must be an eternal being.
(See 1.09)

WITHOUT an eternal being, comparisons would necessarily be made from the perspective of a limited part of space and time. But this would preclude an objective evaluation of all Actualities. Temporally distinct Actualities, if they are to be subject to a single standard of comparison, must be grasped from a position outside the limited time in which they historically are. But to have a grasp of the whole of time is possible only so far as one can stand in the dimension of eternity. To affirm this is not yet to affirm that there is a substantial eternal being, a God; the eternity might conceivably be sustained by a realm of possibility. What is now necessary is the acknowledgment of a dimension of eternity where the sequential parts of time, and what they contain, can be compared as better and worse and perhaps even as longer or shorter. One need not suppose—it is indeed self-contradictory to do so—that eternity already has all the sequential parts of time within it; all one needs to affirm is that when those different times have come to be, there is an eternity which can be imposed on them so as to order and evaluate them.

1.14 No Actuality can be absolutely perfect.
(See 1.01, 1.11, 1.12, 1.13)

THERE ARE various types of perfection. Reference is here being made only to maximum or absolute perfection, complete exhaustive reality. If there is more than one mode of being with a reality of its own, no one of them could, even if it were eternal, be absolutely perfect. Each would be irreducible, defying a complete mastery or absorption by the others, and defining them to be not exhaustive of what is real. To be sure each would have its own kind of perfection, but this can never be the maximal. Only all of them together can be maximally perfect.

An Actuality has a triple concern for other modes of being. It deals with them in different ways, and they in turn provide it with different opportunities to be fulfilled through a use of them. Other modes of being in turn endeavor to make use of Actuality, and what each fails to do is left as a task for the others. Only together do they exhaustively make use of whatever is Actual.

The references here to the other modes of being are all anticipatory. (See below, 1.15, 1.19, 2.21, 2.104, 3.13, 4.01, 4.04, 4.59, 4.93.)

1.15 Beings condition one another.
(See 1.14)

THE TOTALITY of being cannot be contained in any one mode, but only in all of them together. Only together do they constitute a whole reality. While constituting that reality with the others, each stands over against them, preventing them from being all there is or could be. Since the others have some reality of their own, each is necessarily imperfect, incomplete. To be complete, and thus fully to be, it must possess the reality possessed by the others. It can truly be, though incomplete, only so far as its reality is supplemented by the rest. It therefore holds on to them as that which it needs in order to be fully. As so holding on to those others it is conditioned by them, enabled to be. Could one be torn away from the rest, it would, self-contradictorily, at once fully be and be less than all there is. Each mode of being is real in itself only because it is interlocked with others, enabled to be by virtue of the fact that its reality is inseparable from theirs. Only because each is conditioned by the others is each able to be at all.

This thesis, too, like the foregoing, is anticipatory, serving primarily to make evident the persistent need of Actualities to take account of beings other than themselves.

II   THE TASKS OF PRIMARY ACTUALITIES

1.16   Each Actuality is unified.
(*See 1.05*)

AN ACTUALITY is a unity in space, a unity in time, a private unity within, a public unity on the outside, and a unity of its private and public sides. It is all of these at the same time. This means that an Actuality is always more than a mere "numerical" or designable unit. If simple, it is nevertheless extended in space and time, has a substantial core, and an outside or shape. All these are "synthesized" in the Actuality, kept together in it. If the Actuality is complex it must, in addition, confine, order, and control the natures and activities of its parts.

1.17   Actualities engage in acts of self-adjustment.
(*See 1.15, 1.16*)

SINCE AN Actuality's outside is conditioned by beings which are external to and independent of it, that public outside will not cohere with its inside or privacy unless the Actuality modifies that outside, changes its import. Actualities are thus in a tension, particularly with respect to their private and public sides. This tension can increase and can decrease; the unity of an Actuality is a matter of degree.

But there is a limit to the possible increase in tension in an Actuality; forced beyond that limit the being will break into bits or be forced to alter its inward nature. Faced with the threat of dissolution, but without yet losing its unity, an Actuality endeavors to overcome the effects and sometimes the conditions of that threatening dissolution. If it fails, a new unity replaces the old; if it succeeds, a greater degree of unity replaces a lesser.

1.18   Actualities affect other beings.
(See *1.15, 1.17*)

AN ACTUALITY strives to adjust itself to the affects of other beings. It also affects these others. The more it affects them in such a way as to reduce its need to adjust itself, the less it risks dissolution. To remain itself it must so determine others that they permit it to retain the unity it had. Self-maintenance, like quiescence and rest, is thus an achievement. It is not, as Whitehead supposed, an achievement which must immediately end in failure, in the perishing of the being. If there could be such perishing, produced without external pressure, it should be possible for there also to be a passage from absolute nonbeing to being, also produced without exterior aid. The distance from nonbeing to being is the same as the distance from being to nonbeing. Yet Whitehead insists on the occurrence of the latter while implicitly denying the possibility of the former. Hume was more consistent.

Self-maintenance has an indefinite duration; the selfsame Actuality continues to be for a length of time, which, except in very special circumstances, cannot be determined in advance. Persistence is the outcome of an adventure of unity over against threatened dissolution. The threat is perpetual. Sooner or later the unitary Actuality finds a task too big for itself and is forced to break apart or to change in nature.

There is no Spinozistic conatus, no endeavor to remain what it had been; an Actuality strives to be better, more complete, a fuller and yet more relaxed unity. Since it is faced with other Actualities and even other types of being engaged in similar enterprises, its continuance and its attempted progress towards greater perfection is always being threatened and defied. Sometimes it is even denied.

1.19 To be at its best, an Actuality must adjust
itself to others.
(*See 1.18*)

OTHER BEINGS threaten and sometimes defy an Actuality, and it
reciprocates. They also contribute to it, offering as well as demanding, giving as well as taking. They are best handled by an Actuality
when, while being used to satisfy its nature and needs, respect is had
for their distinctive natures and needs. To be itself to the full it must
take account of them, adjust itself to them.

An Actuality is most complete when it lacks nothing, but this
state it can never attain, in view of the ultimate irreducibility of other
beings. It is most itself when it stands outside and apart from all else,
but this state too it can never fully attain because of the intrusion of
others. The two efforts, the effort to be complete and the effort to be
itself, are partly at variance, for the one leads it to act on, whereas the
other leads it to stand away from others. To be at its best it must
balance the two tendencies, moderate its appetite to master all else
by its effort to remain to itself, and conversely.

1.20 Each Actuality attempts to subordinate and
accommodate others.
(*See 1.08, 1.19*)

AN ACTUALITY attempts to subordinate whatever else there be; it
also attempts to accommodate everything else. These two efforts are
components in a single act which deals with others both where it is
and where they are.

An Actuality adventures beyond the borders where we normally
locate it, and interplays with what it encounters at a distance; it also
remains within itself, and interplays with whatever beings reach to it.
The interplay has a passive and an active side. Each Actuality thus acts
on others both where it is (by adaptation) and where they are (by
action), and each submits to others both where it is (by yielding) and
where they are (by acceptance). This four-ply movement articulates
its effort to adjust itself, to balance its tendency to be complete with
its tendency to remain itself.

1.21   An Actuality seeks to adjust itself to
possibilities.
(*See 1.11, 1.19, 1.20*)

POSSIBILITIES (Ideals viewed from the standpoint of other beings)
are generic meanings. They have a being of their own, and Actualities
take account of this. As a consequence Actualities not only subjugate
possibilities but yield to them, mastering and accommodating them
to make those possibilities into actualized occurrences, or into determinate features.

Unless every nature is generic, there must be natures, such as the
singular nature of an actual individual man, which are more than possibilities. The Scotists seem to recognize the reality of such individual
natures; unfortunately they also treat them as though they were a
kind of universal. It is hard to see how they can explain the exemplification of that universal in individual beings. The Thomists, on the
other side, seem to deny that there are individual natures; they are
therefore incapable of knowing any individuals. Both seem to overlook an alternative. There are individual natures, integral to Actualities, which are the outcome of the realization of generic possibilities.
These individual natures exemplify and specify those possibilities but
are too determinate to be possibilities themselves.

1.22   An Actuality seeks to make the field integral
to itself, and to submit to it.
(*See 1.12, 1.20*)

A FIELD (Existence viewed from the standpoint of other beings),
unlike space, is a domain of comparative relations; unlike time it is
dynamic. It is somewhat like Plato's "receptacle," "the foster mother
of all becoming," Aristotle's prime matter, Schopenhauer's Will, Bergson's *Élan Vital* and Whitehead's Creativity. As part of an Actuality
it makes that Actuality present; as overrunning the borders of Actualities it allows them to be interrelated contemporaries. The Actualities submit to the field as that which will enable them to be co-present
while they in turn allow themselves to be affected by it so as to be
part of a single dynamic movement. In recompense they give it focus
and help determine its geometry.

1.23 An Actuality strives to adjust itself to eternity.
(See *1.13, 1.20*)

ETERNITY (God viewed from the standpoint of other beings) is the locus of the evaluation of whatever there be, no matter what the date. To be as complete as possible, Actualities must take account of Eternity, be receptive to its nature and influence, at the same time that they impose themselves on it. Eternity is not altogether indifferent to what is actual, as Epicurus and Lucretius supposed. It is not a being to which the world refers but which has no concern for it, as Aristotle maintained. Nor is it an absolutely perfect reality, lacking nothing whatsoever, as the Hebraic-Christian tradition holds. More perfect and inclusive than anything else that there may be, it is a being which, precisely because there are Actualities over against it, is not and cannot be absolutely complete. Actualities must act on it and submit to it where it is and where they themselves are.

1.24 An Actuality engages in all efforts at adjustment together.
(See *1.20–23*)

AN ACTUALITY always confronts all the other beings. It must therefore always try to adjust itself to all of them. Conversely, they all at the same time act on and are receptive to it. Whitehead has perhaps, among modern thinkers, most clearly recognized that Actualities engage in this complex effort. However, he did not seem to take adequate account of the fact that Actualities offer themselves to and act on others where those others are. The closest he came to such an acknowledgment is in his doctrine of objective immortality, which holds that what has been assumes the role of a datum for what is to be. But Actualities are also data for one another even when they are contemporaries. Indeed, they are more than data; they urge themselves on one another. They do not merely present themselves to what comes after, allowing themselves to be used in whatever way later beings see fit.

1.25 All four efforts qualify one another.
(See *1.15, 1.20, 1.24*)

AN ACTUALITY is a single being, and its efforts with respect to other beings all express the need of that Actuality to be itself at its best.

Its efforts to deal with any one type of being are therefore infected by its efforts to deal with the others. Conditioned by other Actualities, possibilities, an existent field, and an eternity, it acts on and is receptive to them, all at the same time. Each of these of course in turn is in a similar situation with respect to the rest. Being is divided in a fourfold way and each of the divisions is occupied with maintaining itself over against and with the aid of the others.

III   THE ACTIVITY OF ACTUALITIES

1.26   An Actuality's attempt to deal with other Actualities is qualified by its attempt to deal with possibility.
(*See 1.21, 1.25*)

THE TOTALITY of Actualities requires a convergence on a single possibility in terms of which that totality can act; conversely, the totality of Actualities defines the one possibility as germane to it, as that which alone is open to realization by them all in independent but concordant ways. The Actualities have their positions with respect to one another determined by what it allows them to be and do.

Each Actuality faces the common possibility. Under the pressure of the presence of other Actualities, it makes that possibility specific and relevant to itself as only one of a number of Actualities. Each Actuality specifies the possibility common to them all, and deals with other beings in the light of what its specific possibility allows it to be and do. Since the Actuality, when dealing with other Actualities, is also occupied with adjusting itself to its own specific, relevant possibility, it must face those other Actualities in the light of that possibility. The bearing of each of the Actualities on the others is in part dictated by the nature of the common possibility which they together confront; the nature of the specific possibilities which can be actualized by each of them is dictated by the natures they each have, and by the relations they bear to one another.

1.27   The attempt of an Actuality to deal with other Actualities is qualified by its attempt to deal with the field.
(*See 1.20, 1.22*)

AN ACTUALITY, while dealing with other Actualities, adjusts itself to a dynamic, circumambient field. As the field moves on in time the Actualities in it either move with it, thereby remaining contemporaries at the next moment, or become static facts in the past.

The field offers a frame for the Actualities, a tissue of connections which keeps them contemporary. Were there no such field, there would be no domain where the Actualities would be together. The Actualities would have to leap, as it were, over a region of nonbeing and deal with one another immediately. The field makes them deal with one another mediately. That field is not another Actuality; it lacks their boundaries, individuality, focus, while they lack its relentless persistence, its cosmic spread, and its capacity to penetrate everywhere.

The accommodation of Actualities by one another enables them to raise the level of the field, to make it continuous with them, so that it is tempting to speak of them as mere intensifications of the existent field. But this temptation is readily resisted when it is recognized that the field determines the way in which Actualities are related just as much as they determine its geometry.

1.28   The attempt of an Actuality to deal with other Actualities is qualified by its attempt to deal with eternity.
(*See 1.20, 1.23*)

AN ACTUALITY is occupied both with other Actualities and with eternity. Its stress on the other Actualities is qualified by its adjustment to the eternal, with the consequence that the eternal becomes a kind of frame within which it and the other Actualities are caught. Eternity imposes a unity on them as all together. Because of it they are not merely beings directed towards a common possibility, nor beings which merely keep apace with one another; they are also beings which have their various natures eternally preserved and judged. It is because of eternity that they are capable of being evaluated concurrently.

Actualities deal directly with eternity, but qualify their adjustment to it by their acknowledgment of other Actualities. Such qualification turns eternity into a temporally oriented category, expressing the meaning of the totality of those Actualities.

1.29 Each Actuality attempts to turn all other Actualities into concordant beings under the common aegis of a possibility, a field, and an eternity.
(See *1.26–28*)

IT IS WHEN and as it is occupied with other Actualities that an Actuality attends to the other dimensions of the universe, the other modes of being. These others enable it to form groupings of various sorts with the Actualities which are all about. A possibility enables it to force some things into the foreground and others into the background as more or less relevant to what it is about to do; a field enables it to forge an environment with other Actualities; and an eternity enables it to be more and less involved with them.

1.30 Each Actuality uses other Actualities.
(See *1.26–28*)

EACH ACTUALITY is occupied with the other modes of being. Its efforts in relation to other Actualities qualify the effect which these other modes will have on it. Because of the limitations which these other Actualities permit it to impose on other modes of being, an Actuality encounters a possibility, a field, and an eternity as more or less relevant to it, as more or less continuous with it, and as more or less a part of its very substance.

1.31 Some Actualities can change without losing identity.
(See *1.16, 1.17, 1.18, 1.19*)

AN ACTUALITY is a unification of a private and public side. These are not two distinct domains. If they were, each would itself have an inside and an outside. The unity though can be subject to tension, due to the fact that the being as pressed in from without, and thus as possessing an outside, is affected in ways which do not accord with what the being is in itself and thus as expressing itself at the point where the others affect it. It is in order to overcome such tensions that the being makes an effort, not necessarily conscious and often not successful, to meet the various conditions which the others impose on it. It may be able to reassess its outside, give it another import, or it may have to alter on the inside in order to avoid being so at odds with itself that it must cease to exist. At every moment every Actuality attempts to adjust itself not only to what lies outside it but also to itself as affected by whatever else there be.

1.32   It is not of the essence of an Actuality to occupy a particular region of space.
(*See 1.01, 1.08*)

ACTUALITIES, because spatial beings, always occupy some region of space. That this Actuality occupies this region at this moment is a truth about it. But it is not a truth which touches its essence. The Actuality can, unaltered, occupy some other region. Since motion is the successive occupation of different regions in space, the Actuality is therefore capable of motion.

It is an existent being that moves. That movement is an act in which, without entirely freeing itself from the field, the Actuality readjusts itself to the field over a series of moments. Motion in space is a form of coming to be, a form of the activity of releasing and integrating a part of the whole of Existence.

IV   CAUSALITY

1.33   Not everything is eternal.
(*See 1.06*)

IT IS often said that God is the cause of the universe. If so, he is a cause in quite a different sense from that characteristic of Actualities. Their causality is a temporal affair; his would be nontemporal, an occurrence in the unbroken calm of eternity (which is the paradoxical view of classical theology), or would be an act which would require him to have a temporal side (which seems to divide him in two). In any case in the realm of Actuality, causality relates primarily to spatialized beings in time.

1.34 There is causality.
(*See 1.02, 1.33*)

WE SEE the world in casual terms. The category of causality is in constant use. If nothing is caused in this world that category would not properly characterize the world. But since that category would itself not be caused we could not account for its presence; and since there would be no causal powers possible in the world, there would be no way by which we could get rid of that category. The principle of causality would be inexplicable, unremovable, inescapable, and we would as a consequence—contrary to the hypothesis—be unable to envisage a world in which there was no causality.

1.35 The category of causality is an inexpugnable, unrejectable way of ordering what occurs and what we encounter.
(*See 1.02, 1.03, 1.34*)

THE CATEGORY of causality is either constitutive of the world only as known, or it is also integral to the world as apart from us and our efforts to know. The first of these views is essentially Kantian, the second Aristotelian. Hume never could make up his mind just where he wished to stand. He spoke as if there were no causality in the world, and then went on to give a causal explanation of how we got and used the idea of causality.

If there were no causality in fact, and if the category of causality were not constitutive of the world we know (or what is the same thing, if there were a world outside that which is constituted by means of a category of causality), it would be a world where things just happened. In such a world the idea of causality could pop into a man's head at one moment and leave it the next. But not only could he not do anything but think in causal terms while he had the idea of causality, but he would have to grant that what could pop up next could be a new world in which causality ruled absolutely and everywhere.

Those who would like to maintain that there is no causality in fact try also to hold that this is the way the world always was and will be. But this conclusion is not possible to them; he who has no causality in his world allows anything to happen next, including a world in which causality holds full sway. At best then, the view that there is no causality is an idle fancy, characterizing a world we cannot now encounter and which, were it to occur, could immediately give way and forever to the world we now know. When the noncausal world was in existence, there would be no way of explaining or correcting those who mistakenly thought it was a causal world. To deny causation is thus to deny current evidence, to ignore an omnipresent category, to be faced with an inexplicable world, and to have an inexplicable belief that it is a mistake to say there is causation in fact.

On both the Kantian and the Aristotelian approaches, causality is definitive of occurrences and experience. They differ in that the former supposes causality does not hold apart from the constitutive activities of knowledge, whereas the latter supposes it does so hold. The one is faced with the problem of understanding just what it is that is given to the knower for him to constitute by means of his categories, and why it is that he orders what otherwise would seem to be amorphous in the ways he does. The other is faced with the problem of understanding how it is that one can know what in fact takes place, as apart from our knowledge. But this problem is not like the other, insoluble in principle.

1.36 When a cause is actual, its effect is only possible.
(See 1.02, 1.11)

A CAUSE precedes its effect in time. When the cause is, the effect is not; when the effect is the cause is not. An actual cause then is precisely that which has no effect; an actual effect is precisely that which has no actual cause. The paradox in this remark immediately dissolves before a distinction between an actual and a possible effect. An actual cause cannot have an actual effect when that cause exists, without destroying the temporal gap between cause and effect; an actual effect cannot have an actual cause without destroying the temporal distance between it and its cause. But an actual cause has a possible effect, an effect that *can* but does not yet exist; an actual effect has a past cause, a cause that *did* but does not now exist.

It is often said that some causes at least are simultaneous with their effects. The head resting on the pillow, we say, indents it. The resting head is here treated as a cause, the indented pillow as its effect. But the effect in fact is "head resting on and indenting the pillow," the cause of which is the placing of the head on the pillow as met by a characteristic yielding of the pillow. (Even if one supposed that a pillow were to spring back as soon as the head was lifted, the temporal disparity between the cause and the effect of an indented pillow would have to be acknowledged. A pressing head interacts with a springy pillow, forcing the pillow back.) There is, however, no great harm in extending the idea of causality to apply to cases where it is supposed that a cause and effect are simultaneous, providing one then avoids the temptation of supposing that it might be possible for all causes to be simultaneous with their effects. Were that possible there would be no time and no history, no production, no expectation, no inference, and finally not even the thought that causes and effects are simultaneous. Of course the cause which is simultaneous with its effect is not a cause in the same sense in which an antecedent is. It is what Aristotle called a formal cause; the other is an efficient cause.

1.37 To know a possible effect we must infer to it from its cause.
(*See 1.35, 1.36*)

A CAUSE extends from the present, where it exists as an Actuality, to the abstract future where its effect, in the guise of a possibility, is to be found. Were an effect entirely cut off from its cause, were it only subsequent to the cause, there would be no need for the effect to have the nature that it does, and no thought could possibly tell us what it is, until in fact we encounter it at some later moment. Theories of causation which suppose that what has happened in the past or that the laws which prevailed in the past will certainly or probably occur in the future, tacitly suppose that there is something in the nature of the present or the course of the world or the structure of man's mind which puts some limitation on what in fact will ensue. But this is nothing other than an implicit recognition of the fact that an actual cause in the present allows for an inference to a possible effect, an effect which, precisely because it is inferable from the cause, has pertinence to the nature of that cause.

1.38 At least some effects are deducible from their
their causes.
(*See 1.37*)

AN INFERENCE involves a risk; it moves outside and beyond its
premises. But in some inferences, the deductive, the risk is at a minimum. At times the mathematico-logical sciences infer deductively.
The principle of inference which they then employ is patterned on a
law of nature, grounded in a cause and extending to that cause's possible effect.

A law of nature is no iron bond, no injunction from on high to
which objects must submit. Nor is it merely an habitual way in which
they happen to act. Rather, it is an intelligible connection between a
present and a future happening. That is why there can be successful
predictions made by those who infer along the lines expressed by the
laws of nature.

1.39 An actual effect occurs subsequent to its cause.
(*See 1.36*)

A POSSIBLE effect is future to its actual cause. That future is abstract, possible, not *temporally* distant from the present. In contrast
an actual effect replaces an actual cause; it is an occurrence, something
which takes place in a present subsequent to the present in which its
cause occurred, and thus in a present which is temporally distant from
that cause. One can anticipate an actual effect, and even give a date
when it will be, but as referred to from the vantage point of an actual
cause that effect is only possible, with its actual occurrence still to
take place. An actual effect always occurs later than its (efficient)
cause.

1.40 A possible effect is distinct from itself as
actualized.
(*See 1.36, 1.38, 1.39*)

A POSSIBLE effect is deducible, abstract, universal, indeterminate;
an actual effect is produced, concrete, singular, determinate. Only as
actual does an effect require that its cause no longer exist. Whereas a
possible effect, though distinct from its cause, is compatible with the

presence of that cause, the produced nature of an actual effect requires a replacement, a pushing away of its cause.

It is the possible effect that is actualized. Since the actual effect is distinct from itself as possible, an account of it in the one guise will not be altogether appropriate to it in the other. However, since it is the possible effect which is actualized, the actual effect is not altogether alien to the possible effect. Our inferences, therefore, which follow the route of a law of nature and terminate in a possible effect, though they do not reach to, also do not lead us away from the actual effects that in fact ensue on given actual causes.

1.41 What explains a possible effect does not suffice to explain an actual effect.
(*See 1.40*)

A POSSIBLE effect is to be explained by taking account of the nature of the cause and the manner by which, through the laws of nature, it extends to the abstract future. There is no separate date in real time for that possible effect. It is shadowed forth by the cause now. But the actual effect takes place. To explain it we must go beyond the explanation provided by an abstract science or even an expectation, for these proceed, along quite general "law-like" routes, to terminate only in what is possible. One must actually move through time in order actually to get to the actual effect. What is added to the mere law in this movement, the actual production, must be taken account of if we are to understand and explain the occurrence of the effect.

1.42 Production is intelligible but not deducible.
(*See 1.02, 1.40, 1.41*)

A PRODUCTION has no definite nature except when it occurs, and it occurs only over a course of time. Given its antecedents, only its possibility is determined. As concrete, as a genuine activity taking time, it is more than that possibility. It is not a thing of surds and irrationalities, but of what exists and can be known only in a concrete time in which a later occurrence replaces an earlier. A production is thus no combination of universals or laws, but a dynamic and actual sequence illustrating universals or laws.

1.43   An actual effect is produced by that which transcends, is outside the cause.
(See *1.41, 1.42*)

A CAUSE is an antecedent condition, needing supplementation by a production terminating in the consequent actual effect. Since that which is not accounted for by a cause is what is free, a production is a free activity, having its origin in the cause and its terminus in the effect. The production, as confined within these limits, exemplifies laws. Freedom is evidently then no wild uncharterable activity, but well grooved, kept within the area of the predictable possible effect of that cause which begins the production. (One can, of course, term the joint cause and production "the cause," but then one will still have to distinguish between a component which defines the kind of effect that is possible, and a component which brings about the actualization of that possible effect.)

There are two extreme positions that this account precludes. It denies that production—and with it the actual effect—is deducible even by an omniscient intellect, and it denies that it is entirely beyond all prevision, a mere matter of cosmic caprice. The first of the rejected alternatives involves a confusion of the possible with the actual, the abstract with the concrete future, law with occurrence, a relation with an event, the form of time with the movement of time; the second of these rejected alternatives unjustifiably questions and is embarrassed by a host of successful predictions in thought and warranted expectations in practice.

The avoidance of these extremes however, still allows for a spectrum of diverse positions. It could, for example, with some plausibility be maintained that every universal, every mathematically expressible aspect of a production, and thus of an actual effect, is deducible. One will then leave over only the sheer occurrence, the mere sensuousity or immediacy of the production and the actual effect, as that which freely occurs. Or it could with some plausibility be maintained that novel universals are sometimes freely generated in the course of a production, so that only highly generic features of the production and the actual effect could be deduced. It is extremely difficult ot decide between these. The first does more justice to what we know of the mechanical and the inanimate, the second does more justice to what we know of men, particularly in their most creative moods in art and in ethics. Both have many forms, allowing for multiple views, all acknowledging that effects are deducible so far as they are possible but that they are freely reached so far as they are actual.

If we are to avoid, as we ought, the temptation to interpret man in terms of the inanimate, or the inanimate in terms of the human, we ought to recognize that these various views form a single series. The freedom exhibited in the production of an actual effect may vary from the limit of providing only an immediate sensuous ongoing and outcome, to the limit of providing, in addition, unpredictable universals, features, meanings. There is but one type of efficient causality, but the degree of freedom in it varies from case to case.

1.44 An actual effect is necessitated.
(*See 1.36, 1.37, 1.41, 1.42, 1.43*)

AN ACTUAL effect is the outcome of two conditions, the cause and the production, or process of causation. The cause necessitates the possibility of that effect; what is required in order that the effect be actual instead of only possible is provided by the process of causation. Since the process is free, the necessitated effect is in part the outcome of freedom. Just as there is no inconsistency between the idea of freedom and the idea of prediction (for the former occurs within the limits provided by the latter), so there is no inconsistency between the idea of a freely produced effect and a necessitated actual effect (for the process when added to the cause necessitates the effect which the cause made possible). The point has been overlooked because it has been thought that the transcendence of the process of causation beyond the cause meant that there was no limit to where the process might go and what it might achieve. But a production has definite limits. It makes only possible, predictable, and formally necessary effects into actual, not wholly predictable, existentially necessary ones.

1.45 An Actuality makes an effort to change in the face of insuperable obstacles.
(*See 1.17, 1.18, 1.31*)

WERE THINGS amorphous, completely pliable, they would be alterable in direct proportion to the pressures put upon them. But they have natures, and react and adjust in characteristic ways. At every moment each tries to recover its equilibrium, tries to maintain itself despite pressures to make it change. If it cannot overcome the kind of change which others impose on it, give the change a meaning for itself as a unitary being, it will be broken asunder with an outside and an inside in disaccord. It must either allow its privacy to be altered by virtue of the change to which its outside is being subjected, or it must reassert itself so as to master what would otherwise force it to be altered.

The forced alteration of a privacy by virtue of the changes imposed on an outside introduces a vital change in that particular thing. So far as the being reasserts itself by subjugating the change to its original privacy, it persists. When it reasserts itself by changing its privacy in such a way that it is able to master its outside, it undergoes an evolutionary change. That change is of course not a replacing of a being by a nonbeing, but merely a replacing of one being by another. (Destruction thus has not one but two opposites—self-maintenance and evolution—of which the second is the more radical and important.) Evolution, on this view, is the outcome of a strategy, and arises only because the being alters its nature in order to keep control of an altered outside. It is a view which goes counter to the Darwinian account with its supposition that nature is exuberant, throwing off random variations and then being subject to constraining selections so as to yield what might prove helpful to the species. The Darwinian attributes a radical freedom to nature on the one side and a wisdom to a blind process of selection on the other which have subsequently been recognized to have little warrant in fact and little use in theory. He fails also to explain how the living can originate from the nonliving. Nor does he make adequate provision for the difference there is in kind between man and the highest of animals, since he contents himself with noticing only what happened on their outsides and makes no provision for their inward natures, and thus of great differences between them despite their small differences in public features. The eye of a man is quite different from that of an ape, not because it has a different structure but because it is used by one possessing a different kind of inside.

V   THE   NATURE   OF   MAN

1.46 Man is the product of evolution.
(*See 1.45*)

THERE ARE two schools which deny that man is a product of
evolution. One denies that there is evolution anywhere, the other
denies that evolution applies to man. Aristotle takes the first of
these positions, most classical theologians take the second. Aristotle's
view is that the species are fixed, and that they always have been and
always will be so. Discoveries in geology, and biology, in comparative anatomy and in the laboratory have made it unreasonable
to entertain this view any longer. The second school can be traced
back to Augustine. He took the various days of creation to be
more than twenty-four–hour days, and he supposed that God
created the various kinds of things on those days "in their causes,"
which is to say not as full-grown beings but as beings which will
eventually develop to become the beings that now exist. But Augustine made an exception for man. Man, according to him (and all classical theology), is a special creation of God, both individually and as
a species. God, he held, creates each individual man by endowing an
embryonic cell with an immortal, divinely produced soul. Yet man's
body seems close in kind and degree to animal bodies; his embryonic
development, vestigial features, his blood and organs provide most
persuasive evidence that his body represents an evolutionary advance
on the animal. And since a man is a single being, with a human nature
when and as he has a naturally acquired human body, the denial that
his human nature is naturally acquired would involve the supposition
that man is the only species whose natural offspring are of a different
and lower species than that of its parents. Human procreation would
have to be thought of as an act producing subhumans who are to be
transformed into humans only by means of a special divine act. Every
human birth would be a miracle. But caution requires us not to multiply the need for miracles needlessly.

That the human body is an evolutionary product and that men
generate men does not mean that men are not different in kind from
the animals. Much of what the classical theologians insisted on as

characteristic and distinguishing features of men can and ought to be affirmed even when their account of the divine generation of men as a species or as individuals is rejected. Men have nonbodily powers of evaluation; they have minds, wills, and obligations which enable them to function in ways no animal can. The evolution of men from animals does not require that that they should have only animal or bodily powers.

1.47 A man has self-identity.
(*See 1.31*)

NATURAL objects and artificial objects have continuity without persistence or identity. Were a river to change its course and its contents, becoming saline where it had been sweet, dark where it had been light, without fish where it had been full, and so on, we would still speak of it as the same river, for it would have a continuity as a *river* though not a continuity in content. If the timber of a wooden ship were removed and each plank replaced by a new one, and then another ship were made out of the old timber, we would continue to call the first the original ship, for it would have a continuity as a *ship*. The ship using the old timber is a new ship, even though—because of the continuity of the timber—it may look just like the old.

Animals are born and later die. They do not only continue but maintain themselves. Self-maintenance, however, is not yet self-identity. Man alone has this, for he alone has a self which remains unchanged while the body alters, grows, and decays. Among other things that self is the locus of responsibility. It is of man's essence to be responsible, and so far as he fails to carry out his responsibilities he is guilty, whether or not he remembers what he had done or failed to do, whether or not he changes in body or attitude, and even whether or not he is forgiven. This is possible only because he has a self-identical, persistent self throughout his career. And he has that self even when he is not conscious, even when he is just an embryo, not yet in control of its body, unaware of where it is to go and what it ought to do.

1.48 A man can discipline himself.
(*See 1.47*)

HUNGER can be restrained from expressing itself. The art of this restraint is manners; a specific act of this restraint is an act of will.

Imagination can be subdued by reason or made to vanish through exercise. The art of this restraint is habituation; a specific act of this restraint is once again an act of will.

Through the exercise of will men discipline themselves, restrain expressions, impulses, aberrations. Animals can be disciplined, but they cannot discipline themselves. They can withhold, hold back, wait, but they cannot take their minds or bodies as objects, and subject these to conditions of an abstract or ideal nature. This man does not always do. But he *can* do it. It is his power to do this, not his doing it, which is one of the ways he is marked off from all animal kind.

1.49   A man can evaluate himself in terms not exemplified by him.
(*See 1.47*)

AN ANIMAL has likes and dislikes, and can be made to cringe and feel unwanted or in the wrong. But the animal itself takes no measure of itself; it has no standards in terms of which it can ask itself whether what it has done or is about to be done is good or bad. It cannot judge whether or not it is good to be what it is, or to do what it does. A man may not judge himself and very often judges wrongly, exaggerating his virtues or vices, his achievements or failures. He may not be able to say what standards he uses and may misapply those which he acknowledges. What marks him off from animal kind is not his judgment but his capacity for judgment, his ability to look at himself objectively, to estimate his worth in terms of a standard outside and other than himself. He alone can make moral judgments, often about himself.

1.50   A man has a self.
(*See 1.47, 1.48, 1.49*)

THE SELF is a self-identical unity. It has a natural origin, perpetually expresses itself as a life in the body, and sometimes expresses itself as a mind and as a will. Ontologically viewed it is the individual as concerned with, as inseparable from an all-inclusive good to which he might never consciously attend but to which he is always directed. This self is to be distinguished from (1) an Aristotelian form, (2) privacy, (3) the psyche, and (4) the soul. An Aristotelian form is a structure or meaning, a kind of intelligible unity; it has no power,

no capacity to control, and can be said to be self-identical only so far
as it is not in time at all. Privacy is a being as in itself; in the case of
man it is a feature of the self, the self as held apart from its concern.
The psyche is privacy as the source of life and feeling; in the case of
man it is the self as not yet capable of thought, creative imagination,
or ethical responsibility, which is to say as not a genuine self at all.
The soul is what a self would be were it created in each and every
case by God. The self is thus the soul naturalized, the psyche ennobled, privacy engaged, a form endowed with power, control,
concern.

Were there no self a man would not be self-identical from birth
to death, asleep and in a stupor. Were there no self he could not restrain his body and his mind, evaluate what had been done, is done,
will be done, what might be done, and what could not be done.

Norbert Wiener has made popular the idea of a "feedback" in
which not only animals but machines reassess what they are doing in
terms of some set end or result required of them. The idea comes
quite close to that involved in a human judgment, particularly a judgment evaluating what is now being done in terms of some standard.
Still there is a radical difference between a "feedback" and a judgment. A "feedback" is a way of determining whether or not an activity is completed; a judgment is a way of reporting whether or not
an activity is good or bad. The distance between the two can be
enormous, for a completed activity may be completely bad, and an
uncompleted activity may be excellent. A machine cannot tell the
difference; a man can.

1.51   A self is expressed as a life of a body.
(See 1.50)

AN ANIMAL is alive, but has no self; a man is alive because he has
a self. His self makes his body a living, unified body which, unlike
the animal's, may exhibit some other powers, traceable to the same
self. His self charges the body with different degrees of vitality and
interest during the day, and makes it perform on behalf of nonbodily
goods and for objectives which may even have a detrimental effect
on that body. The body too often is driven along routes and towards
goals which court danger and disaster for the body, because the self
insists on it acting in just that way. An animal can endanger itself;

it can have desires which may prove its undoing. But it has no power to envisage an end and evaluate it as desirable, and then quicken and direct the body so that this end is attained. An animal might risk itself for another; only a man can sacrifice himself, deliberately order his body to be endangered for the sake of some goal evaluated by the self.

Occupied with the body, the self is all over it, in every place where the body is alive. Charging the body with more vitality than is necessary to keep it functioning as a living organism, the self makes the body sensitive. Fluctuating in degree of expression in accord with the needs and pressures, the changes and problems encountered by the body, the self makes the individual sensible, ready to act appropriately.

As alive a man can be quiescent; as sensitive he can feel pleasure and pain, and take some account of the prospects that concern other beings; as sensible he can attend to particulars in, on, and around the body. These three capacities he shares with animals. He differs from them because he alone has a self and can alone therefore make his life, sensitivity, and sensibility serve some accepted purpose.

1.52   The self is immortal.
(*See 1.48, 1.49, 1.50*)

A MAN has a self. With the Pythagoreans it could be held that this self was immortal before birth; with classical theology it could be said to be a fresh divine creation, immortal after death; with Plato it could be said to be immortal both before birth and after death; or with most psychologists it could be said to be wholly mortal, with an origin in nature and a short span of activity, to be followed by a complete disappearance with death. No one of these positions does full justice to what we know of man, his powers and his capacities, or to the nature of nature; no one of them is free from difficulties of a seriousness hard to underestimate.

Since the self controls and defies the body, and since it persists while the body changes, and exercises powers which are nonbodily in nature or origin, its career is not necessarily tied down with that of the body. The death of the body does not demand the death of the self. There is no need to suppose, though, that this self existed before the body. If it did it would be a substance separate from the body; the insertion of it in the body would be a miracle which would yet leave it not altogether integrated with the body, thus turning a man into two beings.

The self is no airy spirit, and no hard core of intangible stuff. It is the body itself as private, concerned, and unified, capable of limiting, enlivening, and controlling the various bodily parts and the movement of the body as a whole. It achieves a distinctive being when a portion of Existence becomes integral to it and is held over against the Existence which is integral to the rest of the individual. That is why it can defy the enlivened body and have a career not implicated entirely by that body. At death it cuts off and holds to itself that portion of Existence which once characterized it as the self of the body. Looking back at it as the self of the body, we can say of it that the Existence it takes with it was there overlaid by the Existence of the body. Reciprocally, the body as sustained by the self has a nature which is richer and other than that which it has on death. When sustained by the self the body has an organic unity; it then moves not as a function of its several components but in part in terms of the values, needs, and demands of the self. On death, it loses the nature it enjoyed because of the self, and is left with the nature of a corpse. By dying it loses the enrichment it had by virtue of the self. Looking back at the enlivened body we can say of it that the nature it had as mere body was overlaid by the nature of the self, and that only on death is it able to exhibit the nature which natively belongs to it. The self is immortal only after death, but it is no freshly created being inserted in the interstices of some natural body. It has a natural origin, exists in this life in the body, and yet has a capacity to act and eventually to exist apart from that body.

VI   KNOWLEDGE

1.53   Sometimes the self expresses itself as a mind.
(*See 1.48, 1.49*)

DESCARTES and Kant maintain that man always thinks. Their view is in part a consequence of their double supposition that man persists through time, and that he has a mind but no self. Having denied him a self, they have only his mind, whose essence it is to think, in which to ground his identity. Yet a thinking of which we have no knowledge is hard to term a thinking at all. And in any case the theory begins to sound foolish when it maintains that a man in a stupor is a man thinking. In fact, if mind is viewed as a tissue of thoughts, a plurality of processes of thinking, it seems evident that men do not always have minds, but only the capacity to have or to exercise them.

A mind may be viewed as capable of feeling, imagining, and perhaps even of willing, though the last supposed capacity has difficulty with the fact that one can will to use or not to use his mind. Since none of these capacities may be exercised, however, and since a man remains a man even when he ceases to feel, imagine, or will, evidently a man is more than such a mind. We can speak of him as having an "unconscious" mind, of altering in mood and spirit, and even as moving from one personality to another. But these states and alterations presuppose a persistent life and therefore cannot be equated with the persistent in man.

The mind is one of the self's most signal modes of expression, but it has no being of its own and does not exist except so far as the self expresses itself in just that form. Having expressed itself in one way a number of times, the self may find it difficult to avoid expressing itself in that way again. The expression of the self as mind may limit the self and even subject the self's further expressions to the constraints which habit inevitably imposes. But this does not affect the fact that the mind is still only an expression of the self, without being or power of its own.

1.54   The mind is not a body.
(*See 1.53*)

RECOGNITION of the nonbodily nature of the mind, together with a neglect of the reality of the self, has generated an insoluble "mind-body" problem. The mind of course is unextended, whereas the body is extended; the one is not shaped, the other is; the one is unmovable, the other can move. Were they separate substances they could never meet. And a theory which says that they are parallel risks dividing man or overlooking the ways in which they diverge, affect and at times oppose one another in intent and content. Mind and body often go in diverse directions. Disturbances in the body are sometimes accompanied with thoughts of displeasure, rejection, condemnation of

the immediate and sometimes of the remote causes of those disturbances; thoughts in the mind are sometimes accompanied by bodily
actions which exhibit what one had in mind. Mind and body can function in independence of one another and yet sometimes in accord and
in terms of one another, because they are creatures of the same self.
That self expresses itself as a life in a body and as a mind, sometimes
in independent ways, and sometimes in interrelated ways. It owns
them both and is therefore capable of redressing whatever discrepancies their independent functioning might exhibit.

1.55   The mind is not a function of the body.
(*See 1.05, 1.51, 1.53, 1.54*)

AN INANIMATE thing reacts to outward pressures; its activities are
the activities of its parts. A living being can do more than react. It
can respond. The entire organism, through some specialized channel,
can answer to the disturbance. A man too at times reacts and at times
responds; but there are times when he also reassesses what he encounters. Such reassessment is guided by a concern for self-completion
which, unlike reaction and response, brings to bear the values that
concern the self.

The self is not necessarily occupied with the body and its needs; it
functions in part to keep that body alive, but it also has other powers
and interests in no way limited to bodily needs, and thus not necessarily
confined to bodily problems. As Aristotle observed, there are limits to
what the senses allow us to apprehend; the extremes of heat and cold
destroy the sense of touch; sight is hurt by too much and by too little
light, and so on. There are no such limits for the mind. The senses
may provide it with its initial material but it operates outside their
reach; thinking makes it stronger, more able to think, and this the
harder the thinking is. There is a fatigue of course, but this is bodily
in nature.

The exercise and public expression of the mind requires a body
equipped and freshly prepared in various ways. The self, though able
to attend through the agency of its mind to the good and the evil,
the excellent and the poor without injury, is apparently not able to
express itself as a mind except so far as it can at the same time vitalize
the body, and particularly the brain. This does not alter the fact that
the mind can act independently of the body, and in ways beyond the
capacity of the body. Indeed there would be no harm in saying that

the mind is only the brain, providing that we add that it is the brain only when this functions in response to meanings, values, and implications and not merely to pressures and irritations. The two types of response are independent, even if performed by the same organ.

1.56 The mind can encounter sensuous content.
(*See 1.55*)

THE SENSES by themselves are avenues through which the body is readily affected. But it takes a mind to sense through and by means of them. These senses are customarily held to make a set of five, though most physiologists are inclined to increase the number considerably. Whatever the number be, one must add to them a "common sense" which goes beyond the reach of any particular sense and touches a common sensuous content which the particular senses diversely specialize. Sensuous content is singular and partly exhausted in the experiencing. Not a universal or set of universals, it is no particular either. It has no definite boundary, no sharply demarcated form or nature. It is something undergone, whose presence marks the difference between dreaming or imagining and waking or sensing. Were the sensuous a universal or a predicate or something conceived, we could presumably retain it in our minds and repeat it later, when we were asleep—and thus in fact would be awake. We know when we are awake only when we are awake, for it is then and then alone that we encounter the data which distinguish that state from a dream. The latter falls short of the former, no matter how much more vivid, exciting, or evident it may seem, because it does not and cannot encounter the common sensuous content which is available and enjoyed by the former.

We encounter the common sensuous content when we are awake, and we subjectively exhaust part of it while we are encountering it. We have no capacity to hold on to all of it and we have no capacity to retain or to recall any of it. What we recall and what we remember are at best but phases of it, abstractions from it.

1.57 Perception yields content, which is in part sensuous, is judged and accepted, and may be believed.
(*See 1.55, 1.56*)

SENSUOUS content provides no knowledge of places, kinds, potencies. It is merely undergone. Since it makes no claim to be true, it is never in error. But to perceive is to know something of where the experienced Actuality is, how it contrasts with others, what it has in common with them, as well as something of what it promises to and for them. Perception thus goes far beyond sensing—not necessarily in its grasp of a being, but in what it knows of that being. It divides and analyzes, and then synthesizes that which it has isolated to make a unity claiming to be true of a world beyond.

Inanimate beings do not encounter the sensuous, and thus never perceive; they merely react to others. Low-grade organisms sense but do not judge; they respond to stimuli but do not know the nature of what they encounter. They make errors of practice but no errors of judgment; they err by moving too slowly or too quickly, this way or that, answering a disturbance in a way which does not promote their continuance. The higher animals and man perceive and therefore also sense; they dissect to take account of what they encounter, distinguishing features and aspects in order to be able to deal with the encountered from different angles and for different purposes, and in order to be able to utilize past adventures and to ground expectations. Human perception differs from animal perception by virtue of the fact that it is carried on by a self; human interests, concerns for distant goals, and obligating values infect the perception to make it not merely a report of what is encountered but an estimate of its worth in terms of standards which may be applicable to oneself and others as well.

1.58 Through perception an external world can be truly known.
(See 1.57)

NOT ALL that is perceived can be illusory, for we know that we make perceptual errors. Such knowledge presupposes that there are veridical perceptions of Actualities, for these alone are qualified to reject the perceptually erroneous. It is of course possible to maintain that all perception is unsatisfactory, because it is too vague, too particular, too prone to error, and one might prefer to engage in some other mode of 'knowing,' e.g., by means of the senses, through the use of mathematics, or with the help of revelation. But a judgment about the value of perception as such does not disqualify this or that perception over against any other. When we know that we make a perceptual error, we must know that there is something perceptually veridical. The reason it is an error to judge that this before me is white, is then not that it is, say, a sunflower, but that it is yellow or some other color. What defines it to be an error is the exclusion by something of the same order of being. It is the color of the sunflower—a color which the nature of the sunflower may perhaps preclude forever from being white—and not the sunflower, which makes the perception of the color as white to be in error.

Since our perceptual errors are in a real relation to what can be perceived truly, we are not, when perceiving erroneously, entirely cut off from the world. Our erroneous perceptual judgments are not merely privately entertained, floating in our minds or between our minds and the world. Instead they are in a real relation to a world beyond, which precludes the truth of those perceptual judgments.

1.59 Perception involves the use of nonsensuous content.
(See 1.58)

SENSUOUS content provides no articulate knowledge. It tells us nothing of places, kinds, potencies, of promises or past performances. But perception provides such knowledge. It makes use of the sensuous, but also of what is nonsensuous. The nonsensuous allows for a retention in the mind and the drawing of implications, the sensuous serving to keep the perceiver in touch with what is objective and experienced.

1.60 A perceived Actuality has a location, to be pointed to, indicated, not sensuously undergone.
(See 1.01, 1.58, 1.59)

THE PERCEIVED is an object of knowledge. It can be viewed as the surface of an object related to the perceiver; it can also be viewed as integral to the knower, since it is part of his mind. It is in fact both of these, *something* known, and something *known*. As *something* known it is external to the knower, located beyond him in space but in relation to him. For the knower to perceive he must focus on it as at a position over against himself; he must face it as an "it," as the sensuous content "it-ed," in a one-to-one relation with himself. As something *known* it is the terminus of an act of attending which can be isolated, designated and named. It is then only at a 'psychic' distance from him.

The logical atomists, e.g., the early Russell and Wittgenstein, contend that the substance of things is exhausted in the totality of "its," of mere denoted entities, of the counterparts of true proper names. But if there were nothing but "its," or nothing but perceiveds in the guise of "its," there would be no way of distinguishing one perceived object from another, and thus no predication or qualification or judgment which could in any way claim to be true.

1.61   Perception involves the contemplation of a universal, distinct from but not alien to the sensuous.
(*See 1.59*)

TO KNOW is to possess something from which inferences can be drawn, something which can be thought about, reflected on, analyzed, combined, remembered. In every perception we must isolate a facet of the object which informs us about the nature of the being we confront. This which we isolate is a universal, something which could also be in another situation. It is the sensuous made generic, the sensuous deprived of its singularity and made into a kind or form of which the sensuous is a passing singular illustration. The sensuous is "natured" in the act of contemplation, and while losing concreteness thereby achieves intelligibility and a role in the reflective life of man.

There are Hegelians who seek to acknowledge nothing but contemplateds. For them even the "it" is a universal—and the sensuous is one too, but confused. Such thinkers have nothing to know but congeries of universals. As a consequence they have no way of locating anything and no way of accounting for the fact that there are singular experiences and singular objects.

1.62   Indicateds and contemplateds are had as independent, but also as mutually pertinent.
(*See 1.60, 1.61*)

AN INDICATED and a contemplated are independent of one another; one can be had without the other. Were this not the case there would be only one contemplated or set of contemplateds for a given indicated, or conversely. But we can sometimes correctly perceive where an object is and yet mistake its nature; we can sometimes correctly perceive what an object is and mistake its position. To fasten correctly on an indicated or a contemplated is no surety that we have fastened on the other correctly. Nevertheless they are not necessarily irrelevant to one another. They may have to do with the very same object; this can be approached both denotatively and connotatively.

For knowledge to be possible, the indicated and contemplated must form a unity. Since they are independent they must be brought together, synthesized. Were the unitary outcome of the synthesis of the indicated and contemplated purely external, the result would be arbitrary. Because the contemplated and indicated belong together, are pertinent to one another, despite their independence of nature and their independent functioning they can together express the unitary object.

1.63 The indicated and contemplated are aspects of the object veridically perceived.
(See 1.58, 1.62)

WERE THE indicated and contemplated not aspects of the object veridically perceived, a grasp of them would not be a grasp of the object's place and nature. Those critical realists who insist on forcing a chasm between the content by means of which they know and the object to be known by means of it, are forced to confess that the object to be known is precisely that which they can not know. We are able to know a real objective world through perception only if the content used in the knowing is not only part of the mind but part of the object. The content used in perception is content obtained in perception; we know the perceptual object by means of material we perceptually obtain from it.

1.64 Perception provides knowledge through a union of indicated and contemplated.
(See 1.62, 1.63)

A PERCEPTUAL judgment articulates a perceived object. It first distinguishes the indicated and the contemplated and then unites them in a single claim to truth. Dissecting the perceived object in ways it is not in fact dissected, it reunites the resultant parts in order to represent the unity which the object in fact has. There are no seams in the object, no distinct denotative regions and connotative aspects; there is only a single perceived being in which we distinguish an "it," the object as over against us, and a contemplated, the object in the guise of a generic nature.

The contemplated is not predicated of the indicated. If it were, all judgments would be necessarily true or necessarily false—necessarily true if the "it" had the character which the contemplated ascribes to it, and necessarily false if it did not. But there is no attempt in a judgment to predicate a contemplated of an indicated; the two serve to articulate, analyze, express the object in a way which the mind can handle. The perceiver judges, forges a unity out of the indicated and the contemplated in the effort to have in himself the meaning of the unity of the two. The two as in the object were never divided; they are one there in a way that it is not possible for them to be in the perceiver.

No one, merely by perceiving, can reach that union of singularity and universality enjoyed by the object. But one can know it, forge a counterpart of it, and then see if the conclusions which one draws from this are in accord with the consequences which the object in fact produces in the course of time. Having judged something to be wood I infer that it can burn; the judgment that it is wood is known to be true just so far as the object itself yields the contemplated "burning," or the indicated "here" where and when our judgment permits us to expect them.

1.65   A perception is not identical with its object.
(See 1.56, 1.58, 1.63)

IT TAKES AN actual man to perceive, a man in a real relation to other Actualities. His perceptions are acts of his and presuppose real relations between him and the objects he perceives. If we identify the object of perception with an "it," or with a contemplated, then when we are not pointing out the "it," or not thinking about the object's nature, the object must vanish. Since Actualities do not vanish with the coming of night nor come to be by being perceived, the object must be more than what we synthesize. The indicated and the contemplated are the object only as in special relations to us, and since we can know this, we, in perceiving, must be acquainted with something more than the elements by means of which we perceive.

Perception requires that the indicated and contemplated be combined in a judgment. Since a perceptual judgment is not always in existence, it cannot be identical with its object unless the object could be made to disappear by our ceasing to judge it, e.g., when we fall asleep. The perceptual judgment is distinct from its object. It is about what is perceived, as merging into a real object having a being outside our encounter with it.

1.66 While perceiving, we know that the perceived is not the real object.
(See 1.65)

EACH OF US knows that he is now ignorant and that he will be ignorant in the future. If he did not know this he would allow that he might be omniscient either now or later. There are some thinkers, however, who suppose that everything we know is an induction from experience, yielding only probable knowledge. They are forced to say that their belief that they are ignorant now and will be so later is but the outcome of a swift induction from their past painful experience of learning. Since a low probability is not a zero probability, an impossibility, these men must allow that they might be omniscient now or later. We have then an empiricistic paradox: to suppose we know only inductively, and therefore have only probable and fallible knowledge is to allow that we may perhaps even at the next moment be omniscient and, since we would then know infallibly, have no need to be empiricists any longer.

While holding on to the aspects we isolate in the object perceived, we are aware of it in the shape of a real object beyond these. It is by virtue of this awareness that we know that we are ignorant when we perceive. This is a truth about any perception, for it is the product of the manner in which we judge and of the fact that we do subject the isolated elements to a unity of our own producing. We therefore know, no matter when and what we perceive, that there is always more to the perceived and to the real object than that which we isolate and then unify in a judgment. The perceived has a unity of its own and some depth too; the real object has a privacy and a career not fully manifest in the perceived.

1.67 An Actuality is adumbrated when and as an indicated and contemplated are united in a judgment.
(See 1.56, 1.64)

THE ELEMENTS united in judgment are boundary features, where mind meets the object, where the object blocks the mind. Beyond these elements is a domain of ignorance, the sensuous as the object of a common sense, receding beyond the grasp of the indicated and the contemplated—or alternatively, the private being as enjoying an epistemological role but not yet judgmentally possessed. The adumbrated side of an object is directly had, but only through the help of what is judged. Its sensuous nature, unlike that encountered through the specific senses, is not exhausted in the confrontation; but also it has no definite qualities, being unclassifiable in the terms appropriate to the objects sensed through specific organs. It is a dark recess faintly illuminated by what we judge of it, a unity in a sensuous guise, the object as that which has not yet been judged, the residuum of what is given to perception when we have isolated the indicated and the contemplated, the counterpart of the copula, the real in relation to a perceiver.

Partly because the adumbrated is not characterizable in the terms appropriate to the abstracted indicated and contemplated, and partly because, as a rule, four senses of a proper name have been confused, there has been an inclination in most epistemologies to neglect the adumbrative side of perception. "Socrates" can be used to refer to the real man Socrates, to the perceived Socrates, to the "it-ized" Socrates, and to the adumbrative Socrates. The indicated Socrates is just an "it" correlated with "philosopher," a part of a judgment. The adumbrated Socrates is just beyond the reach of but in relation to a judgment. The perceived Socrates stands outside all judgment and all distinctions made by means of it. And the real Socrates goes his own way in independence of perceivers. We judge a perceived or the real Socrates by means of an adumbrative Socrates integrated with a judgment which makes use of the indicated or "it-ized" "Socrates" and some such contemplated as "philosopher." "Socrates is a philosopher" is a judgment about a perceived or the real Socrates by virtue of its reference to the adumbrative Socrates. It is because there is a perceived Socrates that there is an adumbrative Socrates testing the judgment which has isolated an indicated Socrates in the real Socrates; and it is because there is a real Socrates that there can be a perceived Socrates, to be perceptually judged. To be sure, Socrates is no longer present; the adumbrative side of him is one we now merely take account of in an historical judgment, but it too is quite distinct from the indicated, and of course from a perceived and from the real Socrates.

1.68 The adumbrated conveys knowledge.
(*See 1.64-67*)

WE CANNOT test a judgment by facing it up against the real object as in no way implicated in the judgment. But this does not cut us off from all test. The perceived object is the real object when this is related to the judgment. Because the object is outside the judgment we are cognizant of the fact that there is something more than the judgment—a domain of ignorance inseparable from the judged content.

The perceived object contains part of the adumbrated; it is this which roots the perceived in a reality outside perception. That adumbrated has depth. Every effort to integrate it with the indicated and the contemplated in a judgment ends by leaving some of it outside. To try to include within the sphere of our understanding not only what we judge but also all we adumbrate is a hopeless task; we must be content with holding some of the adumbrated in the foreground and as one with the judgment, while allowing the rest to fade into the background, eventually to be lost in the recesses of the real being beyond. When we do this we have a knowledge that goes beyond the content synthesized in a judgment.

VII   MEANING AND THOUGHT

1.69 Perceptual content grounds generalizations, specifications, and other inferences.
(*See 1.59*)

IF A BEGINNING is made with one mode of being, caution, effectiveness, and precision make it desirable to have no unnecessary recourse to other modes until we are finished with the one with which we began. Since we have chosen to begin with Actualities, we should deal with all else from that perspective until we have as rounded-out an account as we can get. Only then ought we go on to deal with things from other angles. Moreover, the most direct and fruitful source of knowledge is the perceptual. This normally grounds our knowledge in science, history, art, and philosophy. It also grounds a knowledge of the Ideal, of Existence, and of God. (Since these other modes ground a knowledge of the Actual as surely as it grounds a knowledge of them, a satisfactory account of what is will of course require that everything be dealt with in terms of them as well. Only a fourfold approach does *full* justice to all there is and can be known.)

There is nothing to be derived from a bare "it" except such abstractions as that it is in a one-to-one relation to the perceiver, that it has a minimum of meaning, etc. But the contemplated has a structure and can be analyzed and related to other contemplateds, and can, together with the "it," help constitute a judgment from which implications follow and from which inferences can be made. We can obtain more and more generalized forms of contemplateds until we reach some such final form as unity or being; we can imaginatively specify the contemplateds we have, in the attempt to remember or anticipate experience, until we reach a final form, where there are no further specifications imaginable by us; we can also infer to what is and to what is not, the limits being given by whatever laws of inference there may be. Beyond the limits of generalization, there is nothing intelligible; beyond the limits of specification is the concrete being as in itself, not open to our direct experience; beyond the limits of lawful inference is the random and inexplicable. But even what is beyond these limits is inferentially derivable from perceptual contemplateds and judgments. By making use of a fresh principle or process which takes account of the relation of otherness separating what we encounter or accept from what we do not, we can even get to speak of the inchoate which lies beyond the idea of being, of a thing-in-itself which lies outside the reach of any specification we might impose, and of what is itself not formally derivable.

1.70 An idea has an empirical meaning if there is a perceptual contemplated from which the idea can be derived.
(*See 1.69*)

AN IDEA is a contemplated; it might be privately generated or it might be obtained by abstraction from a perceptual contemplated. It has an empirical meaning, if it could have been derived from a perceptual contemplated. The meaning it then has is given by that contemplated as subject to the transformations which would turn it into that idea. The empirical meaning of an early "five-toed horse" is a perceptually contemplated horse as subject to the converse of the transformative process of evolution; the empirical meaning of "angel" is a perceptually contemplated messenger denied a body, identified with a species, and so on.

Peirce's pragmatic principle which affirmed that the meaning of a concept was to be found in the conceived practical effects of that concept ("Consider what effects, that might conceivably have practical bearings, we conceive the object of our conception to have. Then, our conception of these effects is the whole of our conception of the object.") spawned a whole family of doctrines. In essence all of them attempt to give meaning to something by subjecting it to the demands of some alien domain. What that domain does not allow to be distinguished is said to be in fact without distinct meaning, and whatever that domain does distinguish is said in fact to possess a distinct meaning. These doctrines evidently offer a kind of reductionism, asking that items in one domain be evaluated in terms of another. According to James the evaluation is to be framed in terms of particular acts or sensations or beliefs; for Dewey society or democracy provides the measure; for Peirce it is the community of scientific inquirers occupied with observable phenomena.

These doctrines make at least three limitative suppositions: (*1*) they suppose that some special part of experience offers the final test of the meaning or legitimacy of concepts. Peirce, James, and Dewey differ primarily as to just what part of experience one is to use as a test; (*2*) they suppose that only concepts are to be tested, overlooking the fact that what practice distinguishes theory (say, logic or mathematics) might justifiably identify, and what practice identifies theory might justifiably distinguish, so that it would be legitimate to give a kind of "pragmatic" reduction for practice, coordinate with that which these men give for theory; and (*3*) they suppose that the reduction they provide makes the initial distinctions vanish. This supposition, too, is mistaken. The fact that a distinction is not useful in some domain merely points up the difference between that domain and one where it is useful. From the standpoint of a geometry there may be no difference between the line a-b and the line b-a, but for geography there is such a difference. For a religious man much that science, practice, ethics fail to distinguish should be distinguished, and much that they distinguish should not be distinguished.

For an orthodox Hebrew there is no religious difference between pork and ham, but a great difference between the names of God, all equally referring to him and only to him.

All three suppositions must be overcome if we are to have a non-arbitrary, flexible theory of meaning.

1.71   The meaning of an idea is any other, perceptual or not, as qualified by that conceivable transformation which would convert it into the former.
(See *1.69, 1.70*)

THIS PROPOSITION generalizes and extends the foregoing. No longer restricted to empirical meanings, it need not require one to refer to some perceptual contemplated. It therefore enables one to give meanings, for example, to numbers without having to look to some experience. The meaning of "six" is a "four" to which a "two" can be added, a "seven" from which a "one" can be subtracted, and so on. The irrationals, imaginaries, and infinites of mathematics, with their strange properties, are easily shown to be meaningful in analogous ways. Traced back by transformations to familiar numbers, they can of course be rooted in the empirical, since they can be obtained from the empirical by transformations which combine those by which the familiar numbers are obtained and those by means of which the strange numbers were obtained from the familiar ones. He who wishes to remain inside mathematics or would like to relate its items to those in some other nonempirical enterprise such as divinity or metaphysics (as Newton and Pythagoras did) can provide intelligible and useful definitions by attending only to the manner in which the items with which he is concerned are translatable into those he is willing to take as already acceptable, and then qualifying the latter by the manner in which they could be made to yield the former.

1.72   An idea of something nonempirical can be transformed into an idea of something empirical by subjecting it to the conditions of experience.
(See *1.71*)

ONCE IT IS recognized that any idea can be given meaning in terms of some other, when that other is subject to qualifications expressing whatever transformations would in fact change it into the former, it becomes evident that the problem of giving meaning to the non-empirical is but a special case of the problem of giving meaning to any idea. It is presupposed of course that what is nonempirical can be related to what is empirical, and that the difference between them can be expressed by referring to the conditions of experience—a perceiver, an encounter, a category, judgment, etc. If these presuppositions are not allowed there would be no way of making experience intelligible or of giving empirical meaning to what is nonempirical. But, as we saw before, we can give an empirical meaning even for "angel." Those who take the empirical to provide the only test of what is significant will, of course, employ this principle to define the nonempirical as meaningless. But as we shall immediately see, the reverse procedure is just as legitimate—or better, just as illegitimate.

1.73 An idea of the empirical is transformable into an idea of the nonempirical by freeing it from the conditions of experience.
(See 1.72)

WE CAN take our start with a nonempirical idea and understand our empirical ideas in terms of it. The nonempirical idea may have had its origin in, and its meaning defined by something empirical; but whether this is the case or not, when we subject it to the converse of the transformation which would derive it from an empirical idea, we make it into the meaning of that empirical idea. A human messenger is an angel endowed with a body, made into a member of a species, and so on. The account sounds strange for those who think all understand the idea of a human messenger better than they do that of an angel. It is strange for one whose experience is like Abraham's, but not strange for one whose experience is like that of the Mormon, Joseph Smith. For Smith and for others the nonempirical is prior to or independent of the empirical in origin and validity.

1.74 What is independent of experience can be understood in terms of the empirical, and conversely.
(See 1.72, 1.73)

THIS PROPOSITION combines the preceding two. It means that we can give meaning to "God" in terms of "this book," and to "this book" in terms of "God." "This book" is "God" as given location, matter, etc.; "God" is "this book" as freed from time, enhanced in value, separated from its matter, etc. The illustration seems odd, and tempts the denial of the principles which justify it. But when it is recalled that the Bible is but a name for book, and that it is, for some, God made manifest, the strangeness may perhaps vanish. Or, if we take seriously, as the Franciscans do, the idea that everything in the universe is a sign of God, bearing some mark of his presence, not on its surface but in its being, instead of seeming odd our illustration will appear most apt.

Were it not possible to make such transformations and give such accounts of meaning, there would be ideas so cut off from others that there would be no way, not even through negation, that they could be reached. To go from one to the other would be impossible, for even a leap from one to the other can be expressed in the form of a transformational act. Having the one we would not, while remaining single beings, be able to have the other; if we could have the other we would be so divided against ourselves that we could not know that we also had the first. The transition through which we in fact go from one idea to another can always be formally expressed as a mode of transformation of the one into the other. To have two ideas within the same mind is to allow for the presentation of a meaning of the one in terms of the other. The meaning might be vague and incomplete, because we might not have an adequate grasp of the way to transform the one into the other. But we will never be warranted in supposing that in principle no full transformation is possible.

1.75 Different types of transformation provide supplementary ways of defining the meaning of a given idea.
(See 1.71, 1.74)

THERE ARE nonempirical meanings and there are empirical meanings. Most of our nonempirical meanings seem to be the product of transformations of the empirically contemplated. These transformations however can be quite radical, making it more correct to say that the ideas were then and there engendered than that they were derived from something empirically encountered. Be that as it may, we have knowledge of modes of being other than the Actual, and so far as this is true we have ideas which have no necessary empirical origin. These other modes do have bearing on Actualities and have some effect on experience. We not only note objects but evaluate them; not only confront complexities but recognize unity; not only encounter individuals but are aware that they are caught in a process larger than themselves. Since the evaluation, the unity, the process provide standards, impose prescriptions on the way in which the empirical is dealt with, they cannot be completely reduced to what is experienced or wholly located there.

The empirical and nonempirical are intertransformable. The use of one to give meaning to the other is justified by the clarification which it provides. In a way this extends the idea of meaning which Peirce first formulated, freeing it from his limiting supposition that somehow nature is in a privileged position to determine what meanings ideas have. He required all ideas to give an account of themselves in terms of what is conceived to happen in fact, saying in effect that the meaning of an idea is all the consequences into which nature will transform that idea. Instead of asking what one supposed was involved in an idea, one instead thought of what nature might bring out of it, and used this result to define what the idea meant. Meaning thus became a matter not of perception or cognition but of the intelligible processes of nature. But a different stress is equally justified and often more valuable. Instead of attending to nature's transformations one might attend to God's; or perhaps more conservatively, one might take the transformations which a poet in fact imposes on an idea and then judge the transformations that nature produces as being inadequate, obscure, distortive, or incomplete just so far as they fail to match what the poet discerned. These different approaches are equally legitimate. They are in fact supplementary.

The complete meaning of an idea is given by all others as qualified by the possible transformations which can convert those others into it. The complete meaning of the idea of a book cannot then be obtained short of a knowledge not only of how nature but also of how Actualities, Ideality, and God can transform all other entities, empirical and nonempirical, into it.

1.76 Memory reverses transformations produced by the passage of time.
(See 1.75)

MEMORY and recollection are distinct. Recollection reinstates a previously entertained idea. Without it there would be no recognition and thus no reflective use of experience. The reinstatement does of course involve not a literal recurrence of the previous idea but a re-confrontation of the meaning which that idea expresses. It is often quite general and often makes no reference back to a previous time. Memory, in contrast, makes such backward reference. It involves the use of an idea which is more determinate in nature than the future allows, and which at the same time is excluded by what is present. The idea used in memory may be recollected, it may be freely conceived then and there, or it may be produced by some transformation of what is perceived. It may be determinate in fact or it may merely lay claim that a determinateness is essential to its very being. In any case, because denied reference either to the future or the present, it is inevitably referred back to ourselves as experiencing something at some previous time. The idea, entertained by us now, is transformed in an act of memory into an idea characterizing an experience of ours in the past.

What is remembered is quite distinct from what is known to be historically past. The remembered is inseparable from our own experiencing; the historically known past, even when it is something which we have experienced and may even remember, is divorced from us as experiencing it. An objective fact, open to any one, it may involve a reference to us as a participant but not to us as the subject experiencing it.

1.77 Expectation is a waiting for determinations for some idea.
(See 1.41, 1.76)

WHAT IS not yet determinate cannot be referred to either the present or the past. It can, of course, be contemplated, reflected on. Expectation looks beyond such a contemplated idea to what could give it determination. It waits for experience to provide a filling for the contemplated idea.

Prediction goes beyond expectation, not in being more precise, for an expectation may have any degree of precision, but in not involving a necessary reference to oneself, the individual who will have that experience. When an experience is predicted, it is predicted as a public occurrence, as an encounter which others can observe; an expectation is oriented towards the expectant individual.

Hope goes further than either expectation or prediction, in that it involves a desire for something which the expected or predicted object will produce. Fear is a present emotional rejection of something expected to be injurious. Without hope we have no ground for laying plans for the future; without fear there is no adequate alertness to what may prove our undoing. We may be said to be able to hope for what is bad for another as well as to hope for what is good for ourselves. But since we do not really desire evil for ourselves we cannot hope for it. We can only fear it.

1.78 Ideas can be imagined.
(See 1.73)

UNDER THE pressure of the romantic tradition we have today freed the idea of imagination from a necessary association with images. Imagination is a power by which new ideas, not necessarily germane to past, present, or future, are produced. Through its agency we deal with possibilities and situations never encountered, and which we may never expect to encounter. There are no rules for its most fruitful exercise, and no known ways of making it function, unless it be odd stimuli and a readiness to be intelligent.

VIII   INFERENCE

1.79 Thinking is the act of transforming an idea or judgment into another.
(See 1.69)

THINKING has a broad and a narrow meaning. Taken broadly it includes the operations of memory, recollection, hope, expectation, generalization, and so on; taken narrowly it is a specialized act of the mind which makes use of rules in order to transform given ideas or judgments. On the one hand we apply the term to any activity of the mind, and on the other hand we apply it only to mind's most excellent, desirable activity. Most of us use the term sometimes in the one sense and sometimes in the other without attending to the fact.

Pragmatists such as Peirce and Dewey tend to suppose that men think only when they must. Were men in situations which were calm or determinate or satisfying, these pragmatists hold, the men would not think at all. But there is nothing in a state of doubt or in an indeterminate situation which compels one to move away from it. A man can remain ill at ease for an indefinite period of time. Moreover, we often think deliberately, set ourselves to raise questions and to find solutions, and this when all is calm and otherwise satisfactory. The very agreement of men and the agreeableness of a situation may serve the philosophical mind, and surely the sceptical and rebellious mind, to ask questions which the situation tends to keep safely in the background.

The mistake of the pragmatists was to try to explain thinking as a device for avoiding or escaping from what is unpleasant. They neglected its final cause. To be sure, there is thinking when men are in a quandary, but only because they are concerned with going elsewhere. Men also think when not in a quandary. What is present may have little relevance to what in fact interests them; that is why thinking sometimes passes over the entire present to deal only with what had been and what might be, without any necessary benefit or loss to a man, now or later. It is because a man wants more truth than he now has, a truth not now within the reach of his body or mind that he has a need to think, and profits from the thinking. An interest in an outcome, not a disturbance in the present is what primarily provokes him to think.

Thinking as a rule saves time, and often energy and money, since it transcends the sluggish movements of nature and its odd heterogeneity of items that so often block and obscure the things we want to understand. We usually think in order to have an answer now which we could not otherwise obtain in that form, or so readily.

1.80   A sound inference is a thinking which terminates in the warranted qualification of an idea.
(See 1.79)

INFERENCE is a mental act by which one obtains a warranted

characterization of an idea. When most cautious it concerns itself solely with the qualifications or 'values' of "truth" and "falsehood." It is one of the tasks of logic to tell us how to transfer these from accepted ideas or expressions to some others. An inference may, however, not only transfer but may also transform a value; starting with p as true it can, to take the simplest case, end with not-p as false. A still bolder type of inference involves transformations in modal values, from contingent to necessary truth or necessary falsehood or conversely, from possibility to contingency or conversely, and so on.

Ideas and their expressions can be characterized not only as true or false, necessary, contingent, etc., but also as reliable, plausible, legitimate, beautiful, interesting, clear. Any one of these characterizations can serve as the beginning of an act of inferential transformation, ending in a new qualification of the ideas in which we are interested. But logicians have so far been inclined to ignore this fact. The history of logic has so far touched only the borders of the field of inferences that men can and do make.

1.81   Inference is governed by rules, conformity to which determines the warrant of a transferred or transformed qualification.
(*See 1.80*)

A RULE of inference prescribes the kind of outcome which is entitled to some designated transferred or transformed value. The simplest rules are those which relate to nothing more than a transfer of a 'value' such as "truth" or "falsehood." These rules are studied in classical and in modern symbolic logic. As just observed above, there are, however, inferences which involve a transformation of truth values, and others which transfer other types of qualification of an idea or a judgment. Their rules are to be found mainly in the inquiring sciences, but there are some in logic, particularly those having to do with the use of logical constants. One can disjoin two contingent truths, for example, in such a way as to generate the truth value "necessary": "p or –p" is a necessary truth whose constituents are only contingently true or false.

The most productive modes of inference, of which all others can be viewed as limiting cases, engage in radical transformations. These often change the kind and nature of the initial values, and often accompany these transformations with transformations of their qualified ideas and expressions as well. Their rules are to be found in the fine and practical arts.

Each discipline has distinctive interests; it attends only to some types of qualifications and ideas, and is interested in warrantedly moving only to certain definite types of things, which may be identical with or quite different from those to which it initially attended. Each has its own rules, often offering a different type of warrant from that which others do. There is no point in trying to make one discipline conform to the rules characteristic of another. It is foolish to demand that poetry conform to the canons of logic and to dismiss it as invalid or irrational because it cannot so conform, any more than there is a justification for making logic conform to the canons of poetry and dismissing it as vapid or dead because of its failure to function as poetry does.

1.82 All thinking exemplifies rules and terminates in necessitated conclusions.

(See *1.44, 1.80, 1.81*)

THINKING is a mental passage from a beginning or premiss to a terminus or conclusion. The conclusion is *deduced* when the thinking arrives at it; it is deducible through the use of rules which express the structure of the thinking that can arrive at it. These rules are of two kinds: contingent, alterable rules of transformation, employed for some limited purpose, and necessary, unalterable rules which serve only to transfer or transform some qualification in such a way that the outcome is not less valuable to the inquiry than that from which the transfer or transformation was made.

A premiss and a contingent rule together suffice to give the conclusion. Given that "Socrates is a man" and the contingent rule that "all men are mortal," we can rigorously deduce that "Socrates is mortal," i.e., acknowledge it to have the value 'truth' if the premiss has it too. The contingent rule as applied to the premiss transforms it into and transfers its value to just that conclusion.

The conclusion is necessitated in an inference as having begun just where it did and as having been reached in the way indicated. The conclusion is not necessary in itself; it is necessary only in relationship to these others. In an analogous way, the conclusions of the insane or of those who commit logical blunders are rigorously deducible by one who knows the premises from which and the manner in which they think. What is amiss with the insane and the illogical is that they have poor ways of transferring and transforming qualifications and ideas. They end their inferences—which perhaps began with truths—with what does not have the features they ascribe to it. They necessarily end by characterizing as necessary or true or good or important what in fact is usually not so. Following their method of reasoning, they do end, however, with what is inevitable. Their mistake is in using that method as a means of getting to a reliable conclusion from the premiss with which they begin.

When a contingent rule is joined with the original premiss so as to constitute a single larger premiss, the conclusion is as necessitated as before, and continues to remain distinct from the premiss. The connection between the premiss (constituted by the original premiss and the original contingent rule) and the conclusion that is brought about by operating on that original premiss in accordance with the contingent rule adds nothing to the conclusion. Such a connection is a logical connection, and its meaning is given in a necessary rule or law of logic. A necessary rule is thus present in every inference which employs a contingent rule. However, it has no distinct status there, but is embodied in the premiss and the contingent rule as together grounding a conclusion. Charles S. Peirce apparently was the first to see this point clearly.

1.83 A particular conclusion has content, meaning, implications beyond that expressed in a general rule.
(See 1.41, 1.81, 1.82)

THE SCIENCE of logic, among others things, studies necessary, formal implications between ideas and judgments or their expressions. It views all contingent rules as parts of premisses; it allows nothing except necessary rules to connect premisses with conclusions. Nothing happens in the science of logic; there is no movement from one point to another; there are only structures and the relations between them. Logicians of course do work, hard work, but this, though illustrating logic, is done outside the province of the science of logic; that science merely exposes the nature of necessary implications between the most abstract, formally expressed premisses and their conclusions.

When one reasons in strict conformity with the canons of logic, one follows necessary rules. But a rule by itself is quite general; it does not pick out this or that conclusion. From a single premiss, modern logicians have made evident, we can draw an endless number of conclusions; which ones we will pick out, just what the content and meaning of the conclusion may be, awaits our actual decision.

An actual conclusion is concluded to; it is the outcome of an activity. He who deduces asserts the conclusion in place of the premiss. He leaves the premiss behind to take up a new position, one which is warranted by the fact that he began at that point and operated on it in such and such a way.

The process through which one goes in order to get a conclusion, connected with a premiss by a necessary rule of logic, has content, power, a meaning not altogether expressed in such a rule. Though it makes use of that rule over a temporal span, it does so only when and as it also exhibits a contingent rule, for the union of a necessary rule and a process has a nature not expressed by either alone. Every act of reasoning, even the most austere and formal, exhibits a contingent rule even though it conforms to and attempts to do nothing more than use a necessary rule. Accordingly, though one might get rid of a contingent rule by making it part of a premiss, one will nevertheless make a place for some contingent rule when one in fact reasons, even in accordance with logical rules. This contingent rule is a rule for using the necessary rule; it need not affect the fact that the conclusion at which one arrives ought to be accepted by anyone who accepts the premiss.

1.84 A process of moving to a conclusion ends with with what is not wholly predictable.
(See 1.41, 1.83)

EVEN WHEN one infers from a formal premiss to a conclusion related to it by a logical or necessary rule of connection, one obtains a result not fully expressed in the formally statable conclusion. The fact that the conclusion is one of an endless number of possible conclusions which have necessary connections with the premiss means that its presence involves the exercise of some choice, a fact not expressed in either the premiss, the conclusion, or the formal statement of the nature of the relation which connects the premiss and conclusion. To be a chosen conclusion, to be an arrived-at conclusion, is to be more than what *can be* chosen or arrived at. The process of getting to the conclusion is outside the rules it illustrates and outside the area where predicted outcomes are formally necessitated.

1.85 Premiss and rule together define only a possible conclusion.
(*See 1.43, 1.83, 1.84*)

THERE IS no actual conclusion until one has concluded to it. Until then there is only a host of possible conclusions, one of which will be produced when and as we conclude to it. We do not have the conclusion so long as we have only premiss and rule; we must also have a process which illustrates the rule when and as the process gives that rule a temporal form.

Strictly speaking, the various possible conclusions are not distinct enough to be severally possible; what is really possible, given a premiss and a rule, is a type of conclusion, and this type is made concrete, actualized in mind or, in fact, in the process of going from the premiss to the conclusion with which one actually concludes.

1.86 All inference is logically necessitated and creatively free.
(*See 1.44, 1.82, 1.83, 1.85*)

THE CONCLUSION at which we arrive, no matter from where we start and how we proceed, was reached along a route governed by a logical rule. What we arrive at is necessitated, given such and such a beginning and such and such a procedure. The rule which we then exhibit is distinct from the logical rule we follow, the former being contingent and manifest in the process, the latter necessary but only formally relating the premiss to what it gives way to at the end of the process.

A logically necessitated conclusion is arrived at through a process which, though illustrating a necessary rule, exhibits a contingent structure, adding as it does content to that necessary rule when and as it illustrates it. The conclusion at which the most mechanical act of inference arrives, even the concluding to that which is foregone and prescribed in advance, is thus achieved only through a free creative act, since it goes beyond and outside the reach of any formal implication and any antecedent cause.

1.87 All making is rational as well as creative.
(See 1.42, 1.86)

REASONING is an art; it makes a conclusion be. Illustrating a logical rule it nevertheless is creatively free. If we engage in arts which make use of things rather than ideas, the situation is not changed in principle. An art begins with material of a certain nature and subjects it to various transformations; that at which those transformations terminate is, given the initial material, necessitated. It has been made just that way, along just that route.

The nature of a transformation as conjoined with the nature of material constitutes a complex nature which has formally necessary relations with the nature of the outcome at which an art arrives. The outcome is necessary. But it is logical, formal, empty. The outcome of the initial material, when subjected to an actual transformation, in contrast, is concrete and unpredictable, not empty at all.

The traditional antithesis between logic and science on the one hand, and the arts and practice on the other, is based on a stress of one of the two components both sides have. The sciences stress the nature of the rules that processes illustrate, and therefore tend to minimize the novelty in outcomes; the arts instead stress the nature of the outcomes at which one arrives and therefore tend to minimize the formal and necessary structures which one illustrates in arriving at those outcomes. But each contains the other component as well. Sciences are rational and arts are creative; but also, sciences are creative and arts are rational.

1.88 To produce well is to engage in an art; to produce for an enjoyment which awakens an awareness of an adumbrated is to engage in a fine art.
(See 1.67, 1.87)

ART, AS ARISTOTLE long ago remarked, is a making, a producing, a changing of one thing into another. We tend today to give it a more honorific meaning; we tend to say a little more insistently than he did that art is not merely a making, but a good making, a making well, a making, as he at times said, which is in accord with a right rule. Such making well can of course be the making of something evil, regrettable. There is an art to murder, to making gas chambers, to making people miserable, and there are some who practice them regrettably well.

A fine art has a desirable function. It seeks to free man from the blinders of convention so as to enable him to grasp the nature of things, free from irrelevancies and distortions. Literature, e.g., is essentially a tissue of contrary-to-fact conditions, a set of expressions having the logical form "if x were the case (which it is not) then y would be the case." Such expressions are revelatory of the world. To say of a man that he is in fact honest is to claim that it is true that "Were he to be trusted with this money (which will in fact not be done) he would live up to his trust"; "Were he asked to lie (which in fact is not the case) he would refuse," and so on. Literature rephrases such expressions without altering their import and is therefore able to expose something of the essence of what is real without ostensibly affirming that it does so. Other arts concern themselves not with words or meanings but with material of various sorts, ranging from sounds to stones. These arts subject encountered colors, shapes, bodies to various ideal conditions and operations. The resultant whole articulates the nature of the colors, shapes, and bodies (or of what lies beyond them), as they are in themselves, free from the constraints and distortions produced by special human interests and accidental situations.

The task of the master of fine arts is to awaken emotions and expectations which are germane to some fundamental facet of reality. An emotion is pure if aroused by a dramatic case; it is purged by being limited and controlled by the world at which it points.

Art is no mere device for producing pleasures. We do not need the services of genius to provide even lasting or especially delicate pleasures. There is of course pleasure in the apprehension of an art object, even when the theme is tragic, but this pleasure is not altogether separable from the fact that the art object, while it articulates according to the grammar of its medium, then and there directs us, via emotions and expectations, at what is in fact the case beneath the veil of obtrusive, familiar particularity.

1.89 Inquiry is a chain of inferences designed to reach a source of desired judgments or their elements.
(*See 1.69, 1.77, 1.86*)

INQUIRY is sustained, systematic thinking, originating and terminating in something outside itself. Like inferences, it is at once governed by rules and comes to inevitable outcomes, at the same time that it involves a process freely actualizing the prospective outcome which the starting points and rules together determine.

Unlike a deductive chain of reasoning, which need not begin in or terminate in anything outside itself, a genuine inquiry makes at least two contacts with the world beyond. It originates with something in the present, and points to some outcome in which the inquirer is interested. But instead of being content with logically certifying the outcome by means of a valid transferal of the value of some accepted judgment, an inquirer looks beyond the terminal judgment to what can ground it.

Verification is not simply the outcome of a successful expectation that the world will put its mark of approval on something we have previously acknowledged or certified. It is the outcome of an encounter with some reality which can yield a determinate perceptual judgment that is otherwise acknowledgeable only formally, and thus, even if adequately certified, is not yet fully determinate.

1.90 A science is an inquiry well conducted.
(*See 1.88, 1.89*)

A SCIENCE differs primarily from other types of enterprise not by its language, its ideals, its methods, though these are, to be sure, distinctive. It is first and foremost an inquiry, i.e., a way of thinking which is rooted at its beginning and end, and often throughout, in a real world beyond its discourse. Inquiries carried on for short spans are sciences in embryo.

Science, strictly speaking, is ordered knowledge, a knowledge which has been and continues to be mastered by pursuing established and certified methods of inquiry. Today the term seems to be used primarily to apply to empirical systematic inquiries, and secondarily to theoretical inquiries relating to the world dealt with in the empirical inquiries. The empirical inquiries are concerned with discovering those modes of transformation which will enable them to interconnect every perceptual fact with every other; the theoretical inquiries are concerned with transformations which interrelate idealized versions of the perceptual facts—mathematics being concerned with principles governing transformations of all other transformations.

Every science has its element of art, of making and doing something well. This is evidently the case with the experimental sciences, but it is also true of mathematics and the theoretical sciences. Not only do they make occasional recourse to diagrams and thus in an attenuated way make use of material to bring out a desirable outcome, but they specialize in the production of conclusions requiring creative, imaginative constructions.

1.91 Philosophy is at once a science and an art.
(*See 1.88, 1.90*)

PHILOSOPHY is a persistent, resolute, self-critical, speculative adventure seeking to encompass the whole of things, freed from irrelevancy and error; it is an inquiry concerned with achieving an ordered knowledge of the world and of the conditions and principles involved in an adequate grasp of it. Seeking to bring to the fore the presuppositions characteristic of all thought and experience, philosophy thereby illuminates what is daily encountered, known in the sciences, and enjoyed in the arts.

Philosophy's language and its values partake both of science and of art. It uses both technical terms and metaphors; it defines, sharpens, refines at the same time that it forges new expressions and combinations of terms. At once cautious and adventurous, it is concerned with knowing and enjoying, with intertwining truth and insight to constitute an articulate wisdom about man and the world outside him.

There are philosophers today who reject all claim to system. They dedicate themselves to the mastery of some limited domain, to the study of some special project. But since they do not attend to the nature of their presuppositions, since they do not ask how their special inquiry is related to the inquiries which are pursued by others, they are inevitably driven to operate inside a frame of unexamined assumptions. Usually they take it for granted that the categories of ordinary knowledge, the assumptions men normally make regarding what is real, and the accepted beliefs regarding the way in which the various disciplines are related to one another, are on the whole satisfactory. They assume that no critical examination of those categories, assumptions, and beliefs will find them seriously wanting. But they have no way of knowing that any of these suppositions is justified. A nonsystematic treatment of the world, a concentration on some limited field, depends on a dogmatism, the acceptance and use of somewhat questionable assumptions regarding the nature of knowledge, being, and the interrelationships of things. The least dogmatic of philosophies is an all-inclusive system in which its own basic, indispensable principles are critically examined and systematically connected.

1.92   Philosophy's method is speculative; i.e., it infers to presuppositions. Its argument is primarily dialectic; i.e., it infers to what would complete the already known. And its attitude is at once sympathetic and critical.
(*See 1.91*)

AT EVERY moment we presuppose much. We presuppose a body of funded knowledge, for we come into a world which has been going on for some time and which has been partly understood and evaluated by those who educate us. We presuppose good sense, without which we could not live in the world or with our fellows. We presuppose principles by means of which we organize what we encounter, and without which we would have little more than a sad heterogeneity of separate bits of knowledge. And we presuppose an objective world, a world of substantial beings, values, existence, and eternity, which give body to and explain the world we directly encounter.

The historically minded thinker and the conservative philosopher tend to acknowledge only the funded knowledge we all have. They offer a healthy antidote to those who would speculate in a vacuum. But since our funded knowledge is not necessarily reliable, coherent, satisfactory, as the cataclysmic turns in the history of thought make evident, these thinkers evidently have a philosophy which more likely than not cannot outlast the epoch in which they live. A dominant school of English philosophers, on the other hand, tends to devote a major portion of its energies to the isolation of the presupposed common sense from which men often take their theoretic flights. Philosophy, it clearly sees, is no deduction of a universe, no mere play of fancy, but the grasp of what men of good judgment and sound sense know to be the case. But no man is merely a man of good sense; what we uncritically accept is a mixture of the sound and the foolish, of the superficial and the bed rock. Epistemologists concentrate instead on the principles which justify the acceptance of this or that as true, reliable, or real. But if we attempt, as many students of language, semantics, and logic do, to ignore what is the case apart from our epistemology, we will end with a theory of knowledge which has nothing to do with men in fact, and the world they are supposed to know. Finally, there are ontologically oriented thinkers who concentrate on the nature of being; since they do not ask themselves how they might determine which of their assertions are valid, reliable, unbiased, true, they have no way of knowing whether what they claim is fancy or fact, a mere coherent fiction or a report of what is the case. Nothing less than a critical examination of all these presuppositions, with a consequent speculative systematic interrelating of the results, will protect one from a precipitate dogmatism, and permit of an acknowledgment of the purified accumulated wisdom of the race, of the good sense of the day, of sound criteria for acceptable knowledge, and of the being of ourselves and of what we know.

There are many and even conflicting statements of the nature of dialectic. But we come somewhat close to what all have in mind when we observe that dialectic is the recognition and the provision of that which would complete a given datum. Marx was inclined to think of dialectic as a work of nature; Aristotle was inclined to think of it as the work of the intellect; Plato and Hegel were inclined to think of it as both at once. A philosophic system, being the work of the mind, would tend to support Aristotle's interpretation, but only with the additional proviso that what dialectic brings about answers to the nature of what indeed is the case. Dialectic is a method enabling men to understand what in fact lies outside them. It need not, though, be supposed that the universe is dialectical or that dialectic is merely an agency for obtaining probable results. When we generalize from the material of daily life we get to the modes of being as terminal points; dialectic is our way of moving to those beings as in fact substantial, necessary correlates, completing one another.

For most thinkers dialectic is a dynamic process of extricating one-self or what one understands from contradictions and conflicts. According to some systematic thinkers, particularly Hegel and Marx, dialectic exhibits a steady pattern of thesis, antithesis, and synthesis. For them the process of the dialectic is the truth itself; there is no terminus in time towards which the dialectic moves and at which it will come to an end. The process in time for them is in effect an eternity making itself manifest. Much of what they say, particularly regarding the power of negation, the reconciliation of the negative with the positive, the need for a logic which is integral with its subject matter, the error in a divorce of the rational and the passionate, the possible and the actual, the free and the determinate, can be accepted without compromising the view that there is a universe whose rationale is not in complete accord with our own. And with them we can say that this universe can be understood through the use of a dialectical method, provided that we use it to ask after the ideas and the things that would complete what we now have or have accepted.

Most important is the fact that for philosophy there is nothing which can be put beyond the reach of critical examination. All questions, for the philosopher, are legitimate; nothing is to be accepted on any authority, whether this be accumulated wisdom, common sense, reason, or relevation. But criticism degenerates into dogmatic scepticism unless sustained by insight, sympathy, an awareness of others, just as sympathy degenerates into sentimentality unless sustained by criticism.

1.93   Philosophy is a circular enterprise.
(See 1.91, 1.92)

IT IS a common mistake to suppose that there is something invalid in a circular argument. Logically viewed it is unimpeachable. A conclusion which repeats the premiss, conforms neatly to the requirements of the most stringent logic. What is wrong with a circular argument is that it is often uninformative, coming back to its beginning too quickly. But if its circle is all-inclusive, if it encompasses all there is, it does all that a philosophic system demands.

Philosophy has quite often been structured in noncircular ways. The most impressive is perhaps the linear, which begins with one or a few truths and seeks to derive all the others in strict accord with

some straightforward deductive device. This is the method employed by Descartes and Spinoza. Could Aristotle know how to get to
his first principle directly it would perhaps have been the method
which he would have employed. Such a method supposes that its
beginning is self-evident; it also usually involves the imposition of a
logic of deduction on alien content, and thus ends finally with some
kind of dualism. Though Hegel said he was pursuing a circular path
his was, I think, rather linear. But he did avoid the supposition that
the logic of deduction was exterior to or imposed on alien content.
Over against his and the other philosophies are the philosophy of
detached observations, and phenomenalism or descriptive philosophy.
Of these, the former uncritically presupposes a systematic background, while the latter has no tests, limits, or principle of order. But
no philosophy can be satisfactory which does not at least allow for
the examination and justification of every one of its presuppositions
and propositions.

There are thinkers who would like to do nothing in philosophy
until they have made sure of their principles of knowledge. They
turn to a study of the nature of thought, of categories, of language,
and of logic in the endeavor to reach first principles which justify
whatever they would wish to assert regarding the nature of things.
But no theory of knowledge is worth anything if it is not a theory of
knowledge of real men knowing a real world. A theory of knowledge
for angels, or for men knowing what is not the case, is a theory of
knowledge only in name. But on the other hand, an account of the
world which in no way could be known, or which could not be
known with any confidence, is an account of the world indistinguishable from a fiction. An adequate theory of knowledge presupposes a grasp of what is the case, and an adequate account of
reality presupposes an understanding of what is reasonable, certifiable,
and certified, and what is not. An epistemology presupposes an
ontology, and conversely. Many coherent systems are possible, however. Circular systematic philosophies in which an epistemology
grounds an ontology and conversely, must be tested by their capacity
to ground an adequate theoretical and practical ethics, politics, history,
art, and good common sense. The test of a philosophy is the understanding and wisdom it sustains and clarifies.

IX   THE PRIMARY CATEGORY

1.94   The essentials of any cognition are expressed
in a category or principle which is embodied in
whatever is apprehended.
(*See 1.64, 1.75*)

A CATEGORY is an ultimate unifying form. Were there no categories
there would be only a collection of felt items with nothing necessarily
in common, and subject to no criterion or test, no comparison, evaluation, or relation. If there is to be warrant for calling all we know
cases of one knowledge, all must exhibit common categories.

There are many categories relating to many different types of
being and to many different types of knowledge. But all of them must
illustrate some one category, for otherwise they would represent a
miscellany, make up a set of disconnected unrelated items, constitute a number of distinct and independent minds.

When Kant offered his twelve categories as the basic principles of
all cognition and being, he subsumed them under a single "tran-
scendental unity of apperception," his genuinely basic final category;
Aristotle, earlier, when he offered his ten categories, treated them
all under the aegis of his one inescapable principle, the law of contradiction. And the multiple categories of Hegel illustrate his one
final category, the Absolute, appearing now in this guise and now in
that.

It is customary to speak of categories as though they were only
categories of knowledge. This is not the meaning that Aristotle gave
to them, and it is not altogether just to Hegel; it approximates only
the Kantian conception. The primary category is a category of being
as well as of knowledge. Indeed it is because it is a category of being
that it can be a category not of belief or opinion but of truth, of a
world apart from the fact of cognition.

1.95   The primary category is inescapable.
(*See 1.94*)

WHAT IS contingent might be but need not always be. Were the
primary category contingent, it might not be at some time. At such

a time either (*a*) there would not be anything at all, or (*b*) what was could not be known, or (*c*) it would illustrate or be known through some other category.

a) If the supposedly primary category were constitutive of what was in fact it would either be imposed on content, in which case there would be something exterior to it which might remain apart from it, or it would be one with the very substance of what was in fact. Only the latter case allows that the departure of the category might entail an absence of all being. But Nothing is a self-contradictory idea, since it is the idea of what is completely indeterminate, lacking every feature, and yet is determinately what it is, possessed of the feature of being a Nothing rather than a Something. There always is some being or other. And this means that the category must be one with what is. What is alien to, altogether beyond the category defines the category to be so far contingent and defines itself, as case *b* makes evident, to be not knowable.

b) C. I. Lewis, in his *Mind and the World Order*, treated categories as contingent, and as independent of the content to which they were applied. But this requires that the application of a category to a content be arbitrary. If category and content are wholly independent of one another in being and in nature, a category could be applied here or there indifferently. And in any case the view has no category of "content." Without it the content could not, on this theory, either be or be known; but if there is a category "content" there would also, on this theory, not be anything over against the category to which the category could be applied. The same difficulty faces Lewis' master, Kant. The Kantian categories fall short of the data given in experience; they serve to organize, structure, to give intelligibility, but they presuppose something given, whose nature, since it is outside and over against all categories, cannot be known even as "the to be categorized."

c) A contingent category may fail to apply at some time. At that time it might be the case that some other category might be used. Though no category might be necessary, it would be necessary that some category or other be present always, thereby making it possible for whatever there be to be intelligible. But this necessity that there always be some category expresses the very meaning of a more basic and necessary category, whose primary function is to dictate that in every time and place some one of these lesser categories must be present, that there be no time or place when none of these lesser categories will be operative.

A necessary category must be integral to all knowledge if it is to be that in terms of which we know, and is also to enable us to grasp the nature of what is in fact. It must also be integral to all being, express a structure which is exemplified in everything, or fail to be more than one category among many, somehow included in a more inclusive category, embracing all the others.

1.96   The category embodies the law of contradiction.
(See 1.94, 1.95)

THE LAW of contradiction, "for every x, x is not non-x," is a necessary truth. Its structure is illustrated everywhere, in knowledge and in being. What defies it is the self-contradictory, the impossible, what cannot be at all; what neither defies nor illustrates it is too vague to be distinctive or intelligible.

Modern logic makes evident that all laws of logic are on a level, equally true, equally necessary, the denial of one being tantamount to a denial of the others. An insistence, with Aristotle and Kant, on the priority of the law of contradiction would seem then to conflict with the modern temper. We must, however, distinguish between the symbolized laws of logic which concern the logician, and an ultimate law which all these symbolized laws express in diverse ways. There is a symbolized law of contradiction. This is on an equal footing with every other symbolized law of logic. But that symbolized law of contradiction, no more and no less than the other symbolized laws, expresses (and illustrates) in the guise of symbols or thoughts that ultimate law of contradiction which is embodied in the primary category.

There is force, however, in the view that other laws than the law of contradiction are embodied in the one primary category and are expressed by the symbolized laws of logic. The law of identity, "every x is an x," and the law of excluded middle, "every x is x or non-x," have sometimes been held to be as ultimate as the law of contradiction and to be illustrated in it and elsewhere too. And there would seem in addition to be a law of inference which permits of the assertion of a conclusion, given an antecedent and the necessitation of a conclusion by that antecedent. Each of these is in fact basic, but only from a distinctive perspective. The law of identity is most appropriate to God and the rest of reality as expressing the nature of what is essentially a unity overriding all diversity. The law of excluded middle is most appropriate to the Ideal and the rest of reality as expressing the nature of a general or universal which is open to alternative specifications. The law of inference is most appropriate to Existence and to the rest of reality as expressing the nature of a process possessing its own integrity and rationale. In a similar way the law of contradiction is most appropriate to Actualities and the rest of reality as determinate entities over against one another, interrelated by means of a symmetrical relation of otherness.

There are then in a sense four basic categories. If we abstract from all the content of any one of them we get a category neutral to the different modes of being. Such an abstract category is the common denominator of the four categories and can be characterized as the category of "being" or togetherness. Each mode of being deals with it from a biased position. The primary category for the world of Actuality can consequently be described indifferently as the law of contradiction, or as the category of "being" made appropriate, in the shape of the law of contradiction, primarily to the world of Actualities, and secondarily to all else.

1.97 The primary category must be applicable to the contingent as well as to the necessary.
(See *1.94, 1.95*)

A CATEGORY must itself be necessary. And it must apply to what is contingent as well as to what is necessary. If it applied only to the necessary, there would be areas of being and knowledge that it would not encompass. The categories of Kant and the post-Kantians fail to meet this condition; necessary in some way, their categories are either alien to the content to which they are applied or they ignore whatever is individual, particular, contingent, or temporal. We know what is contingent and temporal, and know it in the same mind and for the same self that knows and is concerned with the necessary and eternal. We can compare and even pass from one of these domains to the other, which means that we must be able to stand outside both of them. This we can do by means of the primary category; it enables us to deal with them severally and together.

1.98 The primary category must be applicable to the false as well as to the true.
(See 1.94, 1.95)

THE PRIMARY category contains the essentials of any cognition and expresses the essentials of any being. Since errors occur and errors are known, the very category which is exemplified in the true and the factual must be exemplified in the false and the fictional as well. There seems to be a tendency in modern times, however, to use the term "category" only in an honorific fashion, to express what is worth knowing or what should be. But in making it serve only for what is good, the category is forced to assume an unnecessarily limited role in knowledge and in being. The errors one makes, the appearances one faces are then left in the limbo of unintelligibility and nonbeing, or are subsumed under some new category which will, together with the category appropriate to the true and the factual, constitute or illustrate the neglected primary category.

1.99 The primary category must have at least two parts.
(See 1.96)

WHAT IS other than this x is non-x. For each Actuality the others together function as a non-x for it. When the category serves to relate the domain of Actuality with some other, the non-x is that other domain; in that case the x is identifiable as one Actuality in the role of a representative of the entire domain of Actuality.

From the perspective of the law of contradiction, even the law of identity must have two terms, an x and a non-x; if it did not, it would have nothing to relate and identify. From the perspective of the law of contradiction, identity relates two instances, or two kinds of entity in such a way as to reduce them to an identity.

1.100 The primary category must inwardly make reference to the content which it organizes.
(See 1.94, 1.95, 1.97)

THE DIFFERENCE between "concavity" and "snub-nosedness" as Aristotle observed, and as Thomas Aquinas so brilliantly clarified in his *On Being and Essence*, is that the former gives only a bare form, whereas the latter makes a *formal* reference to the content which is appropriate to that form. "Snub-nosedness" is "concavity in flesh." The flesh which is here being acknowledged is a flesh *for* the concavity; it is not flesh in its materiality, but rather the material flesh in a formal guise. Were it not possible to make a formal reference to such material, it would not be possible to make a distinction between "concavity" and "snub-nosedness," for these differ only by virtue of the latter's reference to flesh. Yet were the flesh supposed to be just another form somehow added to the form of "concavity," "snub-nosedness" would be as abstract and perhaps even as mathematical an idea as "concavity," and there would not be anything in which the "concavity" could be. It is because we can formally acknowledge what is not formal that we can use a category to organize what is other than it, without turning that other into something irrational. The category has inside it a reference to whatever content there be to which the category as a whole will apply.

1.101   The parts of the category and the content for it must already exemplify it.

(*See 1.94, 1.95*)

THE PRIMARY category is all-encompassing; it expresses that unified structure by virtue of which anything can be or be known. The parts of the category are, and are known, and must therefore exemplify the category. This they can do because, firstly, as parts they offer content for the very category which they help constitute and, secondly, whatever content there is must already have the category within it. The category, as used in knowledge, is the barest of structures, the law of contradiction as unaffected by the nature of specific Actualities; the category, as the structure embodied in content, is the law of contradiction submerged, specified, qualified by the very content it orders.

Knowledge is the mental categorization of what is already objectively categorized; the mind by beginning with the category is able to subjugate in a new way the content which in fact had already subjugated the category. We need not then suppose with the Kantians that the content of the category is something blind and alien, exteriorly encountered and given an intelligible nature which it does not intrinsically possess, nor with the Hegelians that the content of the category is the category all over again, but viewed backwards, as it were. There is a distinction between knowledge and being, between the form for knowledge and the content of knowledge. The category as mere structure functions as a form for itself as permeated by content, mental and otherwise.

1.102   The category is a unity, representing an external unity in which its parts are embodied.
(*See 1.65, 1.94, 1.95, 1.101*)

WHEN WE judge we unify, bring together an indicated and a contemplated to make a single judgment exemplifying the law of contradiction. When we perceive, we obtain elements for judgment from what we encounter, and when we engage in other types of cognition we use elements which are derivable from those obtained in perception. Our judgments are oriented towards a world other than ourselves because the elements which we unite have a being apart from our act of unification. They are in fact unified in the object antecedent to our uniting them. Our unification of the elements thus presupposes an antecedent separation, a separation which does some violence to the integrity of the being that confronts us in fact. It is that being, as single and undivided, which we seek to understand by means of the elements we distinguish, analyze out, and finally unify in judgment.

When and as we force the elements into a unity we refer to the unity of the being from which the elements were derived. Otherness, as it were, does not merely stretch horizontally between an "x" and a "non-x." It burgeons out to the encountered content and inward to the perceiving individual. The perceiver feels, experiences, and goes through a process of unifying the indicated and contemplated, at the same time that he relates the unity of the category to the unity of the being from which the elements of the judgment were obtained.

1.103   The category has four facets.
(*See 1.01, 1.11–13, 1.99, 1.100, 1.102*)

THE UNITY of the category is that facet which answers to the divine, which transcends all diversity and has a relation to other unities as they are in themselves; the category's reference to content is the

category as that which exists in relation to further existence; the x
of the category answers to the Actual, the locatable, definite, and
resistant, while its non-x answers to the possible as that which is intelligible and correlate with the Actual.

When we perceive, the indicated serves as a representative of what
is Actual. But, confusing the representative with what it represents,
we often tend to treat the indicated as though it were the object
of our discourse rather than a subject in terms of which we discourse. In perception the contemplated serves to represent the possible which, in the Actual, is submerged and particularized. But once
again, confusing the representative with what it represents, we often
tend to treat the contemplated as if it gave the essence of what was
real, everything else being viewed as irrelevant accident or sheer confusion. When we perceive, that act by means of which we refer to
content serves to represent existence in the world beyond. Again,
confusing the representative with what it represents, we tend to speak
as though existence were a bare abstraction, a mere matter of dating
and placing. When, finally, we make use of the unity of the category
in order to have a perceptual judgment, we make the unity represent
the transcendent unity of the being that is over against us. Again,
confusing the representative with what it represents we tend to
suppose that the thing in itself is identical with our idea of a unity.

The categoreal eternal unity is related to a unity beyond it; the
act of using the category terminates in a dynamic content outside;
x is related to non-x, and non-x is related to x, and both of these are
related to unity and dynamic content. The primary category, at the
root of all knowledge and being, is an othering which connects unity
with unity, dynamic content with dynamic content, x and non-x with
one another.

There is no knowledge unless there are at least two items interrelated. Because the items, to be two, must be other than one another,
the relation which connects them is a form of othering. All relations,
even the relation of identity, because they connect specifications of
an x and a non-x, are specifications of the relation of "is-not." As
part of the category the "is-not" spreads not only between the x
and the non-x but between their unity and the unity that lies beyond
them.

To speak of the category as an othering is evidently to describe the category essentially from the vantage point of existence. We could speak of it in different terms without distortion. When we look at it from the vantage point of eternity, for example, we see it primarily as a unity; when we look at it from the vantage point of possibility we see it primarily as the principle of intelligibility; when we look at it from the standpoint of Actuality, we see it primarily as over against all else.

1.104 The relations of the various guises which the category assumes are themselves cases of the category. (See 1.97, 1.98, 1.101)

IN A MAN the category assumes four primary guises: it functions in its purity as a principle of knowledge; it provides the most abstract meaning or form for his body; it offers a structure for his emotions, desires, and will, which connect the mind and body; and it states the nature of the self as that which can express itself as a mind, as the life of a body, as emotion, desire, and will, and as a unity over against the unities at the centers of other beings.

The category in the guise of a principle of knowledge is matched by the category as abstracted from an object; in the guise of the most abstract meaning of our body, it is answered by the category as submerged in content and thus as constituting a body over against our own; as the structure of our emotions, desire, and will it is answered by the categorized content we experience; and as the unity which is our very self it is answered by the unitary categoreal centers of whatever other beings there are, actual, possible, existential, or divine.

What we know is not merely inside our minds. By means of our minds we know what is over against us. We perceive as selves who not only spread in feeling between our minds and bodies but who terminate at an object having both a knowledgeable and ontological import, i.e., at an object of knowledge which is also an object over against us, whose content we experience and whose center is as unreachable as our own.

Once we find it acceptable to say that we know bodies over against us in perception, there should be little trouble in dealing with the otherwise vexatious question of how we can will to act out what we have in mind. The act of will is the act of focusing on the terminus of knowledge so as to provoke an act of the body with respect to the object known. It is no agency for making the body move by means

of the imposition of spiritual forces, no way of transferring energy
from spirit to matter, but just a way, additional to that of desire and
perception, of focusing on an exterior object possessing a real relation to our bodies.

X   THE   ETHICAL   LIFE

1.105   An Actuality seeks to realize possibilities, and
the Actuality which is man seeks to realize an
all-inclusive possibility.
(*See 1.11, 1.21, 1.47–50, 1.51, 1.53*)

NEITHER knowledge nor action, nor any combination of them
does full justice to the needs of the self, that finite unity which is
the other of whatever there be and which comes to expression as
the life in a body and sometimes as mind, feeling, and will. Like the
mind, the self has an unlimited reach and, like the body which it
quickens, is an Actuality. As unchanging it is unlike either, for they
are perpetually altering in nature, content and objective. It can be
critical of them and also be capable of evaluating all else, because it
makes use of a standard having pertinence to them as well as to what
else there be. That standard is not yet realized, for things are not now
perfect. The standard represents a possibility which ought to be
realized, and man as a being with a persistent, critical self is a being
who is faced with it as that which is forever, and pertinent to whatever there be.

1.106   The all-inclusive possibility which man seeks
and ought to realize is The Good.
(*See 1.105*)

THE ALL-INCLUSIVE possibility is internally one; it expresses a
standard which measures all beings. To realize it is to be enhanced.
The traditional name for such a possibility, initially given to it by
Plato, is The Good. The Good is possibility as pertinent to Actualities, and thus to the self. Since it enhances whatever exemplifies it,
the Good is that which man ought to realize; since it is a reality which
stands outside him and defines him as incomplete, it is that which he

unavoidably seeks to realize in himself as well as in others. Since men do not as a rule set themselves to do even the minor things they ought to do, it is evident that the attempt characteristic of man to realize the Good is not necessarily conscious. Men always seek to do what they ought to do only in the sense that they are in a state of disliked disequilibrium as long as they have not taken adequate account of the nature of the Good and what it requires them to do.

1.107 The Good is specified in the form of limited objectives which men sometimes consciously acknowledge and bodily realize.
(See 1.21, 1.106)

BECAUSE men must take account of the needs and tendencies of their bodies, and because their interests, efforts, and products are affected by other Actualities, by Existence, and by God, they can in this life concern themselves with the relevant all-inclusive possibility only through a veil of more limited concerns for more limited objectives. The self deals with the Good as in the background of more worldly relevant, more consciously conspicuous, and more bodily significant specific forms of that Good. To know the Good that all men seek therefore requires considerable speculation, self-reflection, and abstraction from practical interests.

Not all the goals that men pursue are solely the outcome of their own specifications of the Good. Fellow men, sometimes as individuals and more often as constituting a society, provide them with and even impose on them various goals which they seek to realize. But whether or not a goal be self-defined or defined by others, its realization may not be desirable. The realization may conflict with realizations of better specifications of the Good. The goals that men pursue are perhaps not always recognized to be even apparently good; sometimes men set themselves to bring about what is predominantly evil, even while knowing that its realization makes for disorganization, conflict, and the muting of values, rights, and promise.

1.108 Men have a freedom of preference.
(See 1.107)

MEN HAVE the capacity to take one of a number of means to some adopted goal. A great deal of the historical discussion dealing with the "freedom of will" has to do with the problem of whether or not men can freely take one of these means. Those who deny that there is such freedom rightly point to the fact that the goals men pursue are defined and prescribed in good part by agencies outside the men; they also rightly point out that no one selects anything except so far as this, for some reason, appeals to him. What men select, they say, is determined both by the nature of the prescribed goals and by the nature of the means in relation to the men with such and such appetites, experience, and knowledge. Those who affirm that men have freedom, on the other hand, rightly point to the fact that men sometimes elect their goals from among a number; they also rightly point out that often the means selected have no genuine intrinsic appeal. Men sometimes select what is repugnant in preference to what is attractive. What neither side sees is that freedom of preference is a limited kind of freedom, quite distinct from a freedom of choice (see 1.109) and a freedom of will (see 1.112). But more important, both sides unwarrantedly suppose that a man is faced with a number of distinct alternatives, one side affirming merely that he is already biased towards that one which he finally elects, the other side affirming merely that he could have taken any other. The former rightly charges the latter with confusing freedom and caprice, the latter rightly charges the former with confusing conditions with compulsions.

In any given situation a goal, near or remote, is accepted, and in terms of this a freedom of preference is exercised by relating a set of not altogether clearly distinguished alternatives to the accepted goal, thereby infecting them with some of the appeal which that goal has for one. The means that is finally preferred has the most appeal, but that appeal is the product of the appeal it natively has and the appeal it acquires when it is freely related, with all the other means, to the goal that one seeks to realize. A repugnant alternative, with its low intrinsic appeal, may as a consequence acquire an overwhelming appeal from the goal which it promotes better than any other alternative.

1.109 Men have a freedom of choice.
(*See 1.107*)

MEN ALWAYS do some wrong. At the very least they not only neglect what deserves attention but must use something—muscles, ground, things—to bring something else about. Inevitably they re-

duce the values of some of the things they use for the sake of achieving some good, distinct from those things, which may not benefit
those things at all. But to do a wrong is to be in the wrong. Unless the
wrong can be justified, the act is wanton, indefensible.

Since we possess values both over against and in relation to the
values possessed by others, we must, whenever we do what is wrong,
maintain some hold on the very values which we are precluding from
existing. Otherwise our act would be without warrant. To reduce
values is unqualifiedly wrong; if values are reduced in one way, they
must, in a justifiable act, be preserved or enhanced in another way.
This is possible if, when, and as we do a wrong, we then and there
commit ourselves to an end in which those values are reinstated or
compensated. Our wrongs inevitably compel us, as beings of value
in a world of value, to identify ourselves with ends we must thereafter realize. Inescapably and absolutely obligated to the Good, we
are also inescapably though only conditionally obligated to bring
about the ends to which our wrong acts inevitably commit us. So far
as we fail to live up to the latter obligation we fail to justify the
wrongs we do, and are so far men whose value as men is partially
abstract, not entirely integral with ourselves.

An end is a possibility of an absolute harmonious totality of whatever values there in fact are. We choose it when and as we choose an
act. In itself no ends commends itself; it is the end to choose because
it is the end for the act we choose. The act to choose is the best possible
act for us to choose, no matter how much wrong it involves, because
it is the justified act, the act which is sustained by the end we then
choose. Evidently there must be many ends, all of equal value, each
justifying a different type of act. For every act there is an end, a world
of values in which the loss that the act involves is made good.

Although every act we choose is justifiable, since we then and
there, though not necessarily consciously, commit ourselves to bring
about a compensatory end, not every end is or can be realized by us.
Our acts are justified in the sense that they are the acts of a man
committed to make good his wrongs; they are not necessarily justified
in the sense that they are the acts of a good or wise man, one who
does what is best here and now.

The reason for choosing an act is produced in the choosing; it is
the acceptance of a commitment to a justifying end. The reason for

choosing the end is provided at the same time; it is the acceptance of some act as the best possible. In the production of these reasons a man is free. Choosing, though unavoidable for a man of value in a world of value, is nevertheless a free provision of a reason which both offers a justification for an act and commits us to the justifying end. It starts with not altogether well distinguished alternative acts of different degrees of attractiveness related to their respective compensating and therefore justifying ends; it closes with an acceptance of a justified action which has the role of a means for bringing about its justifying end.

The determinist knows that the various alternative actions have initially different degrees of attractiveness, and that a man *must* choose *just one* of them. His opponent knows that the various alternatives are all equally open to a choice, and that he *could* choose *any one* of them. The first says that the second treats choice as an act of irresponsible caprice; the second says that the first treats choice as a creature of an external amoral pressure. The first charges the second as having no reasons, and he replies that the first has no ethics. Both criticisms are just. But both make the same mistaken assumptions. Both overlook the fact that choice is an act of providing a reason, an act by which an alternative is justified by being related to an end one is thenceforth obligated to realize. A man freely moves from the state of leaning towards one alternative to the state of being compelled to take the one justified by the end he then adopts—or what is the same thing, a man freely moves from the state of being free to elect any alternative to the state of freely relating one of them to a justifying end.

1.110 Desire for The Good is good.
(*See 1.106*)

THE GOOD is not now fully realized; it is a possibility offering a standard in terms of which all things are to be evaluated, but which itself, because only possible, indeterminate, future, is not of great value.

The Good itself is not perfectly good. If it were, the Good would lack nothing; there would be no gain to it if it were realized. He who desired it, as Plato observed, would be bad, for he would lack the very good he sought. But desire for the Good is a way of realizing it, giving it a determination and a place in the universe it otherwise would not have. The Good is a lure, attracting desire; desire, by being attracted to it, infects it with something of the concrete world, and implicates it in the affairs of men.

This view stands in opposition both to the view that the Good is as it were too Good, and overflows and thereby bestows its excellence on what lies beyond, and the view that the Good is just Good and that is all there is to it. The former is the view of those who think of God's creative act, his mercy, and his grace as so many different forms of an overflowing love, a sheer exuberance of being and excellence which must be siphoned off in order that God be what he is and the rest of things be excellent outcomes of his act. But how this excess which is to be passed on to others is possible is a mystery which no fact and no problem seems to necessitate; it also makes it unnecessary for any being to act on behalf of the Good. The latter view seems trivial and harmless in contrast; in fact it raises an enormous difficulty. If the Good were just Good, if the most excellent of beings was the Good itself, all realization of it in this world would be a limiting, a distorting, a corrupting of it. To realize the Good would be to do no good to the Good, and would benefit man only so far as the Good were made into something less than it in fact is. It is possible to avoid these errors by taking account of the fact that the Good is a possibility and therefore as yet indeterminate, but capable of gaining determinateness and value by being realized.

1.111   The Good needs more realization than it gets from preference, choice, or desire.
(*See 1.108, 1.109, 1.110*)

DESIRE expresses something of the entire man, and its nature has an effect on what men are and do. So far as it concerns itself with the Good, it brings the Good to play on human affairs, but more through diffusion than through action. Desire falls short of production; it may end in faint and futile hope.

Preference, since it deals with goals which are specifications of the Good, and is alert to the means for achieving those goals, does more justice to the need of the Good. But goals are good and bad, and means to them may be regrettable. And in preference no attention need be paid to values. Nor need a preference be expressed in act.

Choice goes further. It attends to an end which is good, and relates it to an act as that act's justification. But there are many ends, mutually exclusive and co-ordinate. The acts one chooses may be predominantly bad and their justifying ends may be beyond the competence of man to fulfill. Choice fails to provide a sure and adequate means for realizing the Good.

To be fully realized the Good must be maximally present everywhere. Man, the ethical being, has such realization as his responsibility. This means that he must seek to impose it on other beings. The task may require him to overcome a rather radical resistance on their part to himself, and to the Good.

1.112 Men have a free will.
(*See 1.20, 1.50, 1.111*)

CHOICE CUTS a man off from ends which might have been chosen, and obligates him to the end to which he is committed by the losses his act produces. It prescribes what action is to occur, but does not control the channels through which the action must move; nor does choice take account of things as they are apart from us.

The will is the self expressing its concern for the Good, so far as this is relevant to what now is. It can and should be used as an agency for adopting the Good without distortion and as relevant to all else. So far as it does this it is an ethical will, cognitively occupied with the Good in the form of the common terminus of mind and body, in such a way as to relate it to whatever now exists. A creative power constantly varying its insistencies and directions, the ethical will provokes different types of acts to make them in consonance with what other things need in order to be internally harmonious and harmoniously related to all else. By means of it a man can make the indeterminate Good determinate to a degree not possible in preference or in choice.

A good will, as Kant observed, is precious; but he failed to remark that it is precious only because it serves the Good, and that it is never able to do all that the Good requires. No man can will continuously, nor will in such a way that wrong is never done.

1.113 The values of all beings should be maximized.
(*See 1.14, 1.106, 1.111*)

THE REALIZATION of the Good requires its embodiment everywhere. He who would realize the Good must enhance others. The realization of the Good thus is good for the Good, since it thereby gains determinateness, and good for the things in which it is realized, since they are thereby enhanced. Since men ought to promote the Good, and since the Good has cosmic relevance, men ought to maximize every being. Not to wish to realize the Good everywhere is not to wish to be a man responsible for satisfying the Good maximally; not to wish to maximize all other beings is not to wish to be one who favors the better over the worse. It is to refuse to be ethical. But to refuse to be ethical is to refuse to complete oneself, to refuse to do for oneself what one in fact already blindly and partially seeks to do whenever one uses mind, body, desire, preference, or choice. The ethical man does willingly and in a better way what man inevitably but inadequately always does: concern himself with the realization of good everywhere, for the sake of the Good, for the sake of the other beings, and for his own sake.

1.114   No one can do only what is right.
(See 1.109, 1.113)

TO DO WRONG is to minimize value; to do right is to maximize value. In between is the act which neither minimizes nor maximizes, an act which keeps things as they were. But this act sins by omission; it involves a neglect of other things and what they need. Every act uses things and perhaps uses them up. To do anything, something else must be utilized, if only to provide a foil, a ground, an instrument. Only an act which brings about nothing but good, while neglecting no claim, can be wholly right. Only such an act is defensible in and of itself. But no such act is possible to man.

1.115   No one can do only what is wrong.
(See 1.114)

WHEN VALUES are reduced, something is done. When men use eye and hand, body and thing, they give them a status in a situation larger than themselves, make them function according to their capacities, allow them to be enriched by context and improved by performance. He who benefited nothing in his act would be an incarnate ill will, or would be so inept, so unco-ordinated, so maladroit as to be unable to do anything at all. To act is to be organized, to be directed, to use mind and body with effectiveness, and this, despite the evil that ensues, to do some good in the process.

There are of course acts which are predominantly good and others which are predominantly bad, but no act of a finite man can be entirely good or entirely bad, entirely right or entirely wrong.

1.116 Men are necessarily guilty.
(See 1.106, 1.114)

NO MAN HAS the vision, the energy, the flexibility, or the persistence to benefit all beings everywhere. No one has the ability to benefit fully even the few beings in his immediate family or vicinity, whom he may deliberately want to benefit. No one knows himself or has sufficient control of himself and other things to be able to benefit even himself maximally. There is no one to whom man does or can do good without admixture of evil. But not to do that which one is obligated to do, not to do the whole Good, is to be guilty of a wrong, through commission or omission. Man is inescapably guilty, not because he inherited some sin, not because he violated some divine command, not because he failed to hold on to some redeemer, or because he failed to merit forgiveness. He is inescapably guilty because he is an ethical being concerned with the realization of a Good to whom no being or value is wholly alien, and yet is also one who is unable to bring more than a finite power, a limited span, a flagging attention, a spotted virtue, and a confused mind to his task.

1.117 All rewards are undeserved.
(See 1.116)

MEN AT EVERY moment, due to the bounty of nature and the generosity of others, are benefited. Despite the fact that they are guilty beings in no way entitled to anything but what helps wipe away or at least reduce their guilt, men have moments of joy and satisfaction, serving no purpose whatsoever. Men prosper though they are guilty. Their prosperity is undeserved. The recognition of man's inescapable guilt thus, instead of being an occasion for despair, should be an occasion for thanksgiving. None of the goods that accrue to man in the course of life are his by right, justice, or merit.

1.118 Men can do all the good that ought to be done if they can utilize other powers besides their own.
(*See 1.106, 1.116, 2.14, 2.69*)

THERE IS nothing axiomatic in the Kantian contention, "One can because one ought." One ought, and sometimes one can. The ought does not depend for its being or its power on the fluctuating capacities of men; the ought is determined by the nature of the Good and its distance from full realization. A man, because he has a persistent self, and because no part of the universe is alien to his mind, value, or spirit, is obligated to bring about the Good. He is guilty to the degree that he fails to do good, either through acts of commission or omission.

It is absurd to say that a man ought to do only that which he can, for then the more incompetent a man, the more dissolute and incontinent, the less he would have to do; but it is equally absurd to suppose that there can be an obligation to do that which is impossible. What a man ought to do must somehow be capable of being done, if not by him then by some other being or power.

"One can because one ought" is not true; but "This can be because this ought to be" is necessarily true. What ought to be is that which can be, because what ought to be is the Good, and this is possible. Or, to put it another way, the Good is cosmic in import; its "can be" has a cosmic range. No one being has the ability to realize it by himself. But it could be realized through the use of whatever powers there are. If a man is to realize the Good and thereby avoid the guilt which is inevitably his when he acts by himself, he must accept as his own whatever powers there be which also partly realize the Good. He must treat himself as an essential part of a whole of effective powers working for the Good; he must recognize the forces in nature, the powers of society and the state, and the abilities of other modes of being to provide so many different agencies that can serve his purpose, and must try to make them his own.

The Good is the Ideal as related to the Actual. Since that Ideal is germane to other types of reality as well, even the fullest realization of the Good, one which makes use of all powers whatsoever, will still fall short of a full realization of the absolute Ideal.

CHAPTER 2

Ideality

I POSSIBILITY

2.01 Whatever is possible must be internally coherent.
(*See 1.11*)

THE SELF-CONTRADICTORY is impossible. What is impossible cannot be. What cannot be, cannot be here or there, today or tomorrow, in this realm or that. It cannot therefore be in mind or in language any more than it can be in the realm of things or ideas. The point seems inescapable, yet most thinkers are inclined to suppose that somehow they are at times confronted with self-contradictions, which they thereupon reject or characterize as incapable of being. But if the self-contradictory is really incapable of being in any sense, it could never appear. There is no doubt but that we "contradict" ourselves, or that we can forge expressions such as "round-square." But the fact that we say one thing at one time and the opposite at another, or that we con-join expressions or sentences, does not mean that we thereby generate a self-contradictory entity. We continue to have two distinct items in a genuine relation of opposition to one another; if we try to hold them together they blur into one another to leave us with a content so indeterminate as to be indistinguishable from nothing at all, or from what is altogether unintelligible.

2.02   Some possibilities are ingredient in, i.e., are idealizations of Actuality, Existence, and God.
(*See 1.21, 1.25*)

THE FACT that something is possible is testified by the fact that it is. When it is not, it *may* be possible; when it *is* it *must* be possible. Actu-alities, Existence, and God are realities and as such must all be possible. When we refine them, idealize them, tear them out of their concrete contexts and activities, make abstractions of them, we treat them as possibilities, identify their full being with the possibilities they realized. Those possibilities are not extra facts inside the beings; they are the very beings themselves made indeterminate, as having been subjected to an idealization.

2.03   A real possibility is what in fact can be.
(*See 2.01, 2.02*)

THE IMPOSSIBLE has two forms: the logically impossible, that which could not be in any sense, and the ontologically impossible, that which is precluded from being by virtue of what in fact is. A round-square is logically impossible; the death of Alexander at 50 is ontologically impossible, since it is excluded by his actual earlier death. One can state an ontological impossibility in such a way as to give it the form of a logical impossibility by defining an object in terms of the actual properties it manifests, and then characterizing it falsely. Thus it is self-contradictory to suppose that an Alexander who dies at 32 dies at 50. But if we view Alexander's death at 32 as a contingent occurrence, and thus as not expressing an essential character of him, we are driven to say that it defines his dying at 50 as only an ontological im-possibility, for there then is no logical contradiction in the idea of his dying at that later time.

The ontologically possible is the really possible. If we wish to know what possibilities are real, it is necessary for us to know what the cosmos or parts of it are like. A real possibility is realized as a mode of being or as some feature of it; idealized, that realized possi-bility attains the status of an ingredient possibility.

2.04 Real possibilities have a being exterior to Actualities and whatever else there be.

(*See 2.03*)

ACTUALITIES and Existence are evidently time-dominated; there is that which they are not yet, that which they are to become. Before they have this feature or that, there must be a possibility for the feature which they, in the course of their careers, realize. It is more difficult to see how a possibility could be exterior to God, if he be understood as a being who is all-inclusive, lacking nothing whatsoever. But if it be recognized that God has relevance to Actualities, that he has a role in history, and that he has a providential concern for what the world might do, it is hard to avoid the recognition that God, too, has possibilities before him. One ought in fact to go further; if God be granted thought and will, not only in relationship to other types of reality, but also apart from them, it must be granted that he too confronts possibilities, though in a way different from that in which we do. A God who had no possibilities to realize in himself or in others would be totally static, self-enclosed; he would be without purpose, value, interest, or need, and could do nothing either in thought or in fact.

The logically possible is possibility itself made into an object of thought; it has no being except so far as one thinks of it. There are no happy gryphons really possible, for they are excluded by what is in the world. But the idea of a happy gryphon is logically possible, for it is not self-contradictory, and has just been thought of by me. The logically possible is not to be confused with logic. Logic is the very structure of the realm of real possibility; it is not created by us. The ingrediently possible, as distinguished from the realities of which it is an idealization, also has being in and for thought. But since it is those very realities themselves under limitation, it exists apart from thought as well. We determine the logically possible; we identify the ingrediently possible. Apart from our determination of it the logically possible has no reality; apart from our identification of it the ingrediently possible has some being.

2.05   Real possibilities are relevant to other realities.
(See 1.21, 1.26, 2.03, 2.04)

PLATONISTS acknowledge a domain of possibility, standing over against other domains, but they differ in their claims as to just what that domain of possibility includes. Plato himself thought that what I have been terming 'the possible' was essentially a desirable value, and therefore found himself forced to deny that there was a possible mud or a possible dirt. Yet a possible mud or a possible dirt is as clean and good as a possible light or possible life. But also, since the possible lacks the determinateness and career characteristic of the Actual, it is equally correct to say that a possible light or a possible life is as impoverished, is as incomplete, has as little value as a possible mud or a possible dirt. Others, such as Santayana, suppose that whatever is logically possible is also really possible. Since the logically possible is not relevant to any one state of affairs in particular, such thinkers are forced to say that every realization of a possibility has to be arbitrary. To account for a realization here or now rather than there or then requires the introduction of something extraneous to their logically possibles. Still others, like Whitehead, are somewhere in between these two extremes; they insist that possibilities be relevant, and deny that they are possibilities only of what is excellent. But they offer no principle for determining just what could be and what could not be a real possibility; nor do they recognize that real possibilities need no agent to enable them to have a bearing on things outside them. For these thinkers, all realizations are really instantiations alien and adventitious to those possibilities.

The Platonists have the problem of bringing the possible into relation with realities outside the domain of possibility. Denying any necessary relevance of the possible to what might exemplify it, they are forced to look to a demiurgos, an animal faith, or a divine evaluation to dictate just which possibilities are to be relevant and which are to be held at a distance from the world. Because they fail to acknowledge that the possibilities are themselves relevant to the realities, they are forced to have them made relevant arbitrarily through the decision of some exterior being, divine or human. And since they have to recognize that some possibilities, such for example as Alexander's death at 50, are not relevant to the world as it is, they are forced to hold that some possibilities are devoid of all relevance. But what is in no way relevant is not a possibility for anything. There is no warrant for denying relevance directly to real possibilities themselves, and no warrant for invoking an arbitrary or irrational act to make relevant what was initially treated as irrelevant. Possibilities are involved in states of affairs outside them.

Possibilities have a being of their own, and express prospects which the different realities seek to realize for their own benefit and the benefit of those possibilities. Each mode of being, to complete itself, acts so as to enhance itself and others. This leads it to try to realize the possibilities it confronts.

2.06 Real possibilities change in the course of time.
(See 2.05)

ACTUALITIES are constantly changing. New ones come to be, and old ones pass away. What is relevant to one is not relevant to another. If possibilities are relevant to what is actual, they must change with changes in the furniture of the world.

There is something odd in the idea that there was a possible jet plane explosion in the time of Homer. Such an explosion is possible only when we in fact have jet planes. This means that possibilities must come to be; it also means that possibilities must pass away.

This would be an intolerable position to maintain were it not that there are some permanent possibilities, and were it not that what passes away is not an unrealized possibility but a possibility that had been realized. Without permanent possibilities there would be no possible Good, measuring all occurrences and answering to the constant and common natures of whatever Actualities there be. And if possibilities could pass away without ever having been realized, they would be possibilities which in fact were permanently excluded from the world and thus in fact were not possibilities for that world at all.

2.07 Real possibilities form linkages.
(See 2.05, 2.06)

WHEN Actualities confront a common possibility (relevant to any) they diversely specialize it, qualify it in such a way that it is at once delimited and made relevant to themselves. Individually relevant possibilities are thus a common relevant possibility divided, specialized by the realities beyond, to which they are germane. The single common possibility, which is thus specialized, remains in the background as an unspecialized, limitless, undetermined future which is to be subsequently specialized by the beings which follow on those now in the present. A specialization of the common possibility today dictates what will happen in fact tomorrow, not in detail of course, but in general. What is in fact realized today partly determines what specializations of the common possibility will be made tomorrow.

It is a possibility, realized today, that dictates what will be a relevant possibility tomorrow. But this which will be a relevant possibility tomorrow is not yet a definite distinct possibility. It achieves definiteness only when the relevant possibility for today is realized. Not until we have actual jet planes are there possible jet plane explosions. While jet planes are only possible, jet plane explosions are but facets of those possibilities, without distinct natures of their own. They have no distinctness, are not genuine possibilities until the possibility of jet planes is realized. It is in this sense that the possibilities form linkages, or rather implicate further possibilities; when a given possibility is actualized, some other further possibility is prescribed.

The Platonist, with all his possibilities given in one fell swoop, is faced with the fact that the possibility of the thief being jailed depends on the realization of the possibility of the thief being caught. Were the latter not realized, the former would not be a possibility at all, or, what is the same thing, it would be an idle, merely logical possibility, which is not and may never be actualized, and thus one which differs in nature and function from a genuine real possibility, one that must be realized.

When account is taken of the habits in things, and the fact that despite changes in individuals, situations, and the course of the world, there are such comparatively constant phenomena as motion and rest, day and night, life and death, one can at times indicate in advance the type of possibility which will be open to a being. With the birth of a child, illness may become a genuine possibility. Thus, to say that the child might possibly become ill is but to say that the realization of the possibility it now confronts, no matter what this be, may entrain the possibility of illness, carve this out of the undifferentiated possibility which the child persistently confronts.

2.08 Real possibilities are systematically connected
(See 1.14, 2.05, 2.07)

EACH BEING operates in some independence of the others, delimiting a common indeterminate possibility in its own way. Nevertheless what it does has an effect on the specialized possibilities which concern the others, and what they do affects its possibility. Because the patient is very ill, death in bed from that illness could now be a possibility for him; because the doctor is in town, being at the hospital in a little while could now be a possibility for him. But it is the patient's illness which makes the doctor face and actualize the possibility of being at the hospital in a little while; it is the doctor's presence at the hospital that makes relief a possibility for the patient now. Each affects the common possibility in such a way as to dictate in part how it is to be further determined. Each delimits his own possibility independently, but inside the area of a possibility which has been affected by the other.

2.09 Real possibilities are relevant and realizable.
(See 2.03–6)

REAL POSSIBILITIES are realizable; otherwise they would not be possibilities for the beings in this cosmos. But since they are possibilities *for* these beings, the possibilities must be relevant as well.

The Aristotelian insists on the relevance and realizability, but tends to neglect the exteriority of possibilities; the Platonist reverses the emphasis. The Platonist rightly criticizes the Aristotelian for over-rigidifying the course of nature, for reading definite nature, habits, compulsions into things which are as a matter of fact infected and directed by what is above and outside them. The Platonist is met by the countercharge that he merely doubles the intelligible aspects of the cosmos without thereby improving understanding, that he fails to take account of the fact that real possibilities are never wholly irrelevant to what is going on, and that they must be realized. Each is very perceptive with respect to the weaknesses of the other. Nothing less than the union of their truths will do justice to what is the case.

2.10 The Good is a possibility which ought to be realized.

(See 1.106, 1.118, 2.09, 2.14)

WHAT I individually ought to do I individually may not be able to do. Though I ought I cannot. I continue to owe money even though I cannot repay; I continue to owe consideration to others even when I lose my temper and am unable to deal dispassionately or sympathetically with them. Still what ought to be can be. Hegel goes so far as to say that what ought to be must be, in fact already is; this comes perilously close to allowing anything to happen, to accepting everything as equally valuable, legitimate, satisfactory. But what ought to be is not yet fully realized; the world is not as good as it could be. Yet an ought to be which in fact could not be realized could not be relevant to us or to our behavior.

What ought to be is the Good. It ought to be realized. And so far as a man is ethical, he takes upon himself the task of realizing this which ought to be realized. The ethical man faces, specializes, and realizes the Good. What ought to be beckons to him, as it were, and he, so far as he is ethical, answers. If he cannot answer adequately by himself it is incumbent upon him to make use of whatever other powers there be which can help bring about the realization of the Good that ought to be. If he fails to do this, the Good, which ought to be realized, will become a task for other types of being, while he, since he is one who neglected to use the available agencies, will be an ethically criticizable being, one who throws an unnecessary burden on those others.

The point can perhaps be most readily seen if a careful distinction is made between a primary and a secondary demand by the Good. The Good makes a primary demand to be realized by the being to which it is relevant. This being may fail to do justice to the Good. If there be no other being which does what the first failed to do, the Good will never be realized. It will then be an ought that cannot in fact ever be. The Good must therefore make a secondary demand to another being to do what the first failed to do. This secondary demand must be satisfied.

Since what ought to be *need not be* fulfilled by the object to which it is relevant, it *must be* fulfilled by some other, or cease to be an ought that is possible. What ought to be, then, can be. And what can be, both may not be realized and yet must be realized—the former so far as it makes a primary demand, the latter so far as it makes a secondary demand. The Hegelian is therefore right and wrong: right in insisting that the Good *must be* realized; wrong in supposing that it may not fail to be realized by the being of which it makes a primary demand.

2.11 Real possibilities are to some extent internally indeterminate.

(See 2.03, 2.06, 2.07)

IT IS a minor and perhaps only a verbal matter to decide to say that the possible is determinate but acquires additional determinations in being transported to the realm of Actualities rather than to say that it is in fact partly indeterminate and that this indetermination is overcome when the possibility is realized, given a role in another domain. Still, I have preferred the latter way of speaking, because it does not mislead us into supposing that nothing ever happens to a possibility. Platonists tend to prefer the former.

The Platonic doctrine of "participation" is presumably designed to keep possibilities unaffected by the world and yet to allow the world to benefit by the reflected light of determinate and excellent ideals. But if there be no realization of possibilities, nothing really becomes, and there is no transformation of what might be into what is. Sometimes, though, the Platonist speaks as if the possible were fully determinate, but capable of taking up lodging in a different realm. Thus, Aristotelians in a Platonic mood often speak of "essences"as fully determinate, yet endowed with or attached to existence without being altered in any way. But only when possibilities are transported into another realm or attached to existence does it become true that they are at such and such a place or time, and are involved in such and such situations. They must evidently on such occasions acquire some determination which they did not have before.

No possibility can be wholly determinate; but also none can be wholly indeterminate. It is relevant to and realizable by this being or that. It must have a nature answering to the nature and promise of this or that, and be capable of being filled in, completed in being realized. There is no doubt, as John Wild has remarked, that the snow that actually falls will be moist or dry, and that "a pure snowiness that is neither cannot fall." But from this he illegitimately goes on to suppose that "what is possible is something fully concrete and determinate." Perhaps what is intended is only the legitimate claim that what is possible is that something will occur which will *be* fully concrete and determinate. But from this it does not follow that the possibility itself is fully concrete and determinate. If it were the case that "when a possibility is realized, nothing is added in the order of essence. What is added is the act of existing," then existing would be adventitious, irrelevant, outside the essence. The essence would in fact then not be realized or transported at all.

2.12 The difference between the possible and the Actual, or any other reality, is not merely possible.
(See 2.11, 4.109)

THE DIFFERENCE between the possible and other realities cannot be merely possible. If it were, the possible would be over against those other realities, and would need a relation to connect it with those others. Nor can the difference be Actual, or Existential, or Divine, for similar reasons. But if these are all the realities there be, and if it can be no one of these, the difference would seem to be nonreal. In that case there would be no relation of difference among the various modes. Yet possibilities and the other modes of being are together in the universe. And Actualities, at least, act so as to make that which is not yet but can be, into what is in fact, giving it a determination it did not have before. There seems to be no other alternative left but the view that the relation of difference among the modes is all of the modes together, not as constituting a new entity, but as in fact constituting an unstable combination of them, dissolving when and as it occurs.

The relation of Actuality, Existence, or God to Possibility—and of course the relation of any one of the modes of being to any other— is a dynamic or creative juncture of them all, perpetually coming to be and passing away. The togetherness of the various modes is all of them intermixed. This togetherness can be viewed as a neutral relation connecting each with the rest, or as a togetherness of all which is possessed by each and terminates in the others. We ought to speak in the latter way when trying to deal with the ways the modes severally function.

An Actuality realizes a possible indeterminate prospect through the actual exertion of an existential, unified power which terminates in the prospect. The Actuality is thereby enabled to make that prospect have a spatiotemporal location, be part of the world of Actualities. A converse activity also takes place from the possible to the Actual. And there are also activities which originate with Actualities but which terminate in Existence and in God. These are given a kind of spatio-temporal localization by the Actualities, and they, reciprocally, give Actualities the determination of being items in an existential field or data for a judging God. And in similar ways Existence and God give determinations to one another.

From the standpoint of the Actual the difference between it and the possible is a difference between the individual and the universal; from the standpoint of the possible it is a difference between the normative and the factual; from the standpoint of Existence and from that of God (which provide ways of standing in between both the Actual and the possible) the difference between the Actual and the possible is a mixture of the two. From the standpoint of Existence the difference between it and the possible is a difference between the dynamic and the effete; from the standpoint of God the difference between him and the possible is a difference between a concrete vital judge and a principle of judgment. From the standpoint of the possible, Existence is to it as the unordered is to the intelligible, and God is to it as the perfect instance is to a principle of perfection. There are analogous descriptions of the ways in which the remaining relations of the various modes are to be described.

Each mode of being exerts a characteristic power. Each reaches to-wards another in an act which is primarily like the being itself, and which, at its terminus, is primarily like the being in which it terminates. In between, it is primarily like the other modes. In between all four modes there would have to be all of the modes together, which is being qua being, being which is not a being at all. That togetherness can, however, be described from the perspective of each mode as that mode itself when it is qualified by the juncture of the other three modes, for each mode imposes a different type and stress on the to-getherness of them all.

2.13   Real possibilities must be realized somehow and somewhere.

(See 2.03, 2.05, 2.10, 3.44)

THE VERY OPPOSITE of this position would seem most plausible. After all, the various occurrences in this world are contingent. There is no contradiction in the idea that they might not have taken the form they did. What is happening now need not happen in just that way. The possibility that is being realized need not have been realized; some other possibility might have been realized in its stead. If this were not the case whatever happens would have had to happen in just that way. Nothing then would ever be accomplished in any act, and there would of course be nothing like the realization of future indeterminate possibilities in the present; there would be no common objectives which different beings might diversely realize; there would be no room for freedom in act or will.

Yet, on the other hand, it is surely true that what will not be cannot be. If it never will be the case that I will be standing at eleven o'clock on December 2, 1955, such standing cannot be possible. Now I was sitting at that time and that means that at that time my standing is not a possibility. Perhaps we ought to say that just before eleven o'clock there was a possibility of my standing but that with the coming of eleven o'clock and my actual sitting, the possibility vanished, or became an impossibility? This would require us to say, not that a possibility need never be realized, but that it might be a possibility only up to the time when the question of its being realized is in fact raised. Before eleven o'clock of course neither sitting nor standing is impossible at eleven o'clock. But this does not mean that they are distinct possibilities, awaiting some act of decision at eleven o'clock to bring one of them down into the world, untouched and untainted, to live out a career denied to the other. What is possible for me before eleven o'clock (to stay with our illustration) is the single possibility "sitting-or-standing." That possibility is inevitably realized, no matter what I do. In realizing it I specify it either as "sitting" or as "standing." The specification "sitting," say, acquires the status of a distinct possibility only by becoming an ingredient possibility. I make "sitting" a possibility by making concrete the more inclusive, less determinate, inevitably realized possibility, "sitting-or-standing."

I, as at just before eleven o'clock on December 2, 1955, faced the possibility "sitting-or-standing"; when that moment passed I, at that moment, was followed by myself as a being with the possibility "sitting" ingredient in me. That "sitting" allows for the abstracting of "sitting-or-standing" and thus for the understanding of the fact that at eleven o'clock I realized the possibility "sitting-or-standing" in the guise of a "sitting." There is no distinct "sitting" or "standing" inside the indeterminate possibility. We suppose there are such distinct contained possibilities because we read back into the possibilities the determinations which the act of specification provided. We do of course anticipate the kind of specifications which will be provided in fact. Those anticipations are creative acts making a difference to the possibilities confronted. But the anticipations make a difference, not by specifying the possibilities, but by provoking the behavior which will result in a realization having an ingredient possibility similar in nature to what had been thought about. The specifications need not have taken the form they did. Each is a contingent occurrence, but that does not mean that it once was a distinct possibility over against and competing with other possibilities.

The past does not contain the activities of the present. It does not have room for change, expenditure of energy, the focusing on possibilities, the realizing of possibilities. But it does have room for possibilities which confronted Actualities when they were present. If it did not, the past would lack items which it contained as present. The past, however, has those possibilities only in the guise of ingredient possibilities, i.e., only as already realized in a time subsequent to that when the beings, for which they were real unrealized possibilities, occurred.

The law of excluded middle, when applicable to facts, and thus to what is present or past, has the form, "p or not-p"; as applicable to the future, it has the form, "p-or-not-p." In the former, the components are distinct and determinate; one of them has been realized and the other excluded as false. In the latter, the components are indeterminate, not yet separable from one another, and thus neither true nor false. This latter case presents a minimal structure that must be realized in either a p way or a non-p way. The realization of "p-or-not-p" is the conversion of it into "p or not-p," where one of the components is realized and excludes the other. The realization of either one is a way of specifying the structure, "p-or-not-p," thereby making it assume another shape.

Strictly speaking, a contingent occurrence is a specification of "p-or-not-p," the realization of a subordinate part of, say, "I-am-sitting-or-I-am-standing." What is contingent is the determination of some possibility, the making distinct what is not distinct in that possibility. Such realization requires the possibility to be subject to conditions which it does not control.

In a given possibility itself there are no genuine subordinate distinct possibilities. Contingent occurrences of such subordinates are produced from it by subjecting the possibility to conditions outside itself, thereby realizing it.

2.14 Normative possibilities must be satisfied by a being outside both them and Actualities.
(*See 1.118, 2.10, 2.13, 3.109, 4.93*)

EVERY POSSIBILITY must be realized. But not all realizations are equally desirable. "Living-or-dying" is a single possibility which I cannot avoid realizing at every moment. But right now "living" is a better realization of this possibility than "dying" is. There is a normative nature to the possibility, demanding that its realization take the form of living rather than of dying; so far as this desirable realization does not take place, just so far is there a possibility that ought to be but is not yet realized.

Unless we are to say that the "ought to be" is not possible, or that there are possibilities which may never be realized, we are forced to say that the "ought to be" is necessarily realized. Yet if we acknowledge only possibilities and Actualities we must say with some Hegelians that what ought to be will necessarily be realized in the course of history, in face of the fact that the world, until the very end of time, may be evil, corrupt, ugly. The truth that the universe may not be as good as it ought to be, combined with the recognition that what ought to be is really possible, requires a reference to a being outside the Actual and the possible, who sees to it that what ought to be is in fact realized, somewhere, somehow.

One might hold that what ought to be is wholly realized by just one being, outside the possible and the Actual. That being might be viewed as one which in acts, analogous to incarnation and grace, simply adds to possibilities those actual specifications which Actualities failed to provide. But such a view compromises the integrity of the realm of Actualities. Or one might, instead, hold that such a being redefines the possible all the time, shearing off that aspect of it which was not realized by Actualities. But this allows that the ought might be reduced to what actually is; in the end it denies that the ought, so far as it is unfulfilled by men, is really possible.

The most cautious view is that such a being in its own way, at its own pace, and for its own reasons, realizes in itself what Actualities do not. The addition is recognized by the religious man to be one in which he can share—a sharing which enables him to become the man he ought to be, and to do what ought to be done. A more philosophic approach, such as Hartshorne's, views the addition as occurring inside a divine being in an act which then and there adopts and transforms the Actuality. The two approaches are not incompatible. But both have the consequence that the kind of realization which the being provides for a possibility may be quite different in nature from that which man provides.

If by the ethical norm we mean just that which ought to be done and can be done in nature, then no supplementation by an exterior being is necessary; a man will be able to do all that ought to be done by recognizing himself to be, stoicwise, one with whatever works towards the production of good in this world. Such a man might affirm that there is a God who acts in and through nature, but this God would be indistinguishable from a good-producing cosmic, natural force. But once it be recognized that all Actualities together produce less than they might, that they are not as good as they ought to be, and thus that some possibility which they confront, because never realized *by* them, must be realized *for* them, one is compelled to acknowledge a being outside nature, with tasks and reasons of its own which, in consonance with a long tradition one can properly call "God."

These observations apply in analogous ways to Existence in relation to Possibility and Actuality. It too must provide realizations for the possible additional to what Actualities provide. Unlike Actualities, Existence is as wide as space and as long as time; the kind of realization it can provide for the possible is world-wide. And unlike God, instead of uniting Actualities and possibilities it keeps them apart, allowing those possibilities to have the kind of spatiotemporal character that divine realizations cannot provide.

II   THE INCLINATION OF THE GOOD

2.15   The Good is an all-inclusive possibility, or Ideal, as relevant to Actualities.
(*See 1.106, 1.107, 2.10*)

THE IDEAL or possible is a reality which has the guise of the Good in its relation to Actualities, the status of the Future for Existence, and the role of a Principle of Perfection for God. When we speak with Plato of God looking to the Good, we must distinguish, as Plato did not, the Good which is the ontologically defined objective of Actualities, and the Principle of Perfection, which is the analogue of that Good for God. Were there no world of Actualities, as Plato conceived might have been the case, there would be no Good, but only a Principle of Perfection and a Future. Were there no God, as Dewey seemed to believe, there would be a Good and a Future but no Principle of Perfection. And were there no Existence, as Leibniz held, there would be no Future, but only a Good, and a Principle of Perfection.

The Good is a norm and thus requires some realizations rather than others. It is to guarantee these realizations that reference must be made to other Actualities than man—in fact also to God and to Existence as powers which can supplement man's efforts to bring about the whole Good. The Good is always realized, for every determination is a determination of it. It is therefore the most inclusive, the least determinate, a perpetually fulfilled possibility. But it is realized in specific Actualities, which may themselves be internally in conflict and more often than not will be in conflict with one another. The realization of the Good by diverse Actualities allows for the production of multiple evils.

2.16   The Ideal is incomplete.
(*See 1.14, 1.15, 2.15*)

ABSOLUTE IDEALISM takes the Ideal seriously. It recognizes, as few philosophies do, that the Ideal is real, powerful, effective. It knows that spirit, mind, reason, meaning, truth, value—alternative and perhaps equally good names for the Ideal—are not impotent shadows thrown by passing things across the wastes of human futility; it recognizes that the Ideal has strength and life, clarifying the limited occurrences in the world, and even making Existence and God instance it.

Unlike other philosophies, Idealism takes everything else to be but an illustration of the Ideal; appearance, error, folly are for it forms of the Ideal, delimited versions of it, reconciled and redressed by being reduced to the Ideal from which they have somehow departed. The Ideal, as the idealists so clearly see, is omnivorous. From its perspective all that is lies within its orbit. Everything, for it, is but an instance of it. But this is not, as the idealists suppose, a correct and full description of the universe. It only describes the way in which the Ideal approaches the rest of the universe. Idealism fails to take account of the reality of beings outside the Ideal. It maintains that, but does not really explain how, the Ideal could alienate itself, produce its very other, turn itself into a multiplicity of illusions, errors, modes, appearances. How can any one of these find its way back to the source from which it is supposed so inexplicably to have descended?

There are further difficulties with Idealism, exploited by those who take their stand with some other mode of being. As Existentialists have been quick to point out, Idealism presupposes a singular, actual man engaged in actual work; but the system has no room for him. And as theologians have urged, the Idealistic philosophy also presupposes a creative being who grounds the Ideal, judges in terms of it, and satisfies it. And as process philosophers have observed, Idealism also presupposes time and thus a realm of vital, onrushing, energizing Existence. These opponents of Idealism are of course in no better position than the idealist, so far as they themselves get no further than the acknowledgment of Actualities, God, or Existence. But this does not invalidate their criticisms of it.

2.17 The Ideal presupposes Actualities.
(*See 1.14, 1.15, 2.15, 2.16*)

IN ITSELF the Ideal is all, all promise. It is most itself when its promise is fulfilled. For this it needs a plurality of occasions, diverse loci in which it can be expressed. Hegel thought that the Ideal produced these out of itself. This is, of course, what he ought to have supposed on his idealistic theory, hard though it is to see just how it could be made intelligible. But whether self-generated or not, the fact remains that for him as well as for everyone else short of Parmenides, the Ideal needs a plurality of occasions in order to be able to be all it should. This plurality which the Ideal presupposes is over against it as a many over against a one. Its items stand outside the Ideal as that which the Ideal must master, make its own by encompassing them when and as they accommodate it. Were there no such plurality, the Ideal would remain wholly promissory; it would not have an opportunity to make itself through and through determinate, by an exhibition of itself in a plurality of distinct but related guises.

2.18   The Ideal presupposes Existence.
(See 2.16, 2.96, 3.07, 3.104)

EXISTENCE gives the Ideal a cosmic relevance. A proof of the reality of Existence can be provided by starting with the Ideal and showing how that Existence enables the Ideal to be itself to the full. This proof is deferred until later. But it is important now to observe that Existence is needed for the Ideal to be temporally as well as spatially articulated.

2.19   The Ideal presupposes God.
(See 2.16, 2.97, 4.18, 4.89, 4.90)

GOD gives the Ideal the status of a Principle of Perfection, of a standard by which everything can be measured. One of the proofs of God is in fact provided by starting with the Ideal and showing how God is required in order for that Ideal to be itself to the full. This proof is deferred until later. But it is important now to observe that without a divine power working on behalf of the Ideal there is no warrant for the supposition that the Ideal can ever become fully explicit.

2.20   The Good's attempt to encompass all Actualities is qualified by the Ideal's need to keep abreast of Existence.
(See 1.26, 2.17, 2.18)

THE GOOD is the Ideal in relation to Actualities. As such it is continuous with itself in the guise of the Future, i.e., in relation to Existence. When the Ideal acts to encompass Actualities, it also functions as a Future which, by giving direction to Existence, controls it. The effect of this double-pronged activity is, on the one hand, to make the

Actualities part of a single-purposed temporal whole, and on the other
hand to make Existence into a field for the interplay of idealized Actualities. (Conversely, the Ideal's attempt to keep abreast of Existence
is so qualified by its efforts to encompass Actuality as to make it in
effect an attempt to turn Existence into a field for the expression of
the Good.)

What Actualities do not do on behalf of the Ideal, severally or together, the whole of Existence might. The Future is the richer, the
less Actualities realize the Good. The failure of Actualities to realize
the Good adds a burden to Existence, facing it with a Future more
determinate than it need be. In realizing that Future, Existence can and
does help Actuality, but it never succeeds in doing all that is needed
if the Good is to be perfectly fulfilled. It is only God who inevitably
realizes whatever part of the Good that Actuality fails to realize and
Existence may not realize. Were Existence to realize whatever part of
the Good Actuality does not, God would have no necessary work to
do on behalf of the Good. But Existence fails to satisfy fully that part
of the Good which Actualities failed to realize.

The Good as absorbed into the Future is part of the Future for Existence. It does not there exist as a separate unit. Existence never acts
ethically. But what it does on behalf of the Good as absorbed in the
Future could be adopted by Actualities as their own work, with the
consequence that they will then offer a better satisfaction to the Good
than they otherwise would. Nor does God act ethically. Actualities,
to give full satisfaction to the Good, must adopt as their own the non-
ethical work that God does on its behalf.

2.21   The Good's attempt to encompass all Actualities
is qualified by the Ideal's need to accommodate a divine
intent.
(See 1.28, 2.17, 2.19, 2.20)

THE GOOD is continuous with the Principle of Perfection, i.e., with
the Ideal as relevant to God. When the Ideal acts to subjugate Actualities, it also functions as a principle of value which, as accepted by God,
evaluates him. The effect of this twofold effort is, on the one hand, to
make the Actualities subject to an evaluation, and thus to be ordered
in a hierarchy, and on the other hand to make God a being concerned
with the fulfillment of the Good. (Conversely, the Ideal's attempt to

accommodate the intent of God is so qualified by its effort to encompass Actualities as to make it in effect an attempt to make the intent of God essential to the Good.)

The Good is an obligating objective; the Principle of Perfection is a measure of excellence. What Actualities fail to do on behalf of the Good remains over to become part of the Principle of Perfection. Conversely, the Principle as not wholly embodied in God remains over as part of the meaning of the Good. What the one fails to do is left over for the other. Because Actualities fail to exhibit the entire Good, God must use it as part of the Principle for judging what things are like. Because God never fully submits to the Principle of Perfection, the Good stands before men as a measure as well as an objective.

If all the Good is to be done, Actualities must be made one with God as the being who inevitably realizes whatever part of the Good is not realized by Actualities and Existence. And just as the Principle of Perfection is accepted by God as incorporating the Good that men ought but do not and cannot realize by themselves, and which may not be realized even when they adopt the powers of Existence as their own, the Future is faced by Existence as incorporating the Principle of Perfection that God ought but does not and cannot realize by himself. For God to be all he ought, he must make himself one with Existence, that mode of being which inevitably realizes whatever part of the Principle of Perfection is not realized by God and Actualities.

Because God refuses to submit himself entirely to the Ideal in the shape of a Principle, both the Good and the Future acquire the status of measures. Because Actualities are measured by the Good, God can morally judge them; because Existence is measured by the Future, God can guide the course of the world.

2.22 The Ideal's effort to keep abreast of Existence occurs together with its effort to accommodate the intent of God and its effort to encompass all Actualities.

(*See 2.18, 2.20, 2.21*)

EACH of the other modes of being satisfies the Ideal in part, imposing on the remaing two modes the need to do what has not yet been done on behalf of the Ideal. The Future is partly made into a present by Existence; what is left over can, as ingredient in the Principle of Perfection, be realized by God, and as in the form of the Good is inevitably realized by Actualities. The Principle of Perfection is partly satisfied by God; what is left over can be realized by Actualities as a measuring Good, and is inevitably realized by Existence as absorbed in the Future which it realizes. And finally the Good is partly realized by Actualities; what is left over can, as ingredient in the Future be realized by Existence, and as ingredient in the form of a Principle of Perfection is inevitably realized by God.

No one mode realizes the Ideal wholly, but each realizes it to some degree—a realization that takes care of the residuum which the other modes neglected. The three modes together, by transferring part of their burdens to one another, and accepting the outcome as their own, satisfy the Ideal. From the perspective of the Ideal this is but to say that it subjugates them all in different ways and through different strategies.

The Good as infected with the Principle of Perfection measures the worth of every occurrence, and as infecting the Principle is embodied in God. As infected by the Future the Good attains cosmic relevance, and as infecting the Future it perpetually qualifies the course of Existence. The Principle of Perfection as infecting the Future is providence, effective and world-wide; as infected by the Future it is embodied in God as his will.

The Ideal treats the other modes as loci; it seeks to encompass all Actualities, to control all Existence, to evaluate God. To each mode it shows a different face, and it attempts to master each in a special way. The incursion of the Ideal into the domain of Existence results in the achievement of a purpose for the whole of history; the embodiment of the Ideal in God results in his becoming an excellent being; the idealization of Actualities results in the achievement of a harmony in and among the spatiotemporal beings of this world.

The Ideal makes a threefold effort, to which corresponding modes are receptive in varying degrees. But the Ideal always shows the same face—the Good, the Future, or the Principle of Perfection—to a given mode. The face it shows to a mode, however, varies in content and burden, depending on how much justice the other modes do to the Ideal's distinctive demands on them.

A successful incursion of the Ideal on a mode of being is compatible with a failure of that mode to do justice to that face of the Ideal which it confronts—an outcome which is manifest in the actions by that mode which fail to conform to the Ideal. Although, for example, the

Good may subjugate Actualities, and thereby harmonize and perfect them, it never does it to such a degree that it prevents them from being in some conflict with one another.

2.23 The Good encompasses Actualities to some degree by making them desirous.
(See 1.29, 1.45, 1.110)

VIEWED from the side of Actualities, desire is an Actuality primarily seeking for satisfaction. It begins as a lack or need and terminates in a possible outcome, the attainment of which completes or quiets the being. Since a desire may not be satisfied, the prospect in which it terminates is only possible, not yet fully good. If we start from the side of the Good, the Good, in contrast, becomes foundational, and the objects in which it terminates are seen to be only data or occasions which enable it to become more effective. From that side, desire is an instance of the Good; it is the Actuality epitomized in the form of a tendency to bring about more good. Because a desire is the Good as localized but still inchoate, it is a sign that the Actuality is less good than it ought to and might be. Because it is desirous, the Actuality will thereafter function in terms of a Good which it epitomizes, and for the sake of a more comprehensive, satisfying Good.

The Good does not proceed directly to the encompassing of Actualities as desirous. It first encompasses nonliving beings, beings without the capacity to desire. There is in fact an entire philosophy of nature to be written from the standpoint of the Ideal. The first stage involves the conversion of Actualities into co-ordinate members of the same teleological world, while subsequent stages deal with the transformation of inanimate into animate beings. This account of the incursions of the Good in the world is not, of course, a report of an historical process. It represents only some of the steps which a wholly successful incursion must traverse.

2.24 The Good encompasses more of a man when it makes him into a being who prefers than it does when it makes him merely desirous.
(See 1.108, 2.23)

VIEWED from the side of Actuality, preference is a private act by means of which a goal helps determine the election of a means for attaining that goal. From the side of the Good, preference is an actual being epitomized, but no longer, as is the case with desire, one who is merely ready to act so as to bring about more good, but one in whom the Good, in the guise of the goal, is already operative, forcing a decision with respect to this means or that.

No matter what a man prefers he exhibits the Good in a way he did not before, for he makes his decision in terms of a goal which expresses in a limited way the nature of the Good itself. If the goal is undesirable, it would be better for it not to be pursued. This shows, not that the act of preference is outside the orbit of the Good, but that the Good as exhibited in that act of preference may be less good than it is when exhibited by one who acts without submission to that particular goal. What is felt in preference is the allure of the Good, and this is compatible with the Good actually taking the limited form of a goal not in fact desirable.

2.25 The Good encompasses more of an actual man when it makes him into a being who chooses than it does when it makes him into a being who prefers.
(*See 1.109, 2.24*)

VIEWED from the side of Actuality, choice is an act by which ends and means are made to support one another. From the side of the Good, choice is a man epitomized. But whereas in the case of preference, the goal which a man might then face might be good, bad, or indifferent, the end with which a choice is occupied is always of maximum value. An end is the values of the universe redistributed, the acceptance of which as the terminus of one's obligation rationally justifies the losses in value that are being brought about.

The Good realized in the guise of an act of choice is more fully satisfied than it is when realized in the guise of an act of preference. Through choice it can function not only as an absolute end but as a justification for actions—even for actions which are destructive or bad. It conquers what is other than itself; it transforms evil by making it into an agent for a commitment to an excellent end.

In choice the Good no longer merely lures, as it does in preference. It is accepted as a supreme value, adopted as an end which sanctions and ennobles whatever it embraces. An end, of course, is not identical with the Good. There are many ends and only one Good. An end is the Good, distributed over a whole range of items in some one of many possible ways.

2.26 The Good encompasses more when it makes a man into a being who creatively wills than it does when it makes him into one who chooses.
(*See 1.112, 2.25*)

NOT ALL ENDS are realizable. The kind of redistribution that an end requires may be beyond the powers of a man to bring about. When this occurs a man must fail to do what he obligated himself to do. But when the Good expresses itself as a creative will, it not only brings all of a man's energies into a focus beyond the capacity of desire, preference, and choice to exhibit, but prompts those energies to be spent in such a way as to realize further good.

By expressing itself as a creative will the Good reaches the limit of its capacity to encompass an individual man. The good it thereby brings about is always limited in range. Sometimes the work performed by a man of good will even comes in conflict with the work of others equally endowed with good wills, seeking nothing more than the promotion and multiplication of the Good. The most that the Good can expect is that an individual man will be tempted by it to become ethical, which is to say, to become a man with a good will who does good. When this happens the Good is still not yet fully satisfied, for a man of good will, even when in harmony with others, brings about only part of the Good (and of course fulfills only part of the Ideal).

2.27 It is good for the Good to be fulfilled.
(*See 2.10, 2.26*)

WHEN men work together in some measure of harmony they constitute a society or social group. Such a group may be more or less permanent. The most transitory is a gathering, the least is an institution such as a family, community, nation, or state. In both types and in those in between, men by virtue of their common environment, training, opportunities, and needs, allow room for one another. Without intent or exercise of will they work somewhat in harmony; so far as they do, they are social beings and good.

The Good transforms isolated individuals into parts of a group in a way analogous to that by which it turns all Actualities into co-ordinates—it appears to them in the form of an objective which is germane to a number, and which they realize together. The degree to which the Good is exhibited in a given group, depends on the degree to which the group status of the members is made an integral part of themselves. The transformation occurs at the same time that the individuals are made into beings who desire, prefer, choose, or will.

As exhibited in desire, preference, etc., the Good relates individuals to prospects they are to bring about; as exhibited in a group the Good relates them to one another. In the one case the individual accretes a private virtue preparatory to the possible achievement of a public one; in the other case the individual achieves a public status which he may make more or less integral to his being. The two cases are independent, and one may at times be properly preferred to the other. A group may do greater justice to the Good than even a man of good will, for the latter may actually be in conflict with other men. A merely desirous man might satisfy the Good more fully than a group, since the good of the group may not be a significant part of the individuals who comprise that group. What is desirable is a conjunction of a private and public virtue—excellent individuals in whom an excellent group character is an essential part.

2.28 Men, as forming a community, can encompass a wider range of goods than is possible in a group.
(*See 2.27*)

LIKE the group, a community contains only a limited number of men. Like the group too, it has a common nature and mode of functioning which may be distinct and even opposed to that of other groups and communities. Most important, it may, because its members are not properly absorbed within it, be in conflict with its own members at various times.

The common character of community is an ideology, a common set of interlocked objects of belief, not necessarily consciously entertained but nevertheless evident in the thought, speech, and actions of the members, and in the institutions, history, and divisions of the community. An ideology is a kind of synthesis of group characters. The various groups in a community reciprocally offer, in their different common goods, different analytic divisions of the ideology. There is no reason to suppose that the ideology is prior in time to the group characters, or conversely.

2.29   A class is a group in which the common character controls the activities of the members.
(*See 2.27*)

A GROUP has a restricted task and objective, having only a tangential or incidental effect on the men who are members of it. It attains the status of a class when the thought, emotions, and behavior of the members are affected by the common group character. The members of a class constitute it; the class is part of their substance, whereas the members of a group only belong to it, since the group character merely collects them and does not dominate or control them. Consequently, though a group may have the very same features as a class, it will nevertheless lack its vitality and substantiality.

The idea of a class came into prominence in two quite distinct areas in the last century—in logic, largely because of Boole, and in economic-political theory, largely because of Marx. Both were in opposition to Aristotle with his theory of real natural classes, of genuine species of beings whose forms governed the activities of those beings apart from all human interest or contrivance.

The logical approach to classes is primarily one which concerns itself with treating entities extensionally, as constituting a collection. Since any items at all can be collected together in thought, the logical approach makes possible the acknowledgment of multiple classes to which the Aristotelian denies reality, and allows for the rejection or division of classes which the Aristotelian takes to be permanent fixtures of the universe. The economic-political approach to classes, in contrast, recognizes that men at least are governed by common forms, patterns, features, or goals. But unlike the Aristotelian, it affirms that they are so governed because individual men were forced together in place, role, and destiny by the work they do and by their society's traditions, needs, and pressures. From this perspective the class is as real as Aristotle's, but it is not a part of nature. While individuals are viewed somewhat in the way they are in logic, as units, not as beings embodying a common form, they are recognized to be as the Aristotelians claim they are, under the dominance of some common form.

One need not give up the Aristotelian view that there are real natural classes, classes which exist even apart from the pressure of society. But if one had to give up that view, one ought not to go further than the position of those who recognize that society can keep men so together that they function as if they were part of a real Aristotelian class. A community, a society, a state are real, though not natural classes; inside them we can sometimes find representative subclasses. It is these subclasses which I will, with Marx, hereafter refer to simply as "classes."

Men can shift their membership from class to class, and from group to group. Belonging to a class at one moment they, by relaxing or retreating, may even make themselves into just members of a group. The converse process also occurs.

2.30   There ought to be classes functioning on behalf of the community.
(*See 2.28, 2.29*)

THE CLASSES in a community are so many different analytic parts of it, in which subdivisions of the ideology are made integral to some of the members. Some of the classes are *essential*, vital to the very continuance or prosperity of the community. They are classes in which some restricted but essential function is performed. An essential class represents the community, doing for other groups, classes and individuals in that community what they need to have done in order that they may exist, function at all, or function better than they otherwise could.

2.31   The community should contain a number of classes.
(*See 2.30*)

A COMMUNITY may have any number of classes. Some of these may not be necessary for doing anything important. They may have no repercussions on the rest. Other classes than these might have provided a better division of labor, made up a more organic community.

A community should contain at least those classes whose members are engaged in activities essential to the continuance or the welfare of the whole. It will fail to achieve all it should if some of these classes are lacking. Additional classes might have important work to do on behalf of limited portions of the community; still others might work on behalf of something good which does not redound to the benefit of the rest. Or they may make for flexibility, color, ease. Such additional classes make the community less neatly organized than it might be, but they do not necessarily involve any loss in efficiency or value. It is a strong temptation, nevertheless, for the philosophic creators of states to suppose that there are only essential classes. This gives their communities an austere look, and makes it hard to relate them to existent communities. But once it be recognized that essential classes are not the only classes which exist or even which ought to exist, it is proper for the philosopher to attend only to the essential, since the others are too many and too multiform to make their study profitable for one engaged primarily in determining the Ideal's persistent needs, vital operations, and ultimate satisfactions. It is to be noted, however, that no society is exhausted by its classes, essential or otherwise. In addition to classes, a society encompasses a public or people, the men as unorganized and without definite roles.

2.32   A class of reasonable men is one whose members' grasp of causal processes and whose adjustments are accepted as representative by the rest.
(See *1.17, 1.43, 2.31*)

REASONABLE MEN are not necessarily rational men. They may not know what is the case, they may not have good minds, they may not be interested in inquiry, they may not be highly critical, and they may have no adequate or proper explanation for what takes place. They may be traditionalized, conventional men, responding to situations without reflection or insight. But they are reasonable if they are expectative of what might most likely result on given conditions, have adjusted themselves in belief, thought, and act to certain outcomes rather than others, and do define in attitude and acts what is probable and plausible for the rest of the community. Most of the men in most communities seem, as a matter of fact, to have some degree of the representative reasonableness, enabling them to go about their tasks in harmony with other members of the community.

Despite the strangeness of the terminology, it is most appropriate to term those who live in consonance with the superstitious practices and foolish expectations of a community, "reasonable men" in that community. Our own community professes to believe that the reasonable and the rational man are identical. We try to ignore the fact that in many communities, and even in our own, not only the rest of the community but the rational man himself often lives reasonably but not in terms of what he knows to be the case. The rational man may have firm and certified knowledge; what he says might benefit the rest if only they would heed him. But since they do not, he is not a practically wise, reasonable man in that community so long as he insists on living only in consonance with what he surely knows.

2.33   A class of prestigious men is one whose members' behavior, values, or standards of what is important are models for the rest.
(See *1.49, 2.31*)

THE PRESTIGIOUS MAN has the respect of the rest; his values are the values the others accept as ideal. They look to him, not necessarily consciously and rarely deliberately, to provide guides enabling them to determine what in that community is right and wrong, worth doing, having, and being. His values may not, in an objective sense, be defensible; it might have been better for the community if others had been taken as models. Nor is the prestigious man necessarily a reasonable one. He might be a prophet, a priest, a saint, a hero whose standards the rest honor in the breach, and conformity to which by the rest might be ruinous to all. Conversely, the reasonable man might be without prestige. His expectations might be acknowledged as models, but his values, his understanding of merit and defect disowned.

The prestigious man is not necessarily prized as a person. He has prestige by virtue of his status, his position, his office. Even when he is recognized by the rest to be of little worth, however, his judgments and his behavior in his office are treated as expressing a standard to be used to measure all. There is perhaps no individual member of a community who does not enjoy some prestige, if for no other reason than that he submits to accepted standards and in this way exemplifies accepted values.

2.34 The members of a class of empowered men have control of the might of a community.
(*See 2.31*)

A COMMUNITY is made up of men each with some degree of strength. And through them it makes use of the forces of nature. Inside a well-formed community there is in fact a class primarily occupied with the organization and use of the power that is available to that community.

The members of the empowered class may not have much power of their own. Not only may they be weaklings, but they may not be able to possess or use for themselves the power they direct and control. Nor need they be men of much prestige. They may be functionaries, men who are thought to do comparatively menial work, while the prestigious either do no work at all or are engaged in supposedly superior types of activity, such as contemplation, worship, or artistic creation. Nor need empowered men be particularly reasonable. They may arbitrarily spend the power which they control; they may not be aware of the consequences of this or that use of power; they may do violence to the desires, needs or structure of the community. Or they may even use power most intelligently, but not in a way that the others accept as wise.

The empowered class represents the others so far as they accept its use of power. Such acceptance may be sullen or joyous, wise or foolish. The power might even be employed to the detriment of all. But the class remains representative just so far as its manipulation of the power is at least allowed by the rest.

2.35 A mature community contains at least three harmonized classes of men.
(*See 2.28, 2.31, 2.32-4*)

ONE and the same man may be maximally reasonable, prestigious, and powerful. He will nevertheless usually belong to three distinct classes, for he will function in the community in three somewhat independent ways. But so far as the acts of men are at once reasonable, prestigious, and expressive of power, the three classes tend to collapse into one. This is not a desirable result, for each type has a proper range which is partly outside the scope of the others.

The three classes are essential and have different ranges. The reasonable class encompasses all grounded acceptable expectations, many of which are too minor to have a community value, and some of which should make no use of public power—manners, for example. The prestigious encompasses the entire domain of standard, acceptable values, some of which may relate to an afterlife and thus are outside the reach of reasonable expectations and may have no bearing on current uses of power. Might encompasses the entire field of acceptable usages of social energy, some of which may not be properly grasped in expectation or thought, and which may rightfully challenge what has been taken as deserving respect.

The classes are not always kept distinct and do not always work in harmony. A community in which they do not function independently is undeveloped. A community in which they function in opposition is diseased, in internal conflict. A mature community is one in which they operate in independence and in harmony, related by an unorganized body of people. It represents the maximum encroachment of the Good in relation to a limited number of unified men who are separated off from the rest of mankind by virtue of a common ideology.

2.36 A model community makes provision for the good of men outside it.
(*See 2.28, 2.35*)

EACH COMMUNITY is limited in scope. To do justice to the Good each should be articulated in independent but concordantly functioning, essential classes. But if a community ignores the other communities it will fail to be fully at the service of the Good. Sooner or later it will be bound to come into conflict with some of the others. Even if it is as excellent as a community can be by itself, it will not be a community which brings about as much good as a community can.]

A model community recognizes in its ideology the presence, rights, and needs of men outside the community. Such a model community is not fully mature and thus not a genuinely model community until its ideology has become an integral part of its members when these are distributed into essential classes. But even then it may not try to bring about the Good which it recognizes to be germane to the others. If it does not try, it will be idealistic. And it may, whether idealistic or active, be opposed by other communities. It will then be ineffective. To have maximum fulfillment in communities the Good must make all of them into model communities which, while pursuing their own characteristic goods, harmoniously promote the good of the rest. Even then there will still be areas which the Good must possess before it can be said to have reached a maximum encompassment of the actual world. (See 2.84 ff.)

III   RIGHT AND MIGHT

2.37 Men are justified in claiming to have their natures preserved or enhanced.
(*See 1.113*)

A CLAIM is a man as resistant or active on behalf of the good he embodies. It is an ontological demand that the good in him continue or increase; it need not be and usually is not consciously urged. It may in fact not even be known. The Good points up this good in a man and sanctions the man's insistence on it.

Destruction of a man goes counter to his claim to be preserved; neglect of him goes counter to his claim to be enhanced. If there were no such claims at all, or if they were not justified, there would be nothing amiss in the elimination of a man, and nothing amiss in the wasting of his talents. But death is always tragic, and unfulfilled promise is always regrettable. This does not deny that death might be desirable at times, because of the greater evil that would otherwise ensue. What is intrinsically tragic, may yet be relatively desirable. The Good is, and what is is good, but some things are better than others, with superior claims to be or to be enhanced.

2.38 Each man makes a number of essential claims to have his nature preserved or enhanced.
(*See 2.37*)

A NEED is a man dealt with from the perspective of a possible satisfaction and thus as essentially *lacking* something. A claim is a man dealt with from the perspective of what he is, and thus as essentially *deserving* something. It is because of what a man is not that he has a need to be preserved or enhanced; it is because of what he is that he claims to be preserved or enhanced. Urging his preservation, his claims presuppose that he already has some value; urging his enhancement, they presuppose that there is some value he should still acquire.

A man's claims express the fact that he is over against other Actualities and other modes of being which he must use if he is to be as complete, as perfect as a man can be. His claims are so many vital demands for that which will enable him to maintain himself or to realize his promise in the precarious world in which he lives. They are himself as capable of being satisfied by this or that type of being, in this or that particular way.

A man makes as many essential claims for what else there be as there are essential parts of him, capable of distinct functioning for the benefit of himself as a whole. Such claims are made on behalf of his mind, emotions, speech, body, etc.—different but interrelated areas in which his single good is in fact essentially divided and exercised.

2.39   A native right is an essential claim defined in terms of others as required to satisfy it.
(*See 2.38*)

A NATIVE RIGHT expresses a limited good, characteristic of some essential division of a man, but requiring a response on the part of other men. The others have a duty towards that right; if they did not, the right would be only a claim or demand which the individual would like to have met but which no one is required to help him or to allow him to meet. Various other kinds of rights and duties will be distinguished in succeeding propositions. A summary table of them will be found in 2.60.

2.40   A right denied is a right alienated, and entails the insistence on some other right having a stronger case because able to satisfy a superior claim.
(*See 2.38, 2.39*)

A MAN'S RIGHT may be challenged from one of three sides: it may be challenged by other rights, by the man himself, or by the beings outside that man. Challenged by other rights it must have a justification greater than theirs if it is to deserve to overcome them. Challenged by the individual, it must have a justification in itself if it would be wrong to absorb it within the unity of the man. Challenged by other beings, it must have a justification greater than theirs if it is to deserve to withstand them.

Rights are denied by being denied expression, either through the removal of opportunities or through the threat of undesirable consequences. Such rights are alienated rights in the sense that they are no longer effective, no longer rights which can be satisfied. The claims they express of course continue to exist; they are still legitimate. But they are no longer operative; they express the intrinsic, but not the viable right of the good that one possesses.

There is no justification for the reduction of a native right to the status of a futile claim unless in that act some greater good is thereby achieved. Such a greater good can be of one of two forms. It can be expressed in some other, quite distinct right, whose satisfaction would otherwise not be possible and which results in the production of greater good. Or it can be expressed in some more comprehensive right whose satisfaction will involve the more ready or complete satisfaction of the initially alienated right.

The United States Declaration of Independence refers to the "self-evident" truths "that all men are created equal; that they are endowed by their Creator with certain unalienable rights; that among these are life, liberty, and the pursuit of happiness." No one of these rights, and in fact no unalienable rights of any kind, are mentioned in the United States Constitution. The closest one comes to such an acknowledgment is in Amendment IX ("The enumeration in the Constitution of certain rights shall not be construed to deny or disparage others retained by the people") and Amendment X ("The powers not delegated to the United States by the Constitution, nor prohibited by it to the States, are reserved to the States respectively, or to the people") of the so-called "Bill of Rights." But there is no assertion in the Constitution that there are rights belonging to the people which are not alienable, *de facto* or *de jure*, by the United States. And this is wise. The right to life is alienated in wartime; liberty is constrained on every side for the proper conduct of common living, transportation, and peace, and the pursuit of happiness is channelized in accordance with the estimate of our society as to what is profitable, desirable, and practical. Every specific right, even though essential, and even though its satisfaction is necessary if a man is to be all he ought, may be justly alienated in order to benefit a superior right or to promote its own eventual satisfaction.

2.41   Not all rights can be justifiably alienated at any one time.
(*See 2.40*)

THERE is no one specific native right which may not be justifiably alienated. But though any right may be alienated at any time, not all can be justifiably alienated at the same time. The warrant for an alienation is the satisfaction of some other right—not necessarily a native one—or the eventual satisfaction of the alienated right. In the former case the alienated right is replaced by another specific right, native or otherwise, then insisted on; in the latter case the alienation is on behalf of a higher order or more general, persistent right to achieve an eventual satisfaction for the alienated right. In both cases the alienation of a right requires the insistence on some other.

2.42   Men with the same type of right may be in conflict.
(*See 2.39*)

MEN have similar essential organs; they have similar basic functions. All of them as a consequence have similar native rights. But the exercise of the rights by one may preclude the exercise of the same type of rights by others. There may be food available for only a few, yet all may have the same right to eat. Acknowledgment that there is an equality of rights may then be but the prelude to a recognition of the imminence of conflict, precisely because the material available does not suffice to satisfy the acknowledged equally legitimate claims of all. When then in Article 2 of the Universal Declaration of Human Rights adopted in 1948 by the United Nations it is said that "Everyone is entitled to all the rights and freedoms set forth in this Declaration" (including such "rights" as "the right to own property," and "of equal access to public service" and "to work") it is apparently not supposed that the United Nations guarantees that every man will be able to exercise or satisfy his rights at all times, or even at the times that others do, or perhaps even ever. Not only is it the case that the United Nations has no power to assure that the exercise of a right will be permitted, but the insufficiency of property or public conveniences or jobs precludes the exercise of the relevant rights by some men if they are exercised satisfactorily by others.

Declarations and tables of rights are pivotal points, or calls to action; they actually guarantee nothing, not only because they lack power, but because such guarantees depend on the provision of appropriate material, and this is outside their control.

2.43   Men have the privilege of ordering and interrelating their native rights.

(See 2.39, 2.42)

A RIGHT expresses a claim by the Good so far as this is embodied in man. So far as the Good is not embodied, men evidently have an ethical duty to exercise their rights. So far as it is embodied, men have not a duty but a privilege to exercise their rights. It is part of the meaning of that privilege that it involves the right of man to determine the way in which their native rights are to be satisfied.

The idea of a privilege is here adapted from law. A legal privilege is a right to act, involving no duty on the part of others. Julius Stone, after Hohefeld, terms it "the kind of 'liberty' which the law tolerates but does not support by imposing a duty on any one else." Viewed apart from a legal context, a privilege is a right to privately order and express specific native rights even in such a way that they achieve a new status and a new kind of satisfaction.

A man's privilege is interior to him; it is a private power enabling him to integrate and express his several specific rights. This privilege may not be exercised, and when exercised may not be exercised consciously or wisely. When a man is destroyed or reduced to incoherence some native rights are directly violated. The privilege which is a man's so far as he is a single being, outside the public arena, articulating the good in him in a number of somewhat distinct and independent ways, is also then incidentally denied.

2.44   Men have the privilege of exercising every one of their rights.

(See 2.39, 2.41, 2.43)

A RIGHT unexercised is a right only in promise. Since a right which is forever denied exercise is not an actual but only a promised right,

men, if they are granted to have any rights at all, must be granted to
have the privilege of exercising them. This privilege is not distinct
from the privilege of ordering and interrelating the rights.

A man has the privilege of ordering and interrelating his rights so
as to be able to satisfy them eventually. But to satisfy a right one
must exercise it. Since a right is satisfied when its demands are met,
the exercise of a right does not necessarily involve any more action
on the part of a man than that of placing himself in a position in which
the right is externally satisfied. The right is a claim contained in the
being that is man; the satisfaction of it is the providing it with what
it by nature but not necessarily through effort demands.

2.45 There is no privilege to exercise all rights at any one
time.
(*See 2.42, 2.44*)

A MAN has the privilege of exercising each and every right that
he has. But he does not have enough knowledge, nor are the conditions opportune for him to exercise them all together. The exercise
of the right to eat may conflict with the exercise of the right to
speak. The privilege to exercise their rights requires men to make an
effective assessment of the rights, and to determine when they can be
best exercised.

Outside the arena of public determination, a man decides (not
necessarily consciously or wisely) to insist on this or that native
right as deserving satisfaction in the face of competing rights, in a
situation where only some of his rights can be successfully exercised.
The privilege, though internally determined, is concerned with
rights whose exercise involves a reference to what is outside the
man. It loses all distinctiveness when held apart from every situation.

2.46 Men have the privilege of alienating any of their
specific rights.
(*See 2.40, 2.44, 2.45*)

TO DETERMINE that this or that right is to be exercised and satisfied,
rather than some other, is to determine that this other is not, for the
moment, to be exercised and satisfied. But to deny a right exercise
and satisfaction is one with alienating it, giving it up, not honoring
its demand. Since a man has the privilege of determining which rights

are to be exercised and satisfied he has therefore the privilege of alienating any right at all. To justify the alienation he must promise in the act to promote the eventual satisfaction of the alienated right, and must then and there urge the satisfaction of some other right which has a superior claim at that time and place. His insistence on some rights and his alienation of others is not necessarily a matter of effort, decision, will, but a matter of adjustment to, and evaluation and acceptance of what the world in fact provides—though of course it is not inconsistent with deliberate effort and the expenditure of energy.

2.47   Men have the privilege of alienating all their specific rights.
(*See 2.46*)

A MAN has the privilege of alienating any one of his specific rights. And he has the privilege of alienating any pair or triplet, or any set of them. Such alienation must be justified. He cannot rightly cancel out a claim which flows from the very nature of the good in him; but he can hold up its satisfaction indefinitely in order that the Good be more fully satisfied.

From the standpoint of privilege there are no specific unalienable rights. Even the right to the integrity of a man's essential organs and functions can be justly alienated and denied.

Were men not to have the privilege of alienating their specific rights, they would not be single, private beings capable of assessing the roles of their essential parts for the benefit of the whole. But if they had the privilege of alienating their rights without forging a new right and without making a compensatory promise to provide those rights with an equal or better satisfaction eventually, they would have a privilege to do wrong. A man has a privilege only so far as he represents the Good; he cannot without self-contradiction have a privilege to do wrong.

If the alienation of a man's rights were to devolve on other men, a man could be denied rights without regard for what he was and needed. If the alienation were assigned to a society, and this acted even only to promote the eventual satisfaction of what was alienated, it still could be true that for any length of time every one of a man's rights might be denied, and this by an outside decision. Only men have the privilege of alienating their own rights, and then they must provide a justification for what they do, in the guise of a superior right, or in a promise to make good the claims now denied.

Statism or Fascism, which is a kind of phenomenology or idealism restricted to political men, denies to men any other nature than that which the political unit provides. Such men never have any rights alienated, but are merely given some at some time, and are denied some at other times. Occasionally they are denied all their rights, and this for the ostensible purpose of benefiting them eventually. But no right can be rightly denied except so far as that right is somehow retained, allowed to make a claim even while denied a satisfaction.

2.48 Men have the privilege of constituting a single unitary right.
(*See 2.41, 2.47*)

MEN can justifiably alienate all their specific native rights so far as they then and there promise a satisfaction of them. But all rights cannot be justly alienated at the same time. The alienation of all specific rights must involve the presence of a right of a different sort. Men have the privilege of holding off the satisfaction of their specific rights only if they incorporate them within a new single right whose satisfaction involves the satisfaction of those encompassed rights. Specific rights are justifiably alienated only in a supervening unitary right which promises their satisfaction.

A man's unitary right is distinct but not separate from his specific rights. Since the rights of a man are functions of his distinct parts and functions, the unitary right cannot annihilate his specific rights; these will remain regardless of how he exercises his privilege to forge the unitary right. But since the satisfaction of a unitary right may involve the deferment of the satisfaction of any of the rights out of which it is constituted, those rights are nevertheless denied the status they had had. The unitary right neither absorbs the specific rights nor stands outside them; rather it orders and unifies them, allowing each some place and expression but denying it the independence, the distinctness, and thus the separate satisfaction it could have had before. It is when and as some of his distinct essential functions are exercised that a man exercises the privilege of estimating whether or not an adequate place is being made for these and other functions.

This estimate is his way of assessing, deferring, and urging his specific rights within the frame of a single unitary right.

2.49 Man's unitary right cannot be justly alienated.
(See 2.48)

THE UNITARY RIGHT of man is achieved through the unification of his specific rights. These are thereby alienated in the sense that they are denied a functioning and a satisfaction which they otherwise could have had. The justification of that alienation lies in the promise of the satisfaction of those rights through the mediation of the unitary right. The alienation of that unitary right would in effect involve the denial of every one of man's rights without compensation, or would bring one back to the state where there were specific rights but no united whole of them. But to deny all rights without compensation is wrong, going counter to the legitimate demands of the Good to achieve a maximum satisfaction; to go back to the stage where one had only distinct rights is to go back to the stage where rights can be in conflict, and thus is once more to go counter to the legitimate demands of the Good. The unitary right which man has the privilege to constitute must find a place for every right in such a way that all are promised a full satisfaction.

2.50 Man's unitary unalienable right is the right to benefit from social existence.
(See 2.45, 2.49)

THERE is a need for a man to carve out a unitary right. External conditions do not permit a satisfaction of all his native rights, taken severally. The unitary right enables him to face those conditions in a more appropriate way. He approaches them with a single demand in which his various specific demands are limited by one another and by the unity they help constitute.

Each man appears on the public scene armed with a unitary right. This is a legitimate unitary claim on behalf of his good, which he has re-established as a unity by transforming and synthesizing its various essential specifications in him. Just how he is to satisfy the unitary right, just what shape that satisfaction will take he does not necessarily know, nor is he in a position to determine. He is caught in a world which is partly alien to him, and he defends the good that is in him and by which he tests the justice of the world, by facing his society with an unalienable right to be satisfied in it and through its help. Instead of confronting the society with a number of co-ordinate distinct claims, he thus confronts it with a single overarching claim to the effect that in some way or other his various specific rights, as encompassed but not absorbed within a single coherent whole, are all to be satisfied in that world, somehow, somewhere, some time.

2.51 Society dictates in part which specific rights are to be satisfied, when they are, and how.
(See 2.29, 2.50)

A SOCIETY or social group is a collection of men illustrating and occupied with some common objective. Each man, as part of the group, is interlocked with others, sent along certain paths, and blocked through threat, tradition, and obstacle from going along other paths. He is a public being who does things and fails to do things which are distinct from those which he could do or might fail to do as a private being, freely initiating acts. The society offers him satisfactions for some of his rights and denies them to others at different times, and often without regard for his preferences.

2.52 Society should satisfy a man's unitary right to benefit from social existence.
(See 2.50, 2.51)

A RIGHT deserves satisfaction. When society denies a satisfaction to a right it does wrong. That wrong is justifiable only so far as there is a promise in the denial that the satisfaction will eventuate, and this without detriment to it because of the delay. The delaying of the satisfaction cannot be extended at the same time to all man's rights, however, without paradoxically making him into a bare instrument for the eventual just treatment of him as a man. This means that when and as the society denies a specific right, it must so satisfy a man's unalienable more basic right to profit from social existence that it then and there also must somewhat satisfy some specific right.

Because the only right a man insists on without qualification is the unitary right to benefit from social existence, and this because he thereby answers most adequately to the claims of a single Good which his essential functions and organs articulate but do not fully express, a society has the unavoidable task of satisfying his unitary right. And because he inevitably yields to the society the determination as to just which rights are to be satisfied at a given time, the society owes him not only the eventual full satisfaction of his unitary right but also a partial satisfaction of some specific right.

A man offers society the good he has; this he allows it to gear and interrelate according to its own designs. And he offers himself to society as a being who should gain from that adventure at least as much as he offers it. To be sure, he does not have a choice in the matter; society has him in thrall from the moment of his birth. Still, he is a substance, a being with a private nature and legitimate claims. Though he cannot escape its control, he rightly judges it as good or bad to the degree that it satisfies him or fails to satisfy him both as a public and as a private being whose essential functions subtend a single unitary demand that his good be preserved and enhanced.

2.53   Society is justified in denying satisfaction to some rights.
(See 2.48, 2.51, 2.52)

WHEN a man forges a unitary right he in a way denies to every one of his specific rights an autonomy it otherwise would have. He subjects all of them to a more inclusive and superior claim. That claim he makes against society, and society in turn decides how it is to be satisfied.

The satisfaction of a man's unitary right involves the satisfaction of specific rights as well, for not only does the unitary right allow place for each of the specific rights, but each is integral to organs and functions which operate to some degree in independence of the unitary being they help constitute and in which they are. But just which rights are to be satisfied, and thus which ones are not to be alienated by society at that time, is determined by the nature of the satisfaction which the society gives to the unitary right.

The way society benefits a man determines the specific rights he then publicly has. Those rights evidently change in nature from time to time, and man as a consequence must be said to have no unalienable publicly expressible rights, except the right to benefit somehow from being a part of a social whole.

2.54   Civil rights are correlate with duties in others to do or forbear.
(See 1.109, 2.39, 2.48, 2.51)

AN END, whose promised realization justifies the wrongs committed in an act of choice, entrains *ethical* duties, the performance of acts serving to realize that end. A *public* duty is distinct from this. It is what the publicly supported rights of one man require of other men if those rights are to be satisfied. These two kinds of duty are independent, and what is most germane to one may be indifferent to the other. An ethical duty may of course involve the performance of a public duty; a public duty may support the fulfillment of an ethical duty. It is always an ethical duty to promote some kind of social existence; it is always a public duty to allow for an ethical life.

Men have ethical duties towards the rest of mankind and nature which no social group can express in the shape of public duties, since such public duties are related only to rights possessed by those who are within the reach of the powers of the social group. On the other hand, a man acquires a public duty as soon as his group defines other men to have a publicly supported, or *civil* right. If a man is given the civil right to some honor in a society, the rest have a public duty to respect it.

By exercising their privilege to alienate their native rights on behalf of a superior unitary right, men preclude the existence of the corresponding specific public duties, but at the same time make a demand on the social group that the unitary right be satisfied. Answering to the single unalienable right of a man to profit from social existence there must, then, be a single unavoidable *group* duty to do or forbear so as to have that right satisfied. This unavoidable group duty is expressed in the form of specific *service* duties to be performed by the members of the group. Some of these service duties may not answer to any specific right; they are the duties which the group imposes on its members so that the group duty, answering to man's basic unalienable right, can be fulfilled.

For every right there is a duty. Civil rights are matched by public duties, and the basic unalienable right of man is matched by a group duty. But there can be duties for which there are no answering rights, e.g., some of the ethical duties defined by an obligating end, and those service duties which the society assigns to its members so that the group duty can be fulfilled.

2.55   Rights are satisfied by the aid of a might outside themselves.

(See 2.51, 2.54)

PUBLIC DUTIES are inseparable from socially imposed liabilities of some sort in case of failure. Apart from such liabilities there would be no relation between the duties and the rights, no support of the demand for the satisfaction of the rights. But a right which need not be satisfied is not a right in fact. Genuine rights are viable rights, rights related to a duty whose performance is required. Such relating it is the function of the social group to provide.

A group's embodiment of its objective is one with the group's relating of its members to one another in such a way that socially acknowledged civil rights are matched with the socially required performance of public duties by others. The social group on behalf of its group duty imposes *essential tasks* on its members, subjecting them to liabilities should they fail to do what it demands. Apart from such liabilities the service duties would be mere social assignments to be ignored if one so desired. The liabilities make the tasks into expressions of genuine service duties.

A social group relates public duties to civil rights and service duties to essential tasks. It does this primarily and persistently through threat, which is no less real for being habitually yielded to, or for being left unmentioned. Threat is the promise of action of an undesirable sort, and operates in hardly discernible ways through hint, fear, slight restraints, and disdain, as well as through ostensible pressures, clear pronouncements, and definite predictions of what will ensue on failure to do what is asked, or on a refusal to stop doing what is forbidden.

A threat is an undesirable use of might, serving to make the use of further power unnecessary. It has power in it and behind it. A threat with no power in it would exert no compulsion, and would then be indistinguishable from a recommendation flavored with a disapproval. Did it not have power behind it, a threat would be indistinguishable from a disagreeable demand. An agency employed by society to satisfy rights by bringing them into relation to duties whose performance is compelled, a threat compels in itself and entrains the use of further power, should the threat be ignored. The presence of the threat is not incompatible with a volitional performance by men of the very acts which the threat is intended to elicit. One can voluntarily accept and perform what would entail undesirable consequences otherwise.

Public duties with their corresponding civil rights, and service duties with their compelled essential tasks, are related through the exercise of a force imposed on both. The connection between the group duty and the corresponding unalienable unitary right possessed by the members of the group is somewhat different in character. The relation between a group and its members, and thus between a group duty and a man's unitary right, is an ontological relation of abstract justice, dictating what each is to do in relation to the other and testing what each in fact does. There is no threat in it, but there is pressure. This pressure is the outcome of an expression of the tendency of the group to use its strength in its own way. The actual linkage which holds between the group as having a duty and its members as having rights against it, is thus a product of the kind of use to which the group puts its power. If there were no such tendency of the group to use its power in its own way, the group either would be just its members, or would be unrelated to them. But a group is more than its members, having a rationale, history, structure peculiar to it. And if it did not have an actual relation to its members, it would not have a real duty towards them, and they would not have a real right in relation to it. The unalienable right of man to benefit from social existence, then, no less than his specific civil rights, must be brought into relation with its corresponding duty. That duty is lodged in the group rather than in other men, and there is no real imposition of force, but otherwise the two cases, the unitary unalienable and the specific civil rights, with their respective correlative group and public duties, are alike.

2.56 Might has the right to be preserved or enhanced.
(See 1.113, 2.37, 2.55)

MIGHT is Existence socialized. It is an unorganized people habituated so as to carry the structure of the whole society, and in this way limit the expression of the classes. It presents us with the social group as a unity, obligated and able to relate both civil and unalienable rights to their respective duties. It may be expressed as force, or it may be expressed as pressure. In the one case it is exerted on and against others; in the other case, it implicates, affects without necessarily attending to or being directed at that which it affects.

It is neither indifferent nor good that there be no might, even if it never acts on behalf of the right of anything else. Might has a nature which instances the Good, and which therefore makes a legitimate claim to be and to be improved. And, since might is needed if there is to be satisfaction of man's civil and man's unalienable rights, might is not only good in itself but good for others.

2.57 The right of might can be alienated only by might.
(See 2.56)

THE RIGHT of might is the right to be itself, which is to say to exercise, to make itself manifest, to compel. To alienate its right is to prevent it from being itself. Such prevention requires the use of superior might. This superior might, whether or not it prevents the exercise of the inferior, has a right proportionate to its superior strength. The right of might is one with its very being.

2.58 The right of might can be justly alienated.
(See 2.40, 2.56, 2.57)

A RIGHT can be justly alienated in favor of some superior right. That superior right must in the end entrain the satisfaction of the alienated right, since that alienated right urged a claim on behalf of a good.

There are rights, however, which are superior to the right of might but which do not have the power to withstand the might. They are rights illegitimately denied, rights which have been made to give way to an inferior right. Because might has a right of its own, it never does only wrong; but because there are claims superior to its own made on behalf of more complete realizations of the Good, not every exercise of might is justifiable.

Since men have an unalienable right to benefit from social existence, they have a right which it is always wrong to deny. And since other groups have natures of their own, the right of might is faced with rights as proportionately well grounded as its own. These facts set a limit to the legitimate exercise of might.

2.59   Might has rights and duties in relation to men.
(*See 2.54, 2.55*)

MIGHT has a right over against men and over against other cases of might. The right it has over against them requires that they have a duty with respect to it.

In addition to his ethical, public, and service duties, every man has a *functional* duty to provide opportunity for the exercise of the might of his group. In addition to its group duty, every group has the *political* duty to allow room for the politically rightful exercise of the might of other groups.

The political duties of social groups towards one another are analogous to the public duties men have towards one another. In the absence of a world society they require a constraining force on the part of civilization or history if the duties are to be brought into relation with the corresponding rights. The functional duties of men on the other hand, are different in type from those thus far distinguished. Like the service duties, they are imposed by the social group on its own members. But service duties are duties on behalf of man's unalienable basic right, whereas the functional duties are duties on behalf of the right of the social group itself. Also, service duties are related to the corresponding unalienable right of men through the agency of the social group, whereas functional duties are related to the corresponding right of might by means of objectives which men pursue in common. A man's alienation of his specific rights is evidently to be performed not only on behalf of those rights, but for the performance of his functional duty towards the right of might when this has the form of a singular social whole.

2.60   It is the sovereign duty of might to help man achieve an eventual satisfaction of his alienated rights.
(*See 2.47, 2.48, 2.50, 2.59*)

MEN alienate their specific rights in order to be able to satisfy them more effectively. They present themselves in public as demanding satisfaction for a single unalienable right which they have constituted out of a plurality of alienable rights. But the justification for their alienating the specific rights is that these will be satisfied eventually. Since the basic unalienable right of man involves a corresponding group duty to be performed by the social group, the group, in satisfying the unalienable right of man, has to provide for the satisfaction of the specific rights of man as well.

Sovereign duty is the form which a group duty assumes when a social whole functions only as a locus of public energy, that is, as might. Might has a sovereign duty towards each man as possessed of a single unalienable right. That might ought to be so manifest that it satisfies the unalienable right of man. It can do this by providing him with occasions, lures, and obstacles, and by giving him the opportunity to use it so as to bring about results no individual by himself could attain.

The following table summarizes the main relations between rights and duties.

RIGHTS	DUTIES
I specific, native, alienable rights (*see 2.39–47*)	correlate with unspecified duties (*see 2.39*)
II privilege (governing I) (*see 2.43–48*)	not correlate with any duties
III unalienable unitary right (product of II) (*see 2.48–52, 2.54*)	correlate with a group duty (*see 2.54, 2.55*) and a sovereign duty (*see 2.60*)
IV civil rights (manifestation of I) (*see 2.54*)	correlate with public duties (*see 2.54*)
V mediated unitary right (*see 2.59*)	correlate with service duties (*see 2.54*)
VI right of might (*see 2.56–59*)	correlate with man's functional duties (*see 2.59*)
VII political right of group (manifestation of VI) (*see 2.59*)	correlate with political duties of other groups (*see 2.59*)
VIII no rights correlated with (*see 1.113, 2.54*)	ethical duties (*see 2.43, 2.54*)

2.61   Might must alienate its right.
(*See 2.48, 2.57, 2.58, 2.60*)

MIGHT is a fragment of the domain of Existence; men are distinct Actualities each embodying the Good in an intensive, distinctive, desirable way. Men have rights (I, III, IV, V) which are superior to the right of might (VI), and consequently have a duty (I, IV, V) towards men greater than that which they have towards might. If the might fulfills its sovereign duty (III) it brings about a greater good than it otherwise could. The right which might has as a singular socialized whole of energy, as the social group epitomized in the form of a single agency of compulsion (vi), ought then to give way before the need to perform its sovereign duty (iii) towards men. Its right (vi) is justly alienated when this serves to help it fulfill its duty (iii), providing of course that such fulfillment promotes the eventual satisfaction of that alienated right.

As a single undivided whole of energy, might is not fully appropriate to the individuals whose unalienable right (iii) it ought to help satisfy. Nor is it fully appropriate to the specific rights (i) which must eventually be satisfied. To be able to perform as it ought, might must alienate its right to be and to act as a singular whole (vi), and appear instead in the guise of a set of distinct powers, appropriate to the rights it ought to satisfy.

Man can alienate his right; might can alienate its right. Were man's right alienated from the outside, there would be injustice done; a similar injustice would occur if the right of might were alienated from without. A just alienation is always a self-alienation.

2.62 Might should be divided just so far as this promotes the satisfaction of man's rights.
(See 2.55, 2.61)

NOT every degree or kind of division of might is desirable. Only those are desirable which make possible not only the eventual satisfaction of might's own unitary right but the satisfaction of the unalienable right of men to profit from social existence, as well as the entailed eventual satisfaction of their specific rights. The warrant for the division of might into smaller units is that it thereby is enabled to fulfill its sovereign duty towards men while doing justice to itself. The divisions of might from its own standpoint are made in order that it might be more effective on behalf of its own sovereign duty (iii) and its own right (vi); from the standpoint of man the divisions of might are to be made so that man's rights (i, iii) can be better satisfied.

2.63 Each of the classes of a mature community satisfies part of man's unitary right.
(See 2.35, 2.48)

MAN'S UNITARY RIGHT is the right to profit from social existence. This profit has three dimensions: as part of a public world a man ought to know just what it is reasonable for him to expect, what it is possible for him to do, and what it is that he ought to do. The three classes of a mature community offer him reservoirs of such knowledge. They enable him to make use of the accumulated wisdom and experience of his group—not unmixed, of course, with folly and superstition—thereby enabling him to function better than he otherwise normally could, and in harmony with others. If a man cannot directly participate in all three classes, he ought, while functioning as part of one class, take the others to be representative of him. His unalienable unitary right will then be satisfied partly in a direct and partly in an indirect way.

2.64   The divisions of might should answer to the needs of three classes of men.
(See 2.35, 2.62, 2.63)

IN A MATURE community there are three classes in which men perform essential functions for all. The successful performance of these functions is necessary if the community is to provide a satisfaction for man's right to profit from social existence and if he is to achieve an eventual satisfaction for his specific native rights. Since the division of might is justified if it thereby most adequately satisfies man's rights, its divisions should attempt to answer to the three classes of men into which a mature community is divided.

The divisions of might that are appropriate to the classes of men are *social institutions*. These are limited domains of might, having their own modes of behavior. One institution has as its primary work the provision of effective opportunities for men; it attempts to answer to the requirements of the empowered class. A second has as its primary work the determination of what efforts men should make; it attempts to answer to the requirements of the reasonable class. And a third has as its primary work the determination of the status of men; it attempts to answer to the judgments of the prestigious class. Each of these institutions provides a structure for a part of the public might.

2.65   A political whole correlates self-divided might and the classes of a community.
(See 2.35, 2.64)

CLASSES and institutions are not always in gear. The one is primarily rooted in the habits of men, the other in the structure and interconnection of the things which men might use. So far as they function together, supporting one another, they constitute a *political whole*. This is an accidental product, but may develop a rhythm and career of its own. Since the degree of consonance between classes and institutions varies considerably in the course of history it becomes largely an arbitrary matter whether or not one should characterize a given community as a political whole, at this or that time.

2.66   A political whole has three essential organs.
(See 2.65)

THE CONJUNCTION of a single class and an institution constitutes a *political organ*, a structured area of might. This energizes and orders representative and essential functions performed by some of the members in the society. Three organs, at least, are desirable. To use modern terminology, a political whole ought to have executive, legislative, and judiciary organs embracing members of the prestigious, empowered, and reasonable classes.

Not every political whole distinguishes all three organs, and many have organs in addition to these. Nor will the members of a given class always fit inside one of these organs. In some modern states the executive seems to be a member of all three classes. On the other hand, there often are portions of these classes which are not provided with adequate institutional counterparts.

2.67   A state is a persistent political whole forcing classes and institutions into harmony.
(See 2.65, 2.66)

A POLITICAL WHOLE is an accidental product. It exists whenever there are political organs, i.e., classes matched by institutions. The habits and structures which it interrelates may affect one another to constitute stable organs with their own rationale, careers, and habits. When this occurs, the political whole achieves the status of a state, with distinct organs limiting the function and nature of the classes and institutions out of which those organs issued.

In its most embryonic form the different organs of a state function through habit and institutional routine, and in some independence of one another. As the state develops, its organs become more and more interlocked, at the same time that they are guided and controlled by some grasp of their own nature and purpose, and the dangers they face. At its best the organs of a state are subject to an overriding set of laws, implicit or explicit, limiting what those organs are to do to the institutions and classes which they encompass, and the men which those organs ought to serve.

IV   LAW

2.68   A man ought to acquire the habit of functioning as a man should.
(*See 1.106, 1.111, 1.113*)

ARISTOTLE, well aware that hell is paved with good intentions, that knowledge is overcome by incontinence, and that ideas of what ought to be done might remain ineffective so long as there was no adequate preparation to act, rightly rejected Plato's identification of knowledge and virtue. There seems little point today, however, in reviving Aristotle's distinction between the intellectual and moral virtues, or in reviving his account of moral virtue as a state of character having to do with the choice of a mean. All virtues are moral, though some relate to the use of the mind, and some concern themselves with the election of ends and the production of new goods. But what is at the root of his account, the doctrine of virtue as a habit of acting appropriately, would seem worth insisting on, as alone permitting the relating of an ethics of responsibility to a politics which is alert to the function of might, and to an education which acknowledges the need of discipline and purposive training.

Men are not born with virtues, Aristotle saw; they acquire them by performing desirable acts. Courage is not achieved through will or thought, but by doing courageous things here and now in the little, in preparation for their easier performance later, and for their possible performance in the large. Because virtue is a habit, it can be taught, and can be lost. Because it is a habit, its possession or absence in no way assures that the desired action will or will not be forthcoming at a given time. The courageous soldier may fail to, while the coward may show great heroism at some particular juncture.

Men ought to do good. The good they do without proper preparation is usually less than it can be. Habit enables them to push past
unnecessary and irrelevant details to concentrate on the central issue;
and the habit of virtue enables them to deal expeditiously with the
problem of bringing about a maximum amount of good in a given
situation.

So far as a man is one he has but one virtue, the virtue of being
good by doing good. So far as he has multiple channels for expression, habituatable in distinctive and independent essential ways,
he has a number of virtues. The latter, however, are under the aegis
of the former. It is best therefore to speak of man as having a single
virtue encompassing and controlling a number of subordinate but
essential ones. That single virtue is the habit of his self to use his
mind, body, and will, and whatever else there is available, so as to increase value as much as possible. It is no rigid set of interconnected
movements, no organization of incipient or actual acts subsumable
under a formula or controlled by a rule. It is the man himself, acting
creatively from within by persistently taking account of the structures, capacities, and needs of what lies without.

2.69   Men should be taught virtue and be forced to act virtuously.
(*See 1.118, 2.68*)

SINCE men are not born virtuous, they must acquire their virtue.
The acquisition is the outcome of the performance of acts which
promote the attainment of the Good. Such acts are sometimes performed by accident. But they are most effectively and persistently
performed when men are directed and controlled by trainers, coaches,
disciplinarian teachers in and outside the home. Moral training is in
fact one of the primary tasks of the family, and one of the main
accomplishments of organized sport.

Since no man has ever enough knowledge, since none has perfect
self-control or much control over others, none can be perfectly
virtuous. None has the habit of doing nothing but good everywhere.
But there are some things that ought to be done, not only in order
to acquire virtue but in order that good in fact be achieved. It is
socially wise to encourage selfishness on the one side and to threaten
on the other, ethically questionable though these acts be, for only in

these ways will men at times respect the rights of others, engage in disagreeable but socially necessary work, and attend to the welfare of the group as a whole. And since men ought to do good everywhere, outside as well as inside their own societies, men, if they are to be fully virtuous, must be trained in their societies to interest themselves in enterprises which lie beyond the particular interests of those societies. Only societies, which so train their members, are *civilized*, for to be civilized is to function on behalf of a greater good than that which a society can itself incorporate.

2.70   There is a natural law.
(*See 2.69*)

A LAW OF NATURE is a rational principle structuralizing the activities of space-time things. *Natural law* is a set of rational principles expressing the minimal demands of social justice, essential to the continuance of a civilized society.

Because laws of nature operate in bodies and are intelligible to one having no recourse to values, it is sometimes thought that they exclude the need to suppose that natural law is in nature. Instead of being granted objective status, natural law is therefore supposed to be a fiction, expressing at best the hope and at worse the prejudice of men. But limitation in scope or involvement in value do not compromise the objectivity and reality of any law. There are laws of gases and heat, laws relating only to water, and laws relating only to what is alive. The fact that these can be subsumed under, or interrelated to constitute more inclusive laws does not affect their status as genuine laws of nature. And these laws at times may be laws for the production of what is desirable; sun and rain and wind and soil promote the growth of things, some of which it is good to have flourish. Natural law is in fact a set of such laws of nature, so far as these are relevant to a society and are governed by a socially desirable end, or *social good*.

The social good is the Good made germane to men in society. It demands that all receive their due in harmony, that they be dealt with justly. It and the Good measure particular things and ocurrences, structures, activities, and facts. They make some to be preferred over others. It and the Good have a bearing on the laws of nature, making some one or more of them preferential in a situation—the social good turning the laws of nature into instances of a natural law, the Good turning them into instances of a moral law.

A law of nature expresses a hypothetical: "*if* justice is to prevail, this is to be done." Natural law instead says, "*since* justice is good to realize, this should be done." A law of nature and natural law ask for the very same acts, the one under a condition which may not be satisfied, the other as a consequence of a condition that never was unsatisfied. The one demands no action, has no normative role, and presupposes neither purpose nor value; the other demands an action, has a normative status, and presupposes purpose and value.

Natural law is worldly law; it is natural not supernatural. Natural law is a law of nature conditioned by an exterior social good; it is natural, not artificial. Natural law is public law; it is a law in nature, not apart from it in a private mind or will.

2.71   Natural law is germane to all societies.
(See 2.36, 2.70)

IN EVERY society men are subject to multiple pressures, forcing them to do all sorts of things. It is one of the tasks of sociologists to isolate these. Some of the pressures will serve to make men virtuous. These cannot be ascertained except by one who knows what virtue is, by one who knows what it is for men to do good habitually. This requires a knowledge beyond the power of the instruments of science to discover, not because the laws are not rooted in nature, but because the ends of the natural activities are not in nature, where "nature" is understood to be the domain of space-time occurrences and ends are recognized to be instances of a Good that ought to be but is not yet attained.

Since the same degree but different types of pressure may be exerted in different model societies to produce the same results in all, the same natural law can be expressed in different model societies in a number of different ways. Abstraction from these different expressions permits of the isolation of the universal natural law. That law enjoins the achievement of perpetual peace and human prosperity everywhere. It is fragmentarily and partially exhibited in every actual society and has diverse expressions in different model societies. That is why they can be contrasted and compared.

In actual societies different types of pressure are exerted. These pressures, as more or less effective in promoting virtue, fall into a hierarchy, carrying out, more or less adequately, more or less adequate exemplifications of the natural law. Different actual societies can therefore be said to express the intent of a universal natural law in various degrees, and are criticizable according to the degree they fall short of perfectly expressing it. Any one which did express the law perfectly would have the status of a model civilized society.

The social good makes some law of nature preferential in a situation, which is to say, it makes natural law effectively normative there. Natural law is the social good measuring the worth of the means available in a society for reaching the social good. It is the structure of time, infected by a good that ought to be and relevant to a real class of socialized men. It relates social beings in the present to what they ought to reach in the future, telling all to bring about universal justice justly, with the least loss of present value.

Natural law and moral law urge minimal demands rightfully made of any society. But whereas moral law pays attention to human will, has application to animals and things, insists on an obligation which no incapacity to meet can wipe away, and has application to men when by themselves and when engaged in nonpublic activities such as philosophizing, artistic creation, and religious worship, natural law keeps to the public arena, relating only to what socialized men need and to what they can and must do.

2.72   There ought to be a common law.
(See 2.70)

NATURAL LAW is a set of laws of nature, pertinent to a society, which, through the agency of a socially desirable end, demand activities that serve to bring about that end. Common law is a subdivision of such natural law, encompassing only those desirable activities which make a man virtuous in his own society, as over against, though of course not in necessary opposition to all other societies. This common or living law is only approximated by what goes by that name in Anglo-Saxon law. It supplements natural law, since it relates to what makes men act virtuously in such a way as to promote the continuance of their society. It is primarily concerned, however, not with the society but with the members of it, and relates only to those pressures which make a man act virtuously in that society, towards his fellow men and the goods which the society acknowledges. And in the societies in which men in fact live, societies which fall considerably short of model communities, there is need for common law. Without it men in extant societies would be subject only to that minimal pressure which enables a civilized society just to continue when what they need is to improve and prosper.

2.73 There ought to be positive laws, public declarations of what is to be done or avoided in a given society.
(*See 2.71, 2.72*)

LAW for the usual practicing lawyer and jurist is neither more nor less than positive law, a set of definite enactments by recognized authorities, publicly declaring what is to be done or avoided in a given society. Because natural law relates to present men and present societies, because it promotes an end not necessarily explicitly desired or known, and because it demands that actions follow a certain course, it is somewhat like positive law. In essence, though, it is quite distinct from positive law. There would be natural law even if there were no positive laws or if it were bad to have positive laws. Natural law is not even identical with the positive law as it ought to be. Knowing what natural law demands, however, one can judge which positive laws are good and which are bad, and the direction in which a change must be made.

If only positive laws are acknowledged there is, of course, nothing like good or bad law, right or wrong law. Whatever the authorities decree would be law, and that would be the end of the matter. As F. S. C. Northrop has so eloquently urged, positive law must be tested by living or common law, and living law must be tested by a universal natural law. If we give up the first test we neglect the witness which is provided by the conscience of decent men in a society; if we give up the second, we neglect the witness which is provided by the universal truths that are relevant to all men qua men. We must affirm with T. H. Green that "The only acts which the law ought to enjoin or forbid are those which the doing or not doing from whatever motive is necessary for the moral end of the society." Unfortunately, positive law instead of thus illustrating common and natural law, sometimes goes counter to these, and too often is indifferent to them. As a consequence men as well as classes and institutions are asked to do either what they ought not to do, or what they have no genuine need to do.

2.74 Positive laws threaten realizable punishments for violations.
(See 2.55, 2.69, 2.73)

POSITIVE LAWS are commands directly or indirectly expressed by a sovereign authority in a state. The commands may be tacit, coming into being through a process of legal decisions, or they may be explicitly pronounced or enacted by a ruler or legislative body. Did these not attach a penalty for a violation of what they command, their laws would be laws only in appearance. They would be indistinguishable from recommendations by a sovereign body; they would not express it as a constitutive and controlling power. Should there be an explicit statement of a penalty for the violation of what a positive law demands, which will, however, never be carried out, the law will be a law in promise only. There are then enactments which are only apparently positive laws, either because they are beyond the power of the state to enforce, or because they are not in fact enforced. The prohibition amendment in the United States was ineffective for the former reason; the income tax law in Italy today is ineffective for the latter reason. Neither is a genuine law. To be in force a law must be enforced.

Until he is apprehended, a man suspected or charged with violating a positive law exercises might in an independent way, neither defying nor accepting the law. Apprehended, on the presumption that he is violating a law, he is subject to trial and deserves a lawyer who raises the question as to whether or not his activity is in fact covered by law. The decision of the court rests on the opinion that there is or is not a law embracing those particular activities. If the court decides that the defendent is innocent, it is decided that he is one who has not defied the law but conformed to it; if it decides he is guilty he is treated as one who attempted to defy the law but in the end failed to do so.

The criminal does not define a law to be nonexistent, for he does not actually confront the might of the state. For a while he acts in areas which the state does not occupy, though it may make a claim to do so. Positive law or any other expression of might thus is never defied except by an actual counteracting might which in fact confronts that might. There can, until then, only be an attempt to evade its power, to define its scope, or to provide a contest in which one or the other might give way or be modified.

We seek to apprehend a man for a crime only because we know it is one by common or natural law. We do not know if it is a crime by positive law until there has been a conviction. Since every act can be said to raise a question as to what the scope of the enacted positive laws are, all positive laws are *post facto*. For positive law, the criminal is the man convicted. No conviction, no criminal, no crime.

Positive law is needed because common law and natural law are too general and vague. Every state requires for its prosperity the performance of multiple limited tasks appropriate to the time, the conditions, the needs peculiar to it. It must define multiple limited tasks and effectively demand that they be carried out. Those tasks are at once too narrow in range, too particular in character, too transitory in nature, and sometimes too novel or rare in occurrence to be encompassable by any set of common or natural laws.

In the ideal case positive law supports the common and natural law. Those positive laws which fail to do this are not needed, but are laws nevertheless. The common and natural law are always as they ought to be, but the positive law is only occasionally what it ought to be. Only it is enacted, brought into being by the deliberate decisions of authoritative men.

2.75 Positive laws are backed by might.
(*See 2.55, 2.74*)

A GENUINE positive law threatens a realizable penalty for its violation. Such a threat must have the backing of the might of the state, for otherwise it will be idle, an expression merely of what a legislative body would like to see done. The penalty attached to a violation of a positive law ought then not to demand for its enforcement more might than the state has, or than it is willing to apply.

Men tend to obey laws. Obedience is a habit gradually developed in the course of community existence. Some laws, unenforceable by the state, may be therefore obeyed by the citizens out of habit or out of loyalty. Strictly speaking, those laws are still ineffective positive laws, and thus really not positive laws at all. They are in fact only effective social conventions having the appearance of genuine positive laws.

2.76 Positive laws should be expressed in an official language.
(See 2.34, 2.73)

AN OFFICIAL language is the language of nobody, or of anybody, regardless of class. But the positive law is in good part an expression of the empowered class. If it is to be a law for all, or if it is at least to appear as a law for all, its bias with respect to any one class must be neutralized. Law requires a vocabulary and rhetoric of its own to enable the empowered class to express in neutral terms the requirements of the state for all citizens in all classes.

2.77 Positive laws should be impartial.
(See 2.73, 2.76)

THE OFFICIAL language of positive law permits of neutral expressions of what the state requires to be done or avoided. Such language could of course be used to formulate laws that favor particular individuals or interests. It would then serve to cloak rather than to overcome a bias. But positive laws should be laws for all, anonymously expressing impartial demands, conformity to which will benefit the whole. This does not mean that they may not actually be directed to some limited part, or that they may not be designed to promote the good of some part, even at a cost to others. It means only that, despite their limited reference, they must serve the good of all.

There should be laws on behalf of the indigent, the ill, the weaker. There should be laws taxing the richer and demanding special services from the younger and healthier. The welfare of disadvantaged groups either concerns or is involved in the welfare of others. But laws dealing with them tend to become forms of class legislation, serving to divide and injure, unless framed in terms of the rights and duties of all.

Some thinkers suppose that there can be nothing more than selfish, limited interests, and that the function of law is to balance an answer to one interest with a compensatory answer to others. The theory either goes too far, or does not go far enough. If there could be no common interests, there could be at most only individual ones. Laws would then have the task of assigning to designated individuals specific roles and work. This is both impractical and undesirable. Men come and go, and each is unique with desires and requirements too specific and private to be encompassed in public language. Also, the required public work can be performed by any one of a number of them, and ought therefore to be characterized and demanded without reference to this or that individual. And, on the other hand, the theory does not go far enough once it be recognized that the individual citizens do fall into various groups. If it be admitted that men have enough interest in common to constitute groups of some sort, there would seem to be no reason for refusing to extend the idea of common interests to encompass all the men in a state, or even in a larger whole. A farmer can share the interests of other farmers. For the same reason and in the same way he can have interests in common with all fathers, with all other citizens, and with all other men. It is the common interests of all the citizens that the positive law should impartially promote, even when it concentrates on the needs or duties of some restricted group inside the state.

2.78   Positive laws ought to define a man's civil rights and duties.

(*See 2.39, 2.51, 2.54*)

SINCE a positive law states what men are required to do or avoid in a state, it in effect defines the public duties of the men in that state. Each of those duties answers to a civil right of man, to what men are entitled in that state. These civil rights may be quite distinct in nature and requirement from the native rights which men alienated to constitute their unalienable unitary right to benefit from social existence.

The most satisfactory state is a just state. This is one in which civil rights either reformulate native, specific rights in official language, or it is one in which civil rights so articulate man's unalienable unitary right that it can be satisfied in that state. The first type of formulation is the primary concern of so-called bills of rights. These offer a public meaning to man's just and natural claims, and match them by prescribing appropriate civil duties. The second type should be the concern of the state as a unity having the sovereign duty to satisfy man's unalienable right. If the state is just and thus serves to promote man's right to benefit from social existence it will, through its positive laws, both grant and satisfy whatever civil rights the men need in order that their unalienable right be satisfied, with an eventual satisfaction of the specific rights out of which that right was constituted. It will, in short, make its positive laws promote man's unitary right to benefit from social existence in such a way as to conform to the demands of a bill of rights.

2.79 Positive laws require interpretation in relation to social power, social expectations, and social values.
(*See 2.32, 2.23, 2.34*)

POSITIVE LAWS are formulated by members of an empowered class. If these laws are to be more than injunctions arbitrarily laid down, they will at the same time express something of the expectations characteristic of a reasonable class. If they are to serve the primary purpose of the state, the promotion of the Good as attainable within that political whole, they will also express something of the values characteristic of a prestigious class.

Like all expressions, a positive law stands outside its sources. Unless it is brought into effective relation with the sources which expressed themselves in it, it is the state epitomized only in verbal form. Positive law must then not only be the product of an empowered class but must look to that class for further support. At different times different degrees of power must in fact be invoked to support a given law so as to keep the activities of men in consonance with the needs of the state as a whole.

Positive laws articulate the characteristic expectations of a given community. They ought to have their general terms and demands brought to bear in particular cases. To serve as guides for particular actions they must be made subject to interpretations by reasonable men; apart from these interpretations they can state only the larger connections between things.

Finally the positive laws must express the values characteristic of a state. They ought to have their meanings constantly reinterpreted so that they in effect support and promote those very values in a world where circumstances are constantly shifting. A refusal to impose new interpretations on old formulae will sometimes result in a failure to realize the objective which the law was originally designed to attain. If a man is not to be compelled to be a witness against himself in a criminal case, as the Fifth Amendment to the United

States Constitution affirms, and if the invoking of such a law entrains penalties in fact, so that it is in effect a witnessing of oneself against oneself, it will be desirable to preclude the need for a man to invoke that law. It is foolish to treat that amendment or any other in such a way that the values it would assure are denied rather than preserved.

2.80   Judges interpret the law in a threefold way.
(*See 2.79*)

A STATE can assign to different men, classes, or organs the task of interpreting positive laws. Some governmental officials may take as one of their primary tasks the interpretation of laws so that they answer to what is reasonably expected in a state, others may specialize in the interpretation of the degree of power that is to be invoked on behalf of positive laws, and still others may take as their province the interpretation of laws so that the values they are designed to promote are in fact promoted. These functions are rarely entirely separated; the very same men, classes, and organs may deal with more than one mode of interpretation. If there is to be little or no conflict between the use of power, the reasonable expectations and the objectives of a law, there ought to be an agency which evaluates the different interpretations. This agency is the judiciary.

A judge has at least three roles. He interprets laws in terms of values to be attained; he evaluates the publicly effective use of power; he estimates how reasonable others are. In effect this means that his interpretation of laws in terms of values dominates and serves to test the other interpretations. This would not be possible were the judge not an empowered officer whose expectations are models for the rest. Primarily a prestigious man, he is empowered by those in power and held by the stable elements of the community to be a perfectly reasonable man. In return he judges those who make him judge, and the standards they employ.

2.81   A wise, creative judge guides his interpretations by natural law.
(*See 2.71, 2.80*)

MEN live inside limited communities, and think about, care about, and work for but a limited fraction of all men. It is the function of the judge, as an agent of the state, to interpret the positive law in terms which make men promote the good of all within that state. But men in one state are not altogether alien to those in other states; all of them have the same perpetual peace and prosperity as their final objective. Or, what is almost the same thing, some of the values actually pursued and promoted in and by any one state are open to criticism. It too often fails to take account of what other states and men need and deserve, and therefore fails to provide room for the entire Good and even for that part to which it could give lodgement.

In every state the good of any man should be realized in each man. This is what the wise, creative judge knows. He sees beyond the formulations and visions of his own state to a universal objective, and interprets the positive laws in terms of it. At times this will force him to oppose the explicit intent of his own people on behalf of the intent of all men, and therefore on behalf of the implicit, not recognized intent of his own people.

Unlike the philosopher or reformer the judge does not urge an ideal value in abstraction from the concrete situation in and through which it is to be realized. The universal natural law serves him as a principle for interpreting positive laws. But he seeks to realize it through the mediation of positive laws which he has been empowered as a reasonable and prestigious man to interpret for the benefit of all.

2.82   In the ideal state citizens are law-abiding and law-controlled, and guided by the interpretations of wise, creative judges.
(*See 2.81*)

AN *ideal* state is a just state. It has laws, distinct classes, and wise, creative judges. Not necessarily world-wide, it may encompass only a fraction of mankind. But then it ought to have other ideal states as contemporaries, each with its own set of just positive laws. If those positive laws are interpreted by wise, creative judges, the men in those other ideal states will form distinctive political wholes, and yet be at peace with one another, primarily promoting the good of their fellow citizens while allowing for the good of others.

Judges, since they are the interpreters of all law, would seem not to be encompassed by any laws. But in fact there are laws which apply to them as well as to others, and to which they are subjected by the power and reason that prevails. Indeed it is even quite correct to say that judges are under the control of empowered and reasonable classes and whatever positive laws these promote, and that the judges' interpretations of those laws are confined and structured by the language of those laws and the reference which those laws have to limited situations and periods of time. They are consequently neither men of caprice nor men above the law.

2.83 The Good is most completely publicly fulfilled in a perfect state, a state where all are wise, creative judges.
(*See 2.27, 2.81, 2.82*)

AN IDEAL STATE is guided by creative judges. In the ideal case, the judges decree exactly what they ought to decree. But although the members of that state work in harmony, they are divided into a part which decides and another which responds. Most of the men in it merely accept what the judges decree. In a *perfect* state, in contrast, the creative decisions are made by any and every man, the official known as a judge serving merely to provide sanction and expression for what is done by all.

There is no completely perfect state; but also there is no state which is entirely ruled by positive law. Both a perfect state and a state ruled only by positive law are of course conceivable. But the one would have no well-defined organs, the other would have no place for decisions which, while going beyond the express statements of the positive law, in fact fulfill it. Since men live more or less in the light of the universal objective of perpetual peace and prosperity, and occasionally interpret positive laws in terms of it, all may, however, now be said to live in a partly perfect state.

V   BEYOND POLITICS

2.84 The Good in a state fails to encompass the ethical man.
(*See 2.26, 2.83*)

IN A PERFECT STATE men are virtuous and do good both to themselves and to others inside and outside that state. Justice, peace, and prosperity prevail. Our states only remotely approximate this goal.

But there is no inherent reason why that goal might not be reached eventually. If it were, it would still be the case that the entire Good would not yet be realized either in man or in other things. From the standpoint of the Ideal it is not enough for men to be virtuous in the sense of having the habit of doing what they ought. They must also have the will to do good.

Through his will a man becomes receptive of the Good, gives it lodgement in himself as a private being, before and apart from its exhibition in public and in a state. It is his will which enables a man to pledge himself on the inside to do what the state otherwise must compel him to do in that state. He ought also pledge himself, if he is to be good, to do other things which are outside the state's interests.

If a man uses his will to bring about what he ought, he is an ethical being functioning excellently. But whether he does make such use of his will or not, he has a wider range of concern than just bodily indurated habits would permit. Whether he does make use of his will or not, the Good is his responsibility to realize. Whether he does make use of his will or not, he is not wholly encompassed by the Good so far as this is exhibited only in a state, actual, ideal, or perfect. Whether he uses his will or not, he is an ethical being, an individual with an unavoidable responsibility to realize the Good both in and outside the state. He must be just and kind, useful and sympathetic.

2.85   The good in a state fails to encompass the aesthetic man.

(See 1.88, 2.84, 3.54)

A POLITICAL MAN, no matter how just, virtuous, and considerate, is in the end one who sees all things in terms of their use, and their power to serve a social end. He uses men, sometimes to their detriment, for the sake of benefiting them or others, and of course uses other things without necessary concern for their present or eventual benefit. If the Good does not find lodgement in a man who is aware of the Good in other beings, it will be fulfilled, even by one who is just, as a good which though directed towards the production of further good does not yet make a unity with other goods.

The aesthetic man is the appreciative man, sensitive to the nature of the Good that is partly hidden by convention and accidental accretions. His sensitivity can of course be characteristic of one who is not just. Such a man would be aware that there was good in other beings and would as a consequence give a greater place to the Good than one who was not so aware. But since he would not do anything on behalf of that Good or the goods he discerned, he would fall quite short of a virtuous or an ethical man. He would be roughly on the level of man of good intent who was content merely to desire and to hope. The Good, to be fully realized, must be ingredient in aesthetic men who are also virtuous men of good will, sensitive to the presence of good everywhere.

2.86 The good in a state fails to encompass the religious man.
(See *1.28, 2.84, 3.80, 4.96*)

THERE ARE secular religions and other-worldly religions. The former are primarily directed not towards God but towards the things of the world as worthy of withstanding the ravages of time. They may see things in the light of eternity, but then primarily only as having an import for man and the rest of the world. Religions of the latter type are instead primarily concerned with knowing, enjoying, fearing, or loving God, and only incidentally with the final fate which he metes out for men and other beings. Many theologically oriented discourses, though they seem to be carried on inside the latter type of religion are in fact but instances of the former.

Religion, in either case, is a private enterprise (though often carried out in public) in which men try to be one with the divine. No state, no matter how excellent, can wholly encompass one who has such an interest. The state may encourage him; it may support his institutions and endorse his practices. But in the end his and its interests diverge. Its primary concern is with the transitory; his is with the permanent as it is in itself or as having bearing on the Ideal and on mankind.

To be fully realized the Good must achieve ingredience in a virtuous man of good will who is not only sensitive to the presence of the good everywhere, but who isolates it, tears it away from time, and thus enjoys it in the form of a permanent, undivided being which the actual world can only partially and transitorily exhibit in a plurality of places and times.

2.87   The good in a state fails to encompass the speculative man.
(*See 1.92, 2.84*)

THE GOOD is the Ideal, an irreducible mode of being, dealt with from the perspective of Actualities. The speculative man cuts behind that Good to its presuppositions, tries to grasp it as an Ideal.

The Good, as exemplified even in a perfect idealized state, cannot encompass the speculative man, not only because speculation occurs in private but because he is concerned with the Ideal as that which is expressed only partly in the guise of the Good, and thus as that which can never be wholly satisfied even by being maximally realized throughout the entire range of Actuality. To be fully satisfied the Good must achieve ingredience in virtuous men of good will who are not only sensitive and religious but who can recognize that the Good (together with the Future and the Principle of Perfection, the guises which the Ideal assumes in relation to Existence and God) is a facet of the Ideal. Such a man will, when concerned with the Ideal, recognize it to be germane also to Existence and God. He will know that even a perfect stable universe, where Actualities are mutually appreciative and sustaining, leaves the Ideal still unsatisfied, and that he himself, to be the complete being he ought to be, must accommodate that whole Ideal, if only in the guise of an object of speculative thought.

2.88   Education is the art of reconstituting individuals so that the Good can be maximally achieved in and by them.
(*See 2.51, 2.69, 2.84–87*)

THE GOOD must encompass men as both public and private beings. Every community, on behalf of the Good which it itself instances, must train men for and in virtue, and lead them to deal with what lies outside the province of all habits, social and otherwise.

Born into a social group, a human being is not social to begin with; he must be socialized. The process of socialization never stops, and it can never succeed in encompassing the entire man. It is a process largely haphazard as a rule, a matter of unreflecting imitation, submission and conformity. Only when it becomes an art, which is to say when it does its work well, does it attain the status of an educative process.

Neither schools nor professional teachers are essential to education. The schools are desirable when they function as laboratories where the art of education can be practiced under ideal conditions, but there is education in the home long before the child is able to go to a school. The professional teachers are desirable when they are masters of the art—a role which usually requires that they be ideal beneficiaries of it as well—but there are effective and necessary teachers in the home and in the playground no less important or successful than the professionals.

2.89 Education should include discipline, the subordination of the individual to the group.
(See 2.72, 2.84, 2.88)

THE CHILD must be taught the manners, the customs, the language of his group. So far as he must be taught these he does not belong to the group; the teaching of them is the transformation of him from a not yet socialized into a socialized being. Or, what is the same thing, it is the taming of him, the making him conform to the patterns that prevail. The discipline can be severe and unrelenting without being unkind. Nor need it ever be wholly separated from other types of education. As the child grows, discipline tends to recede in the background. But it should never be entirely absent. Men always need to be brought inside the social whole, no matter how routine, conventional, and submissive they be; the whole has its own rhythms and changing needs to which men must be made to submit. Every one is in fact constantly guided, admonished, structured, transformed by word and gesture in a hundred subtle, hardly noticed ways, both in and out of school.

Disciplinary education is primarily moral in import and should be guided by the common law. Its object is to make men live in accord with those customs of act and thought which make for the promotion of the Good in that society. The work begun by parents and carried on in elementary schools is continued by coaches, fellow students and others in higher institutions of learning, as well as by the police and other governmental officials, and by those with whom one works and plays. And in the end it should produce the just man, a member of that largest of all groups, mankind.

Subjects such as reading, writing, and arithmetic have been traditionally supposed in our society to be choice media for promoting discipline. These subjects are of course taught for other reasons as well. But as is evident from the way they are taught, and when, they are for the most part conceived to be essentially disciplinary subjects. Yet the first gives only a partial discipline of the eye, the second of the hand, and the third of the memory or intelligence. An adequate curriculum includes other subjects as well, such as art appreciation, the use of tools, and the study of logic, which further discipline the eye, hand, and mind, as well as such subjects as music, gymnastics, and cooking, which help discipline other important organs.

2.90   Education should include training, the mastery of techniques.
(See 1.88, 2.73, 2.88)

IT IS one thing to be forced into society, and another thing to have a role to play within it. Training is needed to enable a man to fill an essential role in society, alongside and in concordance with other men filling other essential roles. Because vocational training has so often been assigned to those in economically or socially disfavored classes, and because it has been taught in almost complete abstraction from other phases of education, advocacy of vocational training has encountered opposition by the partisans of an exclusively liberal educational program. Their program in effect amounts to the vocational training of intellectuals, of teachers and college presidents, of discussion leaders and journalists, a fact obscured by the low degree of success their pupils have had. Both they and their opponents are agreed that vocational and liberal education are antithetical in procedure and objective. This need not be the case. Vocational education need not be narrow, directed towards the preparation of young men to perform menial, servile work in later life. It can concern itself with the mastery of tools needed in the home, the use of leisure time, the mastery of discourse, rhetoric, languages. It can provide men with essential equipment for expressing themselves aesthetically, for understanding the economics and politics of their community, for engaging in war, and for acting effectively in crises.

Training is primarily social or political in import; it should be guided by positive law. It ought to help place men effectively in the society in which they in fact live, and to perform the duties that the state requires of them, primarily in some special role and incidentally as a citizen of the whole. At the beginning it merges with discipline, coming to the fore as the child becomes a youth, and then receding into the background as time goes on. It is never completed, nor should it be. But we tend to ignore its presence and its need as men attain a certain degree of skill, or age, or earning capacity.

2.91 Education should include the art of civilizing, the acquisition of professional competence.
(See 2.69, 2.70, 2.85, 2.88)

WE HAVE been accustomed to think of professional education as the education of a favored few who, having had the benefit of a college or liberal education, go on to master such lucrative and socially desirable fields as medicine and law. But much of this so-called professional education is only vocational training, an education in techniques, favoring a special class of men. A broader profession, and one open to all, is citizenship. Every state needs such constitutive members, men who act inside it to promote the good of those within and those without. The acknowledged professions in fact deserve whatever dignity they have only because they are major ways in which the profession of citizenship is carried out.

When aesthetics is taken in its broadest sense so as to include the appreciation not only of what has been made with inanimate objects, but what men are, and what is and can be made of them, professional training can be viewed as a training in the appreciation of the Good, primarily as it is to be found in man and secondarily in other things. Such training usually begins in childhood, merging at that time with discipline and vocational training. It achieves distinctness as a rule only after men have been recognized to have been adequately disciplined and have had some degree of vocational training. Our professional schools as a matter of fact devote much of their first year to the disciplining of students in the language, and in the vocational training of them in the use of the tools of the profession.

Professional training can be made the object of a special curriculum. It should then be guided by an understanding of the nature and demands of natural law, and of how the reasonable man should exhibit it when performing some such essential role in society as doctor, lawyer, minister, teacher, artist.

2.92   Education should include a mastering of values.
(*See 2.71, 2.86, 2.88*)

WE HAVE, for the most part, been content to allow religious truths to be taught in an incidental way by the family and other social groups, or by those who have identified themselves with institutionalized religions. In the one case tradition has been allowed to hold sway when often it might better have been overcome, and in the other, exhortation has been allowed to serve as the vehicle for the communication of what required and deserved rigorous thought, fresh imagination, and an alertness to the nature of the universal Good. As a consequence the sense of importance has been dimmed and dulled. As a result men tend too often to think that only what is valuable in or to society is good, or that genuine values have no true residence in this world.

Religion involves a grasp of things in terms of their eternal meaning. Made part of a system of education, it serves to awaken and strengthen the sense of importance, the ability to appreciate and thus to master for oneself what is valuable.

It is fortunate that there is always, even at the very beginning, some teaching of values. But formal, deliberate teaching of religious truths by means of literature, history, art, comparative studies of society and morality are needed if one is to illuminate the meaning of the Good, particularly as germane to the crucial events in life: birth, marriage, sickness, and death, and to what has excited the spirit of man through the ages—heroism, adventure, great works, and great achievements. Only then will men, while in this world, most sensitively savor something of the meaning of eternity; only then will they, while in a society or state, live in terms larger than those which the society or state, even when perfect, could contain.

2.93   Education should teach men to engage in the creative, intellectual mastery of the total Good, social and nonsocial.
(*See 2.83, 2.87, 2.88*)

DISCIPLINE, vocational and professional training, and religious instruction are given to social men for the sake of making them deal with goods which are richer and more inclusive than those possible in their society or state. These different types of instruction should be interrelated, and should terminate in a man's free creative effort to deal most effectively with the Good. This is possible only if the Good is dealt with in the abstract while it is enjoyed and multiplied in the concrete.

The task of liberal education is to help make men just, effective, sensitive, and wise through the agency of ideas. But what is usually termed a liberal curriculum is largely a miscellaneous collection of courses, accreted without much plan over the years, and serving primarily to discipline, train, and perhaps ennoble in a rather minor key. Rarely does such a curriculum leave room or time for fresh creative effort on the part of men, so that they can give an adequate place within themselves for that Good which can be exhibited only partly in public work and public life.

A genuine liberal education begins with the first encouragement of the child to think independently, and for the sake of being excellent inwardly and outwardly. It continues throughout life, and should acquire its most articulate and formal expression in liberal institutions of higher learning. Here more attention needs to be paid to what promotes the state, and to what must be done to increase sensitivity. No one of these is the special province of some particular subject, or is to be mastered by some special method. All of them can be conveyed in the course of presenting almost any subject and in almost any manner. Perhaps it is almost enough for the young to share something of a mature man's passion to learn, to taste something of his joy, and to be inspired to imitate his honest and manful struggle with great ideas, his own or others. The hope of liberal education is that it will liberate men from education, allowing them to be and to make excellent men.

2.94　Liberal education should terminate in an understanding of the Ideal.
(*See 1.92, 2.15–19, 2.85–87, 2.88, 2.93*)

LIBERAL EDUCATION attempts to convey the full significance of the Good. Since the Good offers a partial specialization of the Ideal, which is at the same time specialized in collateral ways by Existence and God, an understanding of the Good requires a recognition of the fact that the Good does not exhaust the Ideal.

The Ideal, while most succinctly, most neutrally and clearly presented in a philosophic system, is more vividly encountered in art and secular religion. These begin with the Actual as subjugated by the Ideal, where this has been partly affected by Existence and God. They try to get to the point where they can deal with the pure Ideal, the Ideal freed from limitations imposed on it by transitory Actualities. When successful they discern what the Ideal is apart from Actuality, though not yet what it is in itself.

In the guise of the Good the Ideal can be known in a theory of ethics and politics; it can also be directly enjoyed and used by just men. In the guise of the Future (and thus in relation to Existence) it can be known in a theory of art and history; it can also be directly enjoyed and used by sensitive men. In the guise of the Principle of Perfection (and thus in relation to God) it can be known in a speculative theology and theory of religion; it can also be directly enjoyed and used by pious men. What the Ideal is in itself can be known only by means of dialectic; it can be enjoyed and used only by speculative men. A liberal education ought to lead one to the point where he can at once know, enjoy, and use the Ideal in all these ways. It will of course inevitably terminate in a knowledge, enjoyment, and use of the other modes of being as well, since the Ideal cannot be wholly understood without some reference to them.

VI   IDEALITY AND THE OTHER MODES

2.95   The Ideal provides testimony to the reality of Actualities.
(See 1.11, 1.21, 2.17)

IN 2.17 it was shown that the Good requires a plurality of opportunities, to be provided by Actualities, enabling it to achieve a needed determinateness. This thesis is the reciprocal of 1.11, where it was shown that Actualities presuppose possibilities which enable them to become and to continue. These theses do not get to, do not prove that there are Actualities or possibilities, respectively. They do not even point to evidence that there are such modes of being, distinct and irreducible; they serve only to point up what it would be desirable to prove, to indicate what must be recognized to be correlative with an acknowledged mode of being.

It is conceivable that there might be Actualities but no real Ideal. This would then be something like a Humean world where things could be or become without there first having to be a possibility for them to be or to become. All occurrences would then be surd, non-rational, inexplicable. On the other hand, it is conceivable that there might be an Ideal but no Actualities. This would then be something like a Plotinian world where an Ideal One was multiplied although there were no occasions for such multiplication. Plurality in such a case would be surd, nonrational, inexplicable. An understanding of either the Actual or the Ideal requires a reference to the other as pre-supposed. But that this which is presupposed is real cannot be shown without a proof which begins with one mode and terminates in the other through the aid of the remaining two modes.

Actualities provide testimony to the reality of the Ideal. Every Actuality sustains a meaning, a universal which in itself has a greater scope than that which the Actuality provides. Were there no meaning which the Actualities instanced, all classifications would be arbitrary. Because there are such meanings, not wholly reducible to the Actualities, Actualities offer testimony to the effect that there are meanings apart from them. Such testimony questions the truth of nominalism, but it does not go the length of providing the proof that the Ideal enjoys an independent status as a being on a footing with Actualities, since the Ideal could conceivably be the possession of some other mode of being. It could for example, as Augustine thought, be in the mind of God.

Similarly, the Ideal provides testimony to the reality of Actualities. Although in itself it is single and undivided, it is found to be diversified, localized in a number of independent places. It exhibits a relevance to competing and opposed entities—a fact which cannot be explained by attending only to it. Because the Ideal is involved with that which multiplies it, it offers testimony to the falsity of an epistemological monism. But such testimony does not go the length of providing a proof that Actuality is an independent mode of being on a footing with the Ideal, since it might conceivably be a subordinate part of some other mode of being. It could for example, as Descartes, Spinoza, and Schopenhauer thought, be an arbitrary delimited part of Existence.

2.96 The Ideal provides testimony that there is a real Existence.
(See 2.18, 3.07)

THE IDEAL is subject to adventures in this world which cannot be deduced or known in terms which it itself provides. Although in itself it is selfsame and formal, it is found to be transitory and material, involved in the affairs of a cosmos, functioning as its future. This is a consequence of the fact that Existence infects the Ideal, forces it into situations, and makes it followed by consequences which no reason could derive from it. This fact questions the truth of any formalistic view of the universe, but it does not go the length of proving that there is an independent domain of Existence, for the Existence it presupposes might conceivably be an element in some other mode of being. It could, for example, as Aristotle and Bowen thought, be an abstractive aspect of distinct individuals.

2.97 The Ideal provides testimony that there is a God.
(See 2.14, 2.19, 4.18)

THE IDEAL is normative; it measures the excellence of whatever else there be. It can and ought to be realized. But it may not be and need not be realized in the totality of Actualities or even in a cosmic Existence. These are always open to the judgment that they are not yet as good as they ought to be. If the Ideal is not to be an ought-to-be which in fact cannot-be, it must be realized by God, the only remaining mode, and who alone can be excellent always.

The Ideal prescribes what ought to be; at the same time it describes what is in fact, expressing the value which is realized to some extent by Actualities and Existence, and finally in God. This truth questions the claim of a naturalistic view of norms to the effect that the norms are necessarily satisfied in this world. But it does not go the length of proving that there is a God, for the divine and eternal might conceivably be an aspect of some other mode of being. God might, for example, as Nietzsche thought, be but a facet of Existence.

2.98 The Ideal partly satisfies the needs of Actuality.
(See 1.14, 2.17, 2.95)

ACTUALITIES and the Ideal make partial incursions into one another's domain. The Ideal turns Actualities into so many instances of itself; Actualities, reciprocally, turn the Ideal into so many different pertinent possibilities. The one has its limit in an exemplification of itself as a good in a man existing in an excellent world; the other has its limit in a Good, the objective of a good will.

Actualities and the Ideal also make use of one another. The Ideal, in the guise of the Good, is precisely what the Actualities endeavor to realize for their own sakes and for the sake of the Ideal. From its side the Ideal endeavors to do justice to itself and to Actualities by making the Actualities more and more intelligible. But the temporality and individuality of Actualities in the end defy the Ideal. Unless then Actuality is to be basically surd and unintelligible, what in it is not mastered by the Ideal must be mastered by Existence and God. Their own characteristic tasks with respect to Actuality are in turn burdened by what Ideality fails to do on behalf of Actuality.

2.99 The Ideal partly satisfies the needs of Existence.
(*See 2.18, 2.96, 3.13, 3.104*)

THE IDEAL provides Existence with a direction; could it permeate Existence it would make it teleological through and through, governed entirely by the Future it is to attain. Reciprocally, Existence provides the Ideal with a career in time; could it permeate the Ideal it would make that Ideal into the meaning of the entire temporal world. Each only partly intrudes on the other's domain.

Existence endeavors to realize the Ideal, in the guise of the Future, for its own sake and for the sake of the Ideal. Similarly, the Ideal endeavors to do justice to itself and Existence by making Existence more and more stable. In this effort it is defied by the restless movement of Existence. A full satisfaction of Existence requires that the efforts of the Ideal be supplemented by God and Actualities. These are concerned with Existence in their own ways, and what they fail to do for it becomes part of the burden of the Ideal, just as what it fails to do for Existence becomes part of their work.

2.100 The Ideal partly satisfies the needs of God.
(*See 2.19, 2.97, 4.85*)

THE IDEAL presents God with a purpose. Could it encroach entirely on him it would make him into an idealized being. Reciprocally, God presents the Ideal with a substantial inwardness. Could he encompass the entire Ideal he would make it simply the expression of divine intent. But each presupposes the other as that into which it cannot entirely intrude.

The Ideal in the guise of a Principle of Perfection is what God endeavors to realize in himself for his own sake and for the sake of that Ideal. Similarly, the Ideal, in the guise of value endeavors to do justice to itself and God by encompassing him, thereby making him valuable. The Ideal cannot do full justice to God's inwardness. But what the Ideal fails to provide can be provided by Actualities and Existence. Because the one is individual and diversified, and the other endlessly divisible and singular, they can together provide adequate scope for the expressible meaning of God's being. Each of these also has its own work in relation to God; their completion of the work the Ideal should do for God must occur inside the frame of their own characteristic functions in relation to him.

2.101   The Ideal provides Actualities with a desirable permanence.
(See 1.18, 2.98)

GOD could but does not wholly satisfy an Actuality's need to be permanent. He allows it to pass away, on the one side, and on the other, treats it as a datum for himself and then reorders and restructures it in terms of his own needs. Existence could but does not vitalize an Actuality permanently; it passes on, leaving a desiccated Actuality to constitute the factuality of the past. The Ideal inevitably completes the work of both; it turns each Actuality into an instance of itself, thereby permanently preserving it in the form of a delimited subordinated version of itself.

2.102   The Ideal provides Existence with a desirable intelligibility.
(See 2.99)

ACTUALITIES could but do not wholly satisfy Existence's need to be intelligible. Insufficiently occupied with what is cosmic in reach and endless in time, they provide it with only momentary limits. God could but does not wholly unify Existence. Insufficiently occupied with the flux of the world, he stops short with a limiting of the endless self-divisiveness of Existence. The Ideal inevitably completes the work they leave over. It provides Existence with a meaning which is unified but yet capable of being divided at any point.

2.103 The Ideal provides God with a desirable relevance to what else there be.
(*See 2.100*)

EXISTENCE could but does not wholly make God have a spatio-temporal cosmic significance. It destroys when it produces, rejects when it accepts the presence of God. Actualities could but do not give God the full individual embodiment which his nature deserves. He is resisted by them; they oppose his presence to some extent throughout their careers. The primary task of the Ideal is to subsume God under a Principle of Perfection. It succeeds to some degree and thereby provides him with a relevance, and completes the work left over by Existence and Actualities. God by himself of course has a kind of relevance to the other modes. What the Ideal does is to make him effectively relevant, thereby making it possible for them to benefit maximally from his presence.

2.104 The Ideal while guaranteeing the satisfaction of some needs of the other modes fails to do full justice to any mode.
(*See 2.22, 2.101–3*)

FOR PLATO the Ideal needs no realization; it gains nothing from any act, its own or another's. For Kant, Hegel, and Dewey, the Ideal does need and does receive satisfaction. For all of them it needs completion. Kant guaranteed the completion by "postulating" a concerned God who added what was missing. Hegel guaranteed it by supposing that the Ideal progressively and exhaustively articulates itself. Dewey seemed to have held that the Ideal inevitably spends itself over the course of time, so that if time could come to an end the Ideal would be satisfied wholly, without residuum—time for him made the Ideal really be. It has here been maintained, in opposition to Dewey, that there is always a residuum which no action in time could ever exhaust. But in opposition to Kant it has also been maintained that the satisfaction of the Ideal is guaranteed in the very nature of the case. And in opposition to both Plato and Hegel it has also been maintained that the satisfaction is provided by something itself not

Ideal. The satisfaction of the Ideal is not adventitious, having nothing to do with the nature of the Ideal; nor is it one which might conceivably not have been provided. It is an inevitable outcome of the fact that there are three other modes of being with which the Ideal is interlocked, and which together with it exhaust all there is and can be.

The residuum that man's inadequate activities leave over unsatisfied in the Ideal is realized in God and Existence. In the dimension in which the Ideal makes its demand of man the Ideal is not completed; but there is a completion which the very being of the other modes guarantees. Conversely, while providing Actualities with a needed permanence, the Ideal fails to do justice to their need to be intelligible while remaining individuals. This failure is made good by Existence and God, at the same time that they partly fulfill their characteristic tasks with respect to the Ideal. And while providing Existence with a needed direction, the Ideal fails to do justice to Existence's need to have a stable, effective meaning. This failure is made good by Actualities and God at the same time that they partly fulfill their characteristic tasks with respect to the Ideal. Finally, while providing God with an effective relevance, the Ideal fails to do justice to his need to have the status of a being of supreme value. This failure is made good by Existence and Actualities at the same time that they partly fulfill their own characteristic tasks with respect to God.

Each mode has work to do on behalf of the others. Each fails to do all it should, and therefore fails to satisfy itself, and fails to do adequate justice to the others. But what each fails to do is partly made up by one of the other modes, and is finally made up by the remaining mode. Each mode of being thus guarantees that the failures of the other modes with respect to some second are not final. Consequently every Actuality will be preserved (as a kind of being by the Ideal, as an Other by God, and in its effects by Existence); the Ideal will be wholly realized (as a measure by God, as a purpose by Existence, and as possible Good by Actuality); all Existence will be stabilized (as a plurality of regions by Actualities, as a divisible unitary meaning by the Ideal, and as an endless repetition of the selfsame by God); all of God will be made effective (as a cosmic essence by Existence, as a unity of meaning and being by each Actuality, and as the unity of all value by the Ideal).

CHAPTER 3

Existence

I   THE NATURE OF EXISTENCE

3.01   Existence is being, as engaged in the activity of self-division.
(*See 1.12, 2.96*)

EXISTENCE is one of four modes of being, with a nature apparently quite close to what Plato referred to as the Receptacle, the Aristotelians as Prime Matter, classical physicists as Ether, Schopenhauer as Will, Bergson as the *élan vital,* Whitehead as Creativity, and Northrop as the Undifferentiated Continuum. An irreducible mode of being, Existence is sheer vitality, forever passing from one position or guise into another. By encapsulating a portion of Existence within the confines of its own nature, each entity is enabled to stand away from all others at the same time that it is caught inside a wider realm of Existence, where it is kept at a distance from others.

Those who assume that either essences or individual things provide the only means by which anything can be significantly apprehended, inevitably find that Existence is unintelligible, a surd. But then it is a mystery how even this much could be known about Existence. Those, on the other hand, who contend that God is the source of all there be, deprive the rest of the world of its Existence, or suppose that Existence is possessed only on sufferance, with the consequence that nothing other than God can be said really to exist on its own.

To exist is to stand out or away from; it is to be engaged in an act of opposition which is self-opposing. Existence is opposed even to its own unifying essence. Since it nevertheless continues to have an essence, Existence is in a perpetual inward tension, at once holding on to and distinguishing itself from its own essential nature. By holding on to that essence, it is able to maintain a moment of eternity within itself; by separating itself off from that essence it is able to attain a purity of being over against every other mode. In a similar way Existence holds on to and separates itself from an ingredient meaning to make itself at once a sheer energizing and an active reaching to a future. Similarly, it both holds on to and separates itself from Actualities to become a matrix of relations between them as well as a dynamic field for them.

3.02 Existence perpetually divides.
(*See 3.01*)

AS A BASIC MODE of being, Existence has within it sheer Existence, and its own unitary essence, its own meaning, and its own actual divisions. Self-opposing, it is in a perpetual state of separating itself off as sheer Existence while continuing to hold on to its own nature, meaning, and actual divisions.

Existence, as tensionally relating sheer Existence and essence, constitutes a cosmos of energy, the cosmic aspect being provided by the unity and the energy aspect by sheer Existence. The sheer Existence or energy, as over against the essence, is divided endlessly into parts which, as alongside one another, constitute a primordial extensionality. This Whitehead has brilliantly acknowledged and characterized in his *Process and Reality*. It is also partly formulated in the doctrine of world-lines in relativity theory on the one side and quantum mechanics on the other, the one stressing the expanded nature of energy, the other its units in this epoch.

Existence embraces sheer Existence and meaning in a tensional relation, constituting a whole of time. The sheer Existence as standing over against the meaning is a duration which persistently divides the future into succeeding presents, extensionally related to what had been and what will be. Schopenhauer and Bergson have made us all acutely aware of the vital power of this duration. They neglected to note, however, that the Ideal stands over against it and gives it direction.

Existence as embracing sheer Existence and Actualities in a tensional relation constitutes a cosmic contemporary world. The sheer Existence, as over against the Actualities, is a field or region of environing space. This space does not have—nor does cosmic energy or duration—an infinite number of smaller parts in it. Nevertheless it can be endlessly divided, and anywhere. The dividing of energy, duration, or space requires no mathematician; it is the effect of sheer Existence as it separates itself off from other sides of itself, sides where it is affected by the other modes.

If we could intellectually make endless subdivisions in space—or in cosmic energy or the whole of time—and could hold on to the results, placing them alongside one another, we would have an infinitude of small regions, thereby producing an endlessly expanded region. Zeno was right then to remark that the endlessly divisible nature of space is the ground for its endlessly expansive nature. But it is to be noted that when we intellectually divide space we place alongside one another not divided parts of space but distinct acts of ours which we then relate to distinguished parts of space. We thereby exhibit the extensionality of space as an extended sequence in time, in which one isolated finite part of space after another is made to be present. And we act analogously when we intellectually divide cosmic energy and the whole of time.

3.03   The endless expansion of energy, towards which Existence tends, is restrained by Actuality, Ideality, and God.
(*See 1.27, 2.20, 3.02, 4.91*)

THIS is an expanding universe. Were Existence to be entirely sundered from the other modes of being, it would divide itself endlessly, make every part of itself, without end, stand over against every other part. But Existence can never be entirely sundered from the other modes. They restrain its tendency towards self-division, making that division stop at some finite length, thereby dictating a limit to the extent to which the universe can expand.

The primary restraint imposed on energy is that provided by the eternal essence of Existence. This, by limiting the size of the units into which energy can be subdivided, dictates not only how large the universe can be but how that size is to be measured. The Ideal and

Actuality contribute to this result, the one dictating the manner in which the energy is to be employed, thereby grounding causal processes, and the other determining just where the energy will terminate, thereby dictating the area in which the energy will be expended.

The eternal essence, the Ideal meaning, and the terminating Actualities, on their side, by virtue of the Existence within them, also tend to separate themselves off from Existence. This effort at separation, with a consequent retention of their confined Existences, is restrained by Existence itself. This limits the rate at which they can separate off from it. Could any one hold itself off from Existence entirely, it would be subject to peculiar laws; as it is all are subject to the very laws which govern the rest of Existence, though of course subject to qualifications which their partial separations require.

The laws of nature provide a restraining measure for the behavior of withdrawn existing items. As governing meaning they dictate the rational distance to consequences that will occur, and thus the date when they will come to fruition. As governing the essence they dictate the scope of a genuine unifying rationale, uniting every part of the universe. And as governing actual termini they dictate the degree to which individuals must conform to the pattern characteristic of Existence, so as to continue to be part of one universe.

3.04   The endless expansion of time towards which Existence tends is restrained by Actuality, Ideality, and God.

(See 3.03, 3.103–5)

THE IDEAL in the guise of the Future restrains Existence in the guise of duration. By limiting the size of the temporal units into which Existence can be subdivided, it dictates not only how long time will be, but how it can be measured. Time comes in drops because of what the Future does to the duration of Existence. The acknowledgment of this fact makes it possible to explain how it is that there can be an extensive time. It also allows one to resolve the paradox of Achilles and the Tortoise. In each drop of time the faster and the slower occupy positions which overlap comparatively less and more of the previously occupied positions.

The eternal essence and the terminating Actualities contribute to the restraint of Existence in its temporal guise. The one dictates that, despite the perpetual passing of momentary nows, there will be but one single time, and thus only one temporal totality of energy, a "conservation" of it. The other dictates that there will be a plurality of beings, atomically temporalized.

The Existence within Actualities, Ideality, and God tends to make them separate themselves off from Existence. This effort at separation is restrained by Existence itself. The Actualities are thereby forced to become contemporaneous, the Ideal is forced to become extended, and God is forced to assume the role of a relevant organizing form, a "world-soul."

3.05 The endless expansion of space towards which Existence tends is restrained by Actuality, Ideality, and God.

(*See 1.09, 3.03, 3.04, 3.103–5*)

EACH Actuality brings an end to an unbroken continuum of a spatial field or public extended Existence. The smallest Actuality, as a unitary single bit of extendedness, defines the magnitude of the smallest bit of space that is in fact being distinguished. Actualities thus not only dictate just where public Existence will terminate but provide the unit by which that Existence can be measured. The eternal essence and the Ideality with which Existence is also in a tensional relation contribute to the division of spatial existence into units which measure the whole of it: the essence determines the limits of the whole of spatial existence, putting a border, as it were, around the totality of Actualities which severally terminate the spatial existence, while the Ideal defines a common character for that space, thereby enabling the Actualities, all of which exist in the space, to be characterized in similar terms.

The Existence that is within the Actualities, Ideal, and God tends to make them separate themselves off from the rest of Existence. This effort at separation is restrained by Existence itself. Were it not for that fact, Actualities, the Ideal, and God would have contours and dimensions altogether peculiar to them, requiring the use of quite independent geometries for their understanding. Because they cannot free themselves entirely from the whole of Existence, each can provide only a distortion, a kind of curvature of a common

Existence. The space of Actualities is the common space intensified to conform to the demands of finite substances; the 'space' of the Ideal is an arabesque connecting the various delimited parts of it; the space in God is cosmic and undivided, and subtended by an indivisible unity.

3.06   Existence as separated from Actualities is their spatial field.
(See 1.09, 1.12, 3.05)

AS CAUGHT inside Actualities, Existence is distorted by each, made to have a structure of a peculiar sort. This is true even of the lowest grade of things, as is evident from the still-life paintings of Cezanne, which report so splendidly the nature of the space internal to even artificial apples. And as modern relativity physics recognizes, the more the mass the greater the deviation from the pattern of Euclidean geometry. The Euclidean pattern prevails only where the influence of objects in the world is at a minimum. Near objects space is a thing of bumps and turns; further away it flattens out, finally achieving, if the astronomers are right, a Euclidean guise at the regions where there is a minimal mass.

It is a little strange perhaps to speak of Existence as existing. This is due in part to the fact that it is not customary to view Existence as an irreducible mode of being. The strangeness is dissipated if the outcome of Existence, the spatial field, be dealt with as representing the whole of it. We can, then, while speaking with common sense of the spatial field as existing in separation from Actualities, refer to Existence as it exists apart from those Actualities.

Existence is in Actualities, though of course there delimited, constrained, quantified. Because Existence is both in and around Actualities, the Actualities and space are not altogether discontinuous in properties and not at all discontinuous in being from one another.

3.07   Existence as separated from the Ideal is its causal ground.
(See 1.39, 2.99, 3.04)

THE IDEAL in relation to Existence has the guise of a single cosmic Future which is diversely specified and realized by the various objects in Existence. Because of that Future they are enabled to keep apace with one another, despite their diversity in internal rhythm and their independent status as individuals or unified combinations of individuals.

The Ideal in itself is not caused; but the Ideal is caused to have the status of the Future by virtue of the difference which Existence makes to it. Existence stains the white radiance of Ideality by making it into a cosmic Future, which, because Existence is exterior to Actualities, must be exterior to those Actualities as well. The Future is a perpetual effect of the causal power of Existence, converting an otherwise irrelevant (or relative to nature, indeterminate) Ideal into a relevant prospect, thereby providing limits to what nature can become.

On its side, the Ideal has Existence within it, enabling it to stand self-enclosed, withdrawn from the rest of Existence, as that which can never have its being exhausted in its role as Future. One could speak of it as interiorizing the futurity of Existence, just as one might speak of the present being of Existence as the making of a genuine abstract Future into a vital Now. But remaining with the being of Existence, it is proper to say that it is given an intelligible directionality by the Ideal and in turn gives the Ideal a natural career. As a result there is a continuity in the properties and the being of the consequent intelligibilized Existence and the temporalized Ideal.

3.08   Existence as separated from God is his cosmic vitality.

(*See 3.05, 3.105, 4.86*)

According to Thomas Aquinas, each being has an Existence proportionate to the excellence of its essence. According to him, while God's essence *is* his existence, all other beings only *have* their existences, and then only because and while God bestows it on them. The hard question for the Thomist is then whether or not I, with my peculiar fragment of existence, do not in fact stand over against God with his Existence. The Thomists sometimes speak as though they meant to hold that all Existence is God, in him or from him. But it is not clear then how I can exist. In any case it is hard to see how a plurality of places, moments, energies, and beings can be or have their source in an individual eternal unity which is, according to their doctrine, always the same.

If I have my own Existence I stand over against God and his Existence. If I do not stand over against God and his Existence, in what sense can I be said to exist at all? How could I defy God or adore him, blaspheme or worship, accept or reject him, act either as a man in time or as one marked by or for eternity? What could be meant by incarnation if there were no separate domain of Existence over against God in which he could assume a place?

Whether or not Existence has been given to them, whether or not they continue to hold on to it as their very own or have it as a kind of accretion, the fact remains that all Actualities have an Existence over against God. That is why they can move around, act, do things in a way God cannot. But there is also an Existence outside those Actualities, the Ideal, and God. Existence is more than any or all of these other modes can encompass. Divided by these it is not exhausted by them.

God has Existence within him. Existence enables him to withdraw, to hold himself apart from other modes of Being. He eternalizes Existence and it in turn persistently repossesses him as the unity which it needs in order to be at all. There is consequently a continuity in the properties and being of the eternalized Existence, Existence as in God, and existentialized divinity, God as in Existence. As over against God, Existence is a cosmic turbulence, to participate in which is for him to achieve a status as a vital being in this spatiotemporal universe.

3.09 From the perspective of Actualities, Existence is that which makes them contemporaries.
(See *1.27, 3.06*)

THOSE who take up the standpoint of Actualities, as nominalists, personalists, and existentialists do, constantly find themselves coming up against the fact of Existence as that which for them 'mysteriously' operates in and through these Actualities. They find Actualities to have a degree of determination, a power of action, and relations to one another that cannot be accounted for in terms of these Actualities; they are therefore driven to look at the Actualities as playthings of an irrational fortune, an unfathomable history, an unknowable God, or some blind purpose. Acknowledgment of Existence is needed if we are to understand vital functions and features of Actualities.

As over against Actualities, Existence is a cosmic space. But from the standpoint of Actualities, it is the power which enables them to be contemporaries. Existence is never wholly caught inside any Actuality; it sweeps along outside them while holding on to them, catching up the Actualities to make them move together into the future under the aegis of cosmic laws. It relates them all to a single constraining future which they concordantly but diversely qualify, and which enables them, despite their independent inward rates, to act concordantly. It does not completely control those Actualities; they constrain and recondition Existence when and as it controls them.

3.10 From the perspective of the Ideal, Existence is that which adds implications to those derivable from what is merely possible.
(*See 2.96, 3.07*)

HEGEL, in his logics, treated Existence as a category like any other; it was for him part of a single totality of categories or ideas through which the Spirit goes in the course of its relentless movement from mere being to the absolute idea. Kierkegaard, an Hegelian of the right, like Marx, an Hegelian of the left, found this view of Existence intolerable. Existence, for both of them, was more than any idea or category or essence ever could be. Assuming with Hegel that he had written *the* Logic and *the* Philosophy, they had no other alternative but to abandon both logic and philosophy and try some other way of getting to Existence, as that which is forever and utterly beyond all understanding. They became activists, the one rushing headlong to his God, the other throwing himself into the violent currents of history. (Their Hegel is of course in good part a caricature. In his *Phenomenology of Mind* and his *Philosophy of History* Hegel unmistakably underscores the presence of a vital dynamic, even temporal dimension to reality, though, to be sure, he holds that in the end this dimension is derived from Reason or Spirit and has no genuine independent status.)

There is nothing irrational in the fact that this table is next to a chair. But no one who knows the nature of a table and a chair can deduce the fact that they are next to one another now. It is precisely because and so far as this fact is beyond such deducing that we are justified in saying that they exist. One can of course have an idea of a table next to a chair, and draw consequences from this. But draw whatever consequences we like, we will never encompass all that happens to the table and the chair, for these have careers which are in part dictated by what is not themselves, to wit Existence.

Existence stands over against the Ideal, the possible, the logical, the meaningful, as a causal, productive, energizing power. But from the perspective of the Ideal it is a perpetual source of consequences not deducible from the Ideal, or from any illustrations of it. That Existence does not go counter to a logic; it works out its career from moment to moment, within the limits of logical and other laws and subject to the controls of other modes of being, but with a freedom which precludes any derivation in advance of what it in fact produces. Logic is the art of drawing necessary conclusions from meanings or divisions of the Ideal, and anyone who takes up the standpoint of logic is therefore faced with outcomes for which that logic cannot provide. This does not mean that Existence is irrational or unknowable, but only that its rationale is not the rationale of any other mode of being.

To such an account as this there are two favored alternatives. An idealist, such as Brand Blanshard, holds that there are no nonlogical implications stemming from the table and chair. We think there are such implications, he holds, because our ideas of the table and chair are inadequate, partial, unclear. An adequate idea of them would take account of all their relations, and from that adequate idea all that will ever happen to the table and the chair will follow rationally. But such a theory begs a question. The totality of all the relations in which the table and chair are involved includes relations which are grounded in Existence. 'A table' and 'a chair' as such have fewer relations to one another than do 'this table' and 'this chair'; to transfer to the ideas of 'a table' and 'a chair' the additional relations which 'this table' and 'this chair' add to those ideas is but to add to the idea of 'a table' and 'a chair' the idea of Existence. And even if we passed over this point and started with an idea of a table and chair together, and then added to this the idea of all their existing relations, what will in fact occur will be only partially derivable from the resultant complex idea. There is nothing in the idea which *produces* a consequence, nothing in it which compels one to wait for a slab of time to pass before the consequence occurs, and nothing in it which can move or change. There is

more to Existence than is contained in any idea either of it or of anything else.

A more popular alternative is the Kantian view that we can deduce
all the consequences of this table and this chair as next to one another if we take account of the laws of nature as well as of the laws
of logic. This answer also begs a question, for if the laws of nature
yield consequences not taken care of by the laws of logic, they are
but laws of Existence. And even if we grant the point, it still will be
true that no law yields the individual case, and that no law divides
time into finite, extended periods on whose elapse we must wait before the consequences ensue.

The illustration of a table and a chair next to one another is but a
device for enabling us to focus on the fact that Existence has implications beyond those sustained by the Ideal. Strictly speaking reference should be made to the fact that Actuality and God also have
implications beyond those which the Ideal grounds. Actualities, because they have some Existence in them, have careers which no Ideal
can fully encompass. To be an Actuality is in part to go one's own
way, a way which is not fully explicable by means of concepts pertinent to another mode of being. The same thing must be said of God.
There is Existence in him, and because there is, his activities in fact
transcend any idea of him, no matter how complete it be. In addition
both of them produce consequences by virtue of the being they have
apart from Existence—and of course from one another and the Ideal.

3.11   From the perspective of God, Existence is the power to make something become, by making others pass away, and conversely.
(*See 3.08*)

THIS WORLD is a domain of individuals, transient occurrences, and
finite values. Thomas Aquinas held that God knows these. But just
how this is possible is obscurely explained by one who is usually quite
clear. Still the point should be granted, though not in such a way as
to hide the fact that there is something other than himself for God to
know. This other is evidently outside his being and his necessities.
Indeed it often behaves in regrettable ways. What is outside him are
Actualities, Existence, and the Ideal itself, all of which have functions,
rhythms, powers, natures, and implications of their own.

Existence was long ago recognized by Plato to have its own "anankay," or necessity, over against the necessities of the Ideal, and apparently also of God and of Actualities. And he saw too that the passage of time, the giving way of one moment to another, the coming to be of the present occurs outside God, and is not derivable from him, the eternal being. From the perspective of God's eternal unity, Existence by itself is dynamic power whose self-division is expressed as sheer creativity or becoming.

3.12 From the perspective of Existence, Actualities are focal points, the Ideal is future and God is essence.
(See 3.06, 3.07, 3.08)

EXISTENCE has its limits given by the other modes. It is, as it were, terminated by them from the outside, sideways by Actualities, frontwards by the Ideal and from above by God. From the perspective of Existence, they bound it, and are to that extent alien to it, outside its control. But it can satisfy their needs in part. What it fails to do on behalf of each devolves on the remaining two. The failure of Existence to remain inside Actualities and thereby give them a permanence in time, makes it necessary for God to deal with them as his others in the whole of time, and for the Ideal to deal with them as occasions permanently evaluated or measured. The failure of Existence to satisfy God's need to be involved in the universe imposes on Actuality the need to accommodate him, and on the Ideal the need to incorporate his intent. Finally, the failure of Existence to satisfy the Ideal's need to be realized as the Future leaves over for Actuality the task of making that Ideal, in the guise of the Good, have cosmic relevance, and for God the task of making it, in the guise of a Principle of Perfection, express a divine will.

3.13 The failure of Actuality, Ideality, and God to do full justice to one another imposes a burden on Existence.
(See 1.14, 2.20, 2.98, 2.99, 2.104)

THE IDEAL's and God's failure to do full justice to the needs of Actualities means that Existence must not only make Actualities present, but must endow them with some meaning and some permanence in the guise of effects in time. And since both the Ideal and Actualities fail to do justice to the need of God to be relevant to the world, Existence must, in addition to giving him a cosmic field of operation, actually involve him in nature. And finally, since both Actualities and God fail to do justice to the Ideal's need to be realized, Existence must face a future which is at once providential and normative.

3.14   Existence is unified by the other three modes.
(See 2.21, 3.09–11, 3.13)

EVERY MODE of being is involved with every other. Existence exists in all of them, though to be sure as subject to the conditions which they impose on it. There is some Existence in every one, forcing it to withdraw from the rest and to expand, free from their control. Conversely, there is an element of every being in Existence, forcing Existence to withdraw to itself and thereby expand into a cosmic continuum. All of the modes exist in Existence, where they therefore have over against themselves, themselves as distinct irreducible modes of being. And Existence controls them so far as they exist in it, holding on to them while withdrawing from them.

As outside the other modes of being, Existence vitalizes, produces consequences, and is in process. It needs a unity, a nature of its own. Actualities give it one kind of unity by providing it with spatial limits; the Ideal gives it another kind, in the form of an intelligible purpose, and God gives it a third kind, an essence. Together they provide the unity which it needs, but only because the failure of one to do what it ought is inevitably satisfied by the others. God does not altogether succeed in giving Existence an appropriate integrated essence, for he does not occupy himself sufficiently with Existence. But God does provide a permanent boundary for Existence, thereby making up a deficiency of Actualities and the Ideal towards Existence, so as to enable the vitality of Existence to be confined and thereby made into a single permanent though internally restless whole. Actualities do not offer Existence the termini it requires; they are too few and too puny. But Actualities do provide the remainder of the avenues for the expression of Existence which the Ideal and God failed to provide, thereby enabling the productivity of Existence to be properly canalized. And finally, the Ideal does not altogether provide Existence with its needed direction, since it is not entirely keyed to the course of Existence. But the Ideal does provide a meaning for Existence which God and Actualities failed to provide, thereby bringing the process to a kind of closure, as a single completed domain which is divisible anywhere.

II   THE INTELLIGIBILITY OF EXISTENCE

3.15   Existence is intelligible.
(See 2.102, 3.10)

WERE Existence not intelligible, we would not know what it was for something to exist rather than not to exist. But this we know. Not only that, we know what Existence is, both from the perspective of other modes of being, and in itself. This contention stands in opposition to the claims of the existentialist. He, because he supposes both that what can be known is only essence and that Existence has no essence, is forced to hold that Existence is absurd, irrational, unintelligible, in face of the fact that he seems to know it well enough to be able to characterize it in these belittling terms. Our contention also stands in opposition to the position of the Thomists who suppose that Existence can never be known apart from any individual being, in face of the fact that we know it quite well as an independent domain in which Actualities are imbedded and which relates them as contemporaries and keeps them abreast in time.

He who claims to know that Existence is other than essence or reason knows it as the object of the rational category "Existence," or if one likes of "nonreason." If we could know that something was not the object of "reason," we would self-contradictorily know it by means of what would then be the category "not an object of reason."

Of course, what is, is other than the reason by means of which we know it. Every object of a category is other than, though not alien to its category.

There is a difference between knowledge and its object; otherwise knowledge would not be possible. But difference is not negation. What is distinct from reason is not beyond the power of reason to apprehend; the object of reason is distinct from it, but known by means of it. All knowledge is knowledge of what is other than itself. There is no paradox in this unless to know is to repeat, duplicate, represent. Existence is intelligible not because it is an essence, but because it is knowable through the use of essences, categories, judgments, reason.

Existence has an essence. A grasp of that essence is of course not yet a grasp of Existence itself. But the fact that a grasp of an essence is not yet a grasp of that of which it is the essence is not peculiar to Existence. Nothing—not only Existence—is identical with its essence. The essence of an Actuality is distinct from the Actuality. He who with Aristotle holds that knowledge is confined to a comprehension of eternal essences is forced to hold that the Actuality, as over against these, is possessed of incomprehensible accidents. Nor is the essence of an Ideal identical with that Ideal. He who with Hegel views the Ideal as just an essence is forced to distinguish it from itself when it plays a role distinct from that open to an essence —which is the case when it works through time to constitute history. There is for Hegel a "cunning" to reason which makes it operate as an agency and foil for itself, but this is but to say that there is a real distinction for him between the Ideal as having an unchanging essence, and it as having a changing, effective, historically significant Existence. And finally the essence of God is distinct from God himself. God's essence is but a facet of him, his unity as distinct from the whole of him, that being who is one. He who with Spinoza tries to identify God and his essence is sooner or later forced to distinguish between *natura naturans* and *natura naturata*, the essence of God and the expressions of God, and then will have the problem of uniting these so as to portray properly the God who is both and yet is just one being.

The essence of Existence is, like every other essence, an intelligible unity. This is in a tensional relation to sheer Existence, which though not a distinct reality, can be intellectually distinguished as being over against the essence. So far as we do distinguish Existence and its essence, we but make evident that there is a tensional relation, within that separated Existence, between a subordinate Existence and its correlate essence, and so on. At every stage in a movement to analytic components of Existence, we come to an essence which has over against it an Existence differing from that essence not in the possession of some quality or character, but in its being, in its function, in the way it acts and thereby affects that essence and other beings.

3.16 "Existence" is a predicate.
(See *1.67, 2.12, 3.15*)

IT MAKES sense to say that something exists. Of course an existing hundred dollars does not contain the least coin more than a possible hundred dollars. No one ever thought it did, and it is hard to understand why Kant thought this a remark worth making. An existent hundred dollars contains a number of actual coins, and a possible hundred dollars contains the same number, but only of possible coins. To say of dollars that they exist is to say that there are so many actual coins, that they have such and such relations to some other existent and so on. As Kant himself observed, an existent Actuality has determinate relations to what is perceived, which is but to say to something already acknowledged to be existent.

Nothing can be added to the possible to turn it into an existent— unless it be Existence. This Existence is not another possible; it has a mode of being other than that possessed by the possible. To say of something that it exists is to say that in addition to the particular characters (e.g., shape, color, size, etc.) we recognize it to have, it has the inclusive character, the predicate, "having a career other than and partly inclusive of the careers which those particular characters have." This career can be understood; we can note the object's habits and the course of the world, and anticipate with some shrewdness just where it will go and what it will do. The going and the doing is its work, and an outcome of its Existence.

As a rule when we speak of something existing we mean that it has a career in space-time. But the Ideal also exists and so does God. Neither exists inside space-time. The predicate "Existence" strictly speaking then has a threefold use. It marks the fact that an entity, which it characterizes as a totality, (a) is present, (b) is in a process of becoming, or (c) has more implications than those that follow from an idea of it. By recognizing that Existence is a predicate in any of these senses, we do not turn it into a feature of a being alongside other features, nor do we turn the Existence of that being into an essence. Instead we characterize the whole being in abstract terms, which tell us that it has determinations, adventures, and implications not grounded in what Kant calls our "concepts" or limited predicates.

Three primary arguments have been offered in recent times to show that "Existence" cannot be a predicate: (a) to say that something, e.g., sheep, exists, is but to say that "for some x, x has the property of being a sheep," and is thus to reveal both that "Existence" is an eliminable term and that "sheep" is the proper predicate here; (b) while every significant proposition has a significant contradictory, the contradictory of "all sheep exist" is the absurdity "some sheep do not exist," which shows that "all sheep exist" is not significant; (c) to say that "x is not colored" is but to say that "an existent x is not colored." Substituting "existent" for "colored" (which we can if "existent" is a predicate) we get the absurdity that "an existent x is not existent," showing that "existent" and its affiliates are not genuine predicates.

But (a) "sheep" is not a predicate; "sheeplike" or "sheepish" is. And if we insist on treating it as one, and in translating the expression into the language of the *Principia Mathematica*, the very least we can assert as a proper translation of "sheep exist" is, "for some x, x is a sheep and x exists." (b) "Some" does not necessarily refer to something existent. It makes no less sense to say that "some hippogriffs do not exist" than it does to say that "some hippogriffs are not handsome." Just as we can say that "some sheep are not frightened," so we can say that "some sheep do not exist," e.g., those that never make a mistake. Propositions 9.1 and 10.24 of the *Principia Mathematica* assert that if a proposition is true in any case there is some entity for which the proposition is true. If "some" here means "some existing" we are there offered the ontological argument without apology or excuse. (c) To say that "x is not colored" is not yet to say that an existent x is not colored. It makes sense to say "no sea serpents are blue." We do not necessarily predicate a color only of existents. Of all predicates only "Existence" has existential import; only it requires that its object exist. The existence of that object is not identical with the predicate "Existence," which we use when we speak of that existence.

Like any other predicate, the predicate "Existence" can be predicated erroneously. As a rule we say that such erroneous predication occurs when something is held to exist but does not in fact exist in the normative sense of having determinate relations to commonsense

objects. Thus we usually think that it is an error to say that a hippo-
griff exists, even though it may exist in idea. But since every mode of
being has Existence within it, every mode, and derivatively every
feature, is justly said to exist, though to be sure not in the normative
commonsense way characteristic of an actual object.

When we ask for a proof of the existence of God we sometimes
seem to be asking—and this is how Kant seemed to treat the question
—whether or not he exists in the way things do. He does not. "God
exists" is false if it is supposed to say that God exists in the way a
space-time Actuality does, as a being knocked about in a spatial field,
struggling to remain in time. Or we may mean to ask whether or not
he is but a case of Existence. He is not. "God exists" is false if it is
supposed to say that God is entirely subordinate to Existence. What
we really are seeking to know when we ask about the existence of
God is whether he is more than an idea, more than a myth, more than
an object of hope. I think he is. On this question as to whether or
not God exists, whether or not he is an irreducible mode of being,
and whether or not he fully controls, determines, delimits the Existence in him, see 4.52–55, 4.92.

3.17   "Existence" is a predicable of every idea and predicate.
(See *1.67, 1.80, 3.16*)

EVERY IDEA and predicate occurs at some time, in someone's mind
or language. It is just this item, with such and such specific relations
to others; it is a hard brute fact at least in the psyche or in language.
The idea or predicate as a fact is, as Bradley incisively urged in the
first chapter of his great *Logic*, a "that" which is to be contrasted with
itself as a meaning, or "what." This meaning is but one part of the total
idea, the part with which we are concerned when we speak of essences, of categories, of knowledge. As part of a psychical event, this
meaning has existence. It achieves another existence apart from that
event only when it is dislodged from the idea and transported or
referred or used by the mind and thereby given lodgement elsewhere.

An idea's career in a psychical event is the topic of the psychological study of the nature of thought. In contrast, the psychical
event itself, the idea as an occurrence, is more the topic of the psy-

chological or linguistic study of the origin and repercussions of the occurrence. The one study sees that the idea or meaning "dog" is perhaps followed by one of "cat"; the other study remarks that the idea of "dog" is exciting and is followed perhaps by an unnoticed movement of the hand. Neither of these deals with the idea as playing a part in a judgment or act of knowledge. Judgment and knowledge require us first to dislodge the meaning from its original setting and then to give it a new existence through the agency of a cognitive act. Logic concentrates on the idea in this latter sense. It tells us not which ideas in fact follow on given ideas or which acts follow on them, but what meaning ought to follow on a meaning if the former is to inherit some such desirable character as truth or clarity or elegance, and so on.

An idea, then, can be said to exist in at least three senses: it exists as a psychical or linguistic *occurrence*, e.g., in a sentence; it exists as a *meaning carried* by that occurrence, e.g., in a proposition; and it exists as a *meaning in some cognitive whole*, epistemic or logical, e.g., in a judgment. When an idea exists in any one of these ways, it can be correctly characterized through the use of the predicate "Existence." Since the idea of Existence is as respectable as any other idea, it too can exist in any one of these three ways; it too can be characterized by the predicate "Existence" for three distinct reasons.

3.18   To know an idea is not yet to know the career it has.
(*See 3.10, 3.17*)

WE EMPLOY an idea *b* to refer to idea *a*'s meaning. The idea *b* we have of the meaning of idea *a* does not report idea *a*'s career, and therefore does not report the nature of the career to which *a* subjects the meaning that *a* carries.

If we concentrate not on the meaning of the idea *a* but on its occurrence, we will know idea *a* by means of an idea *c*, which is part of a judgment. Idea *c* is distinct from the ideas *a* and *b*, even when it purports to duplicate them. Idea *c* has a career in judgment and will have all kinds of relations and activities in the knowing mind that ideas *a* and *b* do not have.

The idea *c* of idea *a*'s occurrence, at the very best, gives the essence of that occurrence, and this does not go through the career which its object, *a*, does. No matter how precise our knowledge of an occurrence, it falls short of the fact that it is taking place in a world of contingencies, and that it works itself out in time. It is therefore not available for knowledge even to an absolutely omniscient being—who can know, after all, only what can be known, and not what is not yet there to be known. Idea *a*, taken either as an occurrence or a meaning, has a career which no knowledge of that idea can wholly encompass.

3.19 The features of beings are involved in careers not identical with those they have as part of a mind.
(*See 1.63, 1.65, 3.16, 3.18*)

THE ELEMENTS in a veridical judgment of perception—the indicated and contemplated—are derived from an external object. In the object they are not distinct one from the other; the object is a seamless whole. In the act of knowing, the indicated and contemplated are separated from the object and from one another, and are held apart from the object and its career. When one judges he embeds the elements in a cognizing act, which has various relations (not determinable from the standpoint of the elements) to other acts and other functions, parts, and aspects of the knower, and that with which he is in interplay.

No matter how accurate and precise a perception, no matter how successfully it might be possible to recapture in the judgment the unity and thus the nonseparated natures of the indicated and the contemplated as they occurred originally in the object, there is a difference between the adventures to which the object subjects its features and the adventures to which the knower subjects them. If one could, with the early Wittgenstein, make structural pictures of the world, or if one could, with Pythagorean thinkers, view the world as a congeries of mathematical relations which might be perfectly grasped by a detached or clear intellect, it still would be the case that the adventures of the picture or relations would be distinct from and perhaps not in accord with what is outside them.

Similar observations are to be made with reference to any discriminable features of the Ideal and of God. These are sometimes spoken of as though they were absolutely simple; but if this were the case there would be no possible judgment made of them by means of features derivable from them, or even supposed to be in them. Within the Ideal there are creases and foci which precipitate out as limited objectives under the pressure of appetitive beings; within God there are the Ideal and Actualities and Existence as judged by him. When we know the Ideal or God, we separate out what was part of one organic unity, and then give what we isolate a lodgement in finite beings and existent situations, thereby subjecting it to vicissitudes and conditions to which it was not subject originally.

3.20   The passage from what is in mind to the object known goes through Existence.
(*See 1.65, 1.67, 3.01, 3.19*)

KNOWING is an act which, like every other act, is a delimited bit of Existence. Its primary task is to undo the work which was produced in the act of obtaining elements for judgment. Cognition is, then, no mere simple translucent focusing on an objective fact, immediately, without risk of distortion or error. It is an act which begins with the knower and terminates in an object known. That act affects what the knower feels and decides and does. It makes a difference also to the object, for by making the object the terminus of a cognition, the knower forces it into the foreground, thus making it not only a test of his claim to know, but a possible focal point for further knowing and other kinds of action.

Mind and what is not in mind are divided from one another by Existence. In knowing we must therefore pass through Existence to a being existing apart from us and our act of knowing. The Existence through which we pass (as well as the existent object at which we arrive) is other than and more than we possess in our cognition. We exist as men while we existentially know through the utilization of but part of our being; what is outside us has an independent existence throughout the time that it is being existentially known by means of distinguished facets of it.

3.21   Predication produces a change in the meaning of the predicate.
(*See 1.70, 3.19, 3.20*)

"PREDICATION" is really a "judgmentation," an objective orientating of a privately forged unity of an indicated, or subject, and a contemplated, or predicate. However, since the contemplated contains most of the meaning in which we are interested in discourse, logic, and speculation, we usually are inclined to overlook the other element in the judgment and consequently tend to ignore the judgment as a whole and its "predicational" role.

There is no point in attributing a predicate or contemplated to a subject in or outside us. If we did, all our predications would yield tautologies or contradictions, the first if the subject in fact possessed the predicate we attributed to it, and the second if it did not. A predicate is not predicated; it is but a pivotal point in a judgment which, together with an indicated, articulates an object which is also being adumbrated as that which stands apart from us. In either case, whether we suppose there is such an act as predication or not, what we ascribe to the object of cognition is, in the object, distinct from what it is as something to be ascribed to that object. When outside the mind in another existent locus, the known, and therefore the subject and predicate, have careers other than those which they have when in mind.

The predicate as in an object is an *attribute* or quality; this may be quite distinct in nature, structure, as well as in behavior, from what it is in the mind. Still there is a single nucleal element of meaning which can be abstracted from the predicate and recognized to be also in the attribute. The obtaining of that nucleal element may require considerable effort, particularly when the transformation of the predicate is quite radical. But neither the presence nor possession of the nucleal element affects the fact that the predicate is transformed into an acknowledged attribute in the act of knowing, and is thereby altered in meaning because it has then been given a different career from what it had when it was only an item in the mind.

3.22   Attributes are altered by being abstracted from objects.
(*See 1.70, 3.21*)

IN veridical perception contemplateds are obtained from external objects, where they have the role of attributes. To use them in knowledge the knower must make distinctions not found in the objects. Knowledge analyzes before it unifies, and the analysis introduces distinctions and borders which were not in the objects themselves. When those distinguished elements are united in a judgment, they achieve a function and a career in the mind that they never did have in the object. The point has been overlooked by many modern logicians. And where it is acknowledged (see, e.g., W. V. Quine, *A System of Logistic*), the act of abstraction is not recognized to be a transformative act, one in which the attribute is in effect changed in meaning by being given a new location, new implications, and new adventures.

3.23 The perceived is contemporary with the perceiver.
(*See 1.57–60, 3.22*)

WE PERCEIVE what is contemporary with us, and this even if it be the sun or moon or stars. This truth, it is often thought, is contradicted by scientific discoveries in optics, physiology, and the like. But the one thing which it in fact does is to take account of the truths which make any science and any evidence possible.

There seem to be only three real alternatives to the doctrine that perception is of the contemporary: what we perceive (a) occurs only in our minds; (b) is something projected by us on to an environing void; or (c) is distant from us in space and in time. The first alternative denies that there could ever be any objective evidence; in fact it has nothing to know but what is inside one individual's mind. There are no external facts for it, no evidence, no science. The second alternative offers us an objective world, but one of our own making. Once again there are no objective facts for us to know, no evidence for us to attend to, but only a world to construct, governed by no requirements but that we should exteriorize what we somehow have in our minds. The third alternative is the most favored today. It alone of the three says that there are objective brute facts, real evidence on which one can rely, and seems to be the only view which accepts, without cavil, the theory that light takes time to travel from place to place. The theory, however, makes a number of rather strange assumptions. It supposes that one can go backwards in time. Yet past time is precisely a time which is no longer available. In any case past time is unalterable, as are the objects in it, and cannot therefore be open to fresh traversal by the perceiving mind. It supposes too that one traverses the very path over which some photon came, even though there is nothing in the arrived photon which tells where it came from. And it supposes too that the traversal is instantaneous, so that one can do in perception what has been defined to be impossible in fact—traverse a distance in no time.

There is little doubt but that it takes time for a light ray or photon or sound wave to travel over space. Still, it is not the thing that travels, not the traversal, not that from which the travel starts, that is perceptually encountered. These are inferred to be on the basis of something else perceptually known. The arrival of the photon or sound is the arrival of a physical thing at a physical body, where it may irritate, provoke, stimulate a conscious being, the possessor of the disturbed body, to engage in an act of knowledge. That act starts with an existent, goes through Existence, and arrives at an existent.

What is it at which it arrives? Is it a real object? Is it a quality or feature of a real object, separated from that object, but decorating a real objective space? This latter is close to Whitehead's ingenious suggestion. He held that when we look in the mirror we actually see the space behind the mirror decorated by what we see in the mirror. What we see is, as it were, a "what" dislocated from its "that," but located in an objective space. Just as we see "waterness" in a mirage where there is no real wetness, so we see red in the space behind the mirror though there is no real colored object there. Whitehead's sound realism led him to acknowledge the objectivity of perceptual content; his uncritical acceptance of the view that all effects—even qualities—are transmitted through time made him dislocate that content from its "that," and to suppose that in the mind or in a mirror or in a mirage was the very stuff of a past external object.

What we perceive is never entirely dislocated from objects, nor is what is in our minds identical with what is outside them. The "waterness" in a mirage is not identical with the "waterness" of actual water, or even with the "waterness" in an idea of water; it is infected by the being of the sand and air where it is resident. We may mistake the nature of the being which possesses a character; we may misunderstand the nature of the transformation to which a being subjects a character; but we are not mistaken in seeing the character to be resident in something more than mere space.

What is seen in the mirror is a mirror-toned quality which needs a different type of support from that which it obtained from the object placed before it, and a different kind of support from that which an indifferent space could provide. We need not, therefore, in connection with the mirror image go counter to what most common-sense men believe. We need not suppose that the image is actually carried by the space behind the mirror; the mirror provides the needed support for the mirror-toned quality. The mirror is reddened; but it is not red, i.e., the redness is not possessed by the mirror in such a way as to enable the mirror to act as a red thing. But when we look into the heavens we often see real objects. The qualities we then note are ingredient in something more substantial than themselves and surely more substantial than a bare space could possibly be. Just what they are ingredient in is difficult to determine, particularly since our perception involves an abstracting and universalizing of the qualities we discern, and to that extent (but not entirely) involves a loss of what can lead us to grasp the object which subjugated and thus posssessed those qualities in a guise not identical with that which they have in us or in our judgment. When we look up at the heavens we see starlike features ingredient in contemporary beings. Those contemporary beings infect the starlike features, subjecting them to transformations which preclude their being simply identifiable with any images or judgments we may have.

3.24   What is in mind tests what is in body, and conversely.
(*See 1.70, 1.74, 3.21, 3.22*)

EMPIRICISTS take attributes, and any other features as resident in objects, to test the truth, value, clarity, or meaning of what is in the mind. Rationalists take the opposite tack. For them what is in the mind tests what is encountered in perception or experience. There is no ground for insisting on only one of these approaches to the exclusion of the other. Both tests are legitimate. What is in the mind has one career, and what is in the known object has another. Each career is reputable. For one purpose one can serve as a test for the other; for another purpose their roles can be interchanged.

An idea in mind can be separated off from the dross of daily activity, mere contingent neighbors and connections. It can achieve a purified status and be granted a way of existing more appropriate to its intelligible nature. If then it is clarity, purity, or ideal and intelligible connections which we seek or need, the mind must serve as the

measure for the world. But if it is practice, experience, or other existents with which we are concerned, we will test what is in mind by
what takes place in the world of bodies.

Although each view is as sound as the other, both are subordinate
to a third. This I have sometimes termed "Epochalism" because it
calls our attention to those pivotal points in being and knowledge
around which inquiry and speculation should persistently turn. Each
of the four modes of being is an *epoché;* so are the predicates in the
mind and the attributes or qualities in objects. Epochalism is thus that
position of which both the empirical and rational views are limiting
cases. These limiting cases insist on half a truth to the exclusion of the
other, when nothing less than both can possibly satisfy, not only in
view of the effective criticism each of these views makes of the
other, but in view of the fact that what is in the mind has virtues denied to it when it is resident in bodies, and conversely.

3.25   A claim to truth is vindicatable if a consequence in
mind is abstractable from a consequence in nature in a
predesignatable way.
(See *1.67, 3.22, 3.24*)

WHAT is used in knowledge undergoes transformations when dislocated from objects and given residence in the mind. The transformations may affect the very nature or structure or appearance of
the attributes; at the very least they will end with the imposition of
boundaries on those attributes, thereby inevitably giving them new
meanings, new relations, and new adventures. The occurrence of
such transformations stand in the way of the acceptance either of a
naive realistic or a representational theory of knowledge. The one supposes that we perceive things as they are—an attractive theory
were it not for the fact that we do make errors. The other supposes
that what we perceive is in our minds and altogether cut off from
what is as in the object—a persuasive theory but still one which in the
end collapses before the fact that we do know that we make errors
and thus do have some acquaintance with what is the case.

When we perceive we adumbrate, reach to an object; and we can
continue to do this over a considerable period of time. Having abstracted a contemplatable feature of the object we can derive consequences from it through the use of logic and mathematics, or by

guessing, reconstructing, speculating, imagining. The judgment that we formed through the use of elements abstracted from the object is vindicated if, when we engage in the same type of abstraction with respect to some consequence of the initial object, we obtain the very consequence which we ourselves derived from the initial abstraction. To vindicate a judgment we must keep pace with the object at the distance defined by an initial act of abstraction. It makes no difference to the worth or validity of a vindication that we may have initially transformed an item radically (as we do in fact when we deal with it as essentially a mathematical structure) so long as we transform the abstraction, with which we begin, in a way that parallels the transformation to which the initial object is subjected in fact.

This theory of vindication agrees with naive realism in recognizing that we know a real world beyond us; it agrees with representationalism in recognizing that what we have in mind is distinct from what exists outside it; it agrees with pragmatism in recognizing that we must look to the future to verify what we now claim to know; it agrees with empiricism in looking to external objects to test the truth of what we claim to know; and it agrees with rationalism in recognizing that the mind has the power to know in advance what kind of result the object will produce. But unlike any of these it recognizes that what we know now and what we can know in advance can, while distinct from a real external world, still be in accord with it.

3.26 A vindicatable claim to know the Ideal, Existence, or God requires a capacity to repeat the methods by which we obtained our initial knowledge of them.
(*See 1.73, 3.25*)

WE KNOW about the Ideal, Existence, or God, firstly, by direct acquaintance with them in ourselves. We know them, secondly, as limits at a distance from ourselves, limits at which our beings terminate. We know them, thirdly, through the exercise of dialectic and speculation. Finally we know them as we merge into them in our passage from the first to the second and third of the above ways of knowing. In the first way we see that they are tinctures of the self; in the second, we confront them as objective data; in the third, we see them to be cases of philosophic knowledge; in the fourth, we know them to be not altogether distinct from ourselves or from one another.

To vindicate the first and fourth ways of knowing these other modes, we must attempt to encounter them again and again in their guise of sources of intelligibility, vitality, or unity, and see if they then are in consonance with what we inferred from them. To vindicate the second way of knowing them, we must first acknowledge them in their respective roles as a terminus of obligations, a compelling field, or a felt measure of our importance, and then see if we can deduce from these the kind of content we can subsequently abstract from the modes. And finally, to vindicate our dialectic and speculative knowledge of them, we must attend to them in new combinations to see if they then yield the results formally implied by them in other previously acknowledged combinations.

3.27   A unique characterization is not an attribute.
(*See 3.19, 3.21, 3.22*)

IT IS NOT altogether clear whether or not this assertion is in direct opposition to Proposition 14:02 of the *Principia Mathematica*. That proposition says that it is one and the same thing to affirm "there is one and only one value which satisfies a function" and that "there is an existent which satisfies that function." If by "a value which satisfies a function" is meant an "existent value" the *Principia Mathematica* asserts nothing but a strange though harmless tautology; but if it is intended to affirm that if there be one and only one value for a variable that value does in fact exist the way horses or tables do, it surely is in error. Even if one is willing to speak of or symbolize a value for a variable if and only if there is a real entity which in fact exhibits that variable, this real entity, existent in a hurly-burly universe streaked with contingency, will be distinct from itself as symbolized in logic or mathematics, no matter how precise and inclusive the symbolized form may be. A value, a logically proper name, a unique description applicable to a real being, are all distinct from what exists apart from them. In language or logic, characterizations of any sort—be they predicates, descriptions, or whatever— are not altogether determinate; outside language or logic their counterparts are attributes, determinate facets of existent beings.

From this it is evident that, despite the controversies of the last decades, there is no genuine opposition between symbolic logicians and Aristotelian logicians on the question of the legitimacy of the deduction of "some x is y" from "all x is y." Symbolic logicians have held that the Aristotelians mistakenly deduce the former from the latter; Aristotelians have said that the symbolic logicians mistakenly divorce the latter from the former. But in fact neither makes a mistake. Each side employs a special meaning of "all." For the Aristotelian, "all" refers to a "general," an actual totality of existents; for the symbolic logician, "all" refers to a universal, a meaning. The general "all," the Aristotelian sees, allows for the deduction of "some," where "some" means an "existent some." From "All professors at Yale are men," "some (existent) professors at Yale are men" follows. The symbolic logician sees that "all," the universal, does not allow for the deduction of "some" (existent); he rightly rejects the derivation of "Some (existent) gryphons at Yale are men" from "All (non-existent) gryphons at Yale are men." However—and this the symbolic logician overlooks—from "All (nonexistent) gryphons at Yale are men," we can legitimately derive "Some (nonexistent) gryphons at Yale are men." There are, in short, two distinct meanings of "some," paralleling the distinct meanings of "all," of which only one, the Aristotelian, has been recognized even by symbolic logicians. The (existent) "some" which follows from the general "all" refers to an actual subdivision of an actual class; the (nonexistent) "some" which follows from the universal "all" refers to an intellectually distinguished part of an intension or meaning. From the nonexistent "some," of course, the existent cannot be legitimately derived.

3.28   A "collective" disjunction is distinct from a "distributive" disjunction.
(*See 2.14, 3.18, 3.20*)

ARISTOTLE remarked in his *De Interpretatione,* 19a30 ff: "A sea-fight must either take place tomorrow or not; but it is not necessary that it should take place tomorrow, neither is it necessary that it should not take place, yet it is necessary that it either should or should not take place tomorrow." (Perhaps more evidently: Although it is true that I will either die or not die tomorrow, it is not now true that I will die tomorrow, nor is it now true that I will not die tomorrow. There is no definite dying or definite non-dying to which reference can now be made. "Dying-or-not-dying" is definite, distinctive, but its components are not.) Aristotle was here distinguishing between "f (x-or-not-x)" and "f (x) or f (not-x)," although he did not provide the appropriate logical terms with which to do it. "f (x-or-not-x)" makes use of the *collective* disjunction; here the x and the non-x are not separated off from one another; but they are so separated in "f (x) or f (not-x)" which makes use of a *distributive* disjunction.

The collective disjunction occurs in the realm of meanings, mind, ideality; the distributive occurs in the realm of Existence, the discrete, the exclusive. Failure to note the nature of the passage from the one to the other produces paradoxes, to be avoided only through the mastery of the art of anticrasis, the art of disjoining properly. A good logic should use distinct symbols for different types of disjunction. It will then perhaps be more evident that it is not possible to derive the distributive from the collective disjunction legitimately. "f (x-or-not-x)" states a single necessary truth; "f (x) or f (not-x)" makes two distinct assertions, neither one of which is necessarily true. It follows that f (x) cannot be deduced from f (x-or-y), even when y is equal to o, for the elimination of that o requires an illegitimate movement from the collective to the distributive use of the disjunction, from "f (x-or-o)" to "f (x) or f (o)."

3.29   An "extensional" conjunction is distinct from an "intensional" conjunction.
(See 3.18, 3.20)

NOTHING seems so simple a term as "and." Yet it is a term used in multiple ways. It may connect items in a list; it may mark a subordination; it may be used to express a merging: "here's one and here's another," "father and son," "the taste of sugar, cream, and coffee in a cup of coffee." All these are existent, extensional modes of conjunction, and can be divided into two types—an *external*, represented by the first case, and an *infectious* by the other two. These extensional forms of conjunction stand in contrast with similar intensional modes, where the items to be conjoined lack the distinctness, the boundaries, the existential opposition characteristic of the extensional.

To form a logical conjunction of two propositions, we must bring a proposition p *and* a proposition q together, which is to say, we must first make use of a mode of intensional "and-ing." The p and q here are for formal logic indeterminate; when exteriorly but intensionally conjoined as 'pq' they become logically determinate and ready for the operations of logic. Each of these has a counterpart in the world beyond, which I will symbolize as 'X.Y' and 'X,Y', respectively. These two are extensional modes of conjunction, the one expressing an objective merging, the other a mere exterior junction of determinate entities.

The relation between 'p and q' and 'pq' connects entities which are of psychological interest to entities of logical interest, where psychology and logic are, as they need not be, taken to be exclusive of one another. The relation of X.Y and X,Y connects determinate mutually infective beings with the beings as exterior to one another; it makes possible a transition, in the objective world, from the organic to the additive. The relation between pq and X,Y and the relation between pq and X.Y connect mentally sustained conjunctions with objective conjunctions. Semantics, or the art of applying logic, traverses these latter relations in a transformative way. It presupposes a mastery of syndetics, the art of conjoining in thought and in fact. This art is known to painters. They speak, for example, of additive and subtractive mixtures—yellow and blue yield white additively, and green subtractively. Their knowledge deserves incorporation in logic.

3.30 A negation in thought is distinct from a rejection in fact.
(See 3.18, 3.20)

THERE are at least three types of negation: *infectious* negation (–p), in which the negating transforms the idea, meaning or proposition to which it is applied (and therefore precludes the use of double negation as a device for getting back to the original); *simple* negation, –p, which brings us to the opposite of that with which we began, and whose effect can be reversed by being repeated; and *relational* negation, $\times$, which connects opposing entities, p $\times$ q, where q has the form either of an infectious or simple negation of p. For each of these negations there is a corresponding *rejection* of objects possible; one involves a *modification* of a given entity, the second *replaces* a given entity by another, and the third *opposes* distinct items. If "!" be used to express the objective fact these three can be symbolized as, (!–X), –!X, and !(X∼Y).

The transition from one type of negation to another requires transformations which should be but have not yet been made the topic of extended logical inquiry. Nor has the transition from one type of rejection to another received its appropriate ontological inquiry. Infectious negation "(–p)" and modifying rejection "(!–X)" could, however, be taken to be the primary forms; simple negation "–p" and replacement "–!X" could then be treated as limiting cases, and relational negation "p × q" and oppositional rejection "!(X∼Y)" could be dealt with as derivatives which come into being when attention is paid to what is outside a given negated or rejected entity.

The transition from one type of negation to its corresponding rejection is a change from a predicational to an attributional operation. This is no simple change. Firstly, an infectious negation is distinct from a corresponding modifying rejection in that the former changes the meaning of something whereas the latter changes its being. The former change does not seem to allow of degrees, the latter does. If we infect such a term as "horse" with a negation we get nothing more than "non-horse." This is consistent with the nonexistence of everything whatsoever and encompasses anything there might be which is other than horse. But a modifying rejection of a horse may alter it in any one of a number of ways, and then yield a specific object, as concrete and limited as the original horse. Secondly, when we relate entities in the mind through a relational negation we span the entire range of possible being, since we connect contradictory opposites; when we relate through an oppositional rejection we span only what is, and thus relate specific entities with one another in an existential field. Finally, though we can move quite readily in thought by simple negation from one idea or meaning or proposition to its very other, we can make no similar move in the realm of objects, for no one of them has a precise other. To negate "this is a horse" is to refer to some other entity, but is not yet to say anything definite about that entity. But if we are to replace a horse, it must be by something else; a replacement puts a particular entity, with definite traits, in place of a given one. A simple negation cancels a proposition about a given entity and does not replace it with a proposition about an entity of the same sort; the corresponding operation of replacement provides something real, concrete, substantial of the same sort as the entity replaced. To confound a replacement with a negation is to suppose that by an act of thought all of nature could be made to vanish. We can simply negate a proposition about all nature; we cannot reject all of nature but can only replace items in it by other natural items.

3.31 Formal implications are distinct from material implications.
(See *3.10, 3.18, 3.20*)

A FORMAL implication is a structure connecting a given item in mind or language with some required other. The two items it connects are "at the same time," even when they are assigned different dates. The astronomer now implies that the eclipse will take place a thousand years hence; the eclipse as taking place then is now understood by him in the very way that he understands the premiss which implicates that consequence. A material implication in contrast, expresses how a potentiality in a thing will be actualized, by virtue of the structure of the thing and the world in which it exists. (The expressions, "formal implication" and "material implication" are here being used in senses quite different from that characteristic of modern logic, in good part because they are here in some consonance with common usage.) Because his body tends to lose liquid a man will become thirsty. The potentiality of losing liquid is related to a real future in which there is a possibility of a man being thirsty. That future is now only abstract, but to reach it one must go through the extensional structure of Existence relating a present moment to the possibility in that future. This extensional structure is the structure of material implication; it puts limits, imposes conditions on what is formally implicated, framing those implications inside an Existence whose law-abiding nature extensively connects the tendency to what that tendency, in such an Existence, must eventuate as. The distance between the two types of implication is traversed when we go from pure mathematics to physics, from a nonextended connection between meanings to an extended connection between times.

3.32   Inferences and processes are distinct.
(See 1.43, 1.86, 1.87, 3.31)

INFERENCES take time. They can be treated as a species of "making," of producing something, just as "making" can be viewed as an activity, through and through rational. Either approach is legitimate, for in either way it becomes evident that both thought and action arrive at necessitated outcomes, the inevitable products of just the particular activities in which one engages when moving from given starting points. There are differences, however, between thinking and making, between inference and process, not only because the one looks to possibilities and the other to things, but because they traverse different parts of Existence. Inference is a thinking qualifying the Existence which has been caught within the mind; making is a process which qualifies the Existence that environs and is in things.

Inference has many forms; at its simplest, when most precise and reliable, it has the form of a deduction. The idea we arrive at even in a deductive inference, however, has an object which may still have to be awaited, and thus which can now only be anticipated, not known. The arrival of that object depends on actual occurrences outside the mind which in fact move at a pace and over a temporal distance distinct from that traversed in mind.

3.33   Inferences make a difference to what is formally implied.
(See 1.83, 1.84, 1.86)

INFERENCES are valid or invalid. Both types arrive at necessitated outcomes, outcomes which are formally implied by the premisses and the activity of inferring. A valid inference differs from an invalid one in that the very structure which relates the premiss and the inferring to the conclusion, characterizes the activity itself. Given 'p' to be false and 'p or q' to be true, we can validly infer 'not p and q' to be true; this conclusion is formally implied by the exterior intensional conjunction of 'not p' and 'p or q'. Given only 'p or q', we could not validly derive this result; if we do get to it from this starting point, it is because we in fact take some other route than one having the structure of a valid formal implication. If we add the structure of that route to our initial premiss we will of course get the result validly, but this will be because we have first arranged to have the result formally implied by starting point and structure together. A valid inference thus presents us with a conclusion of a formal implication, while the invalid presents us with a conclusion which can be shown to follow formally not from the premiss alone, but from it as together with the structure of the route which was in fact followed in getting to the conclusion.

There are no bare inferences making no difference whatsoever to what is formally implied. A formal implication has the result or conclusion together with the starting point or premiss; a premiss and a conclusion in it form one organic, indeed a necessary unity. An inference in contrast replaces the asserted premiss by the conclusion. We term it valid only because we suppose that the replacement of the premiss by the conclusion, the sundering of the single timeless unity of the two, inflicts no change on the premiss or the conclusion. Yet in the case of the implication the conclusion is demanded by the premiss, whereas in the case of the inference the premiss is first had without the conclusion and the conclusion is then had without the premiss. The one has premiss and conclusion connected by an internal, the other has them connected by an external relation. It is incorrect then to say that a valid inference imposes no change on the premiss and conclusion. For certain purposes or in certain periods the change may, however, be minor, irrelevant, or just ignored. But then many inferences usually termed logically "invalid" could also be treated as acceptable for similar reasons—which in fact is what does occur in the conventional inductions of daily life.

3.34 Inference is an art in which one risks replacing a satisfactory premiss by an unsatisfactory conclusion.
(See *1.82, 3.33*)

A CONCLUSION (even when it can be shown to follow formally) is, as concluded to, quite distinct from itself as organically related to its premiss. Even if, e.g., it were the case that "this is the word of God" formally implied "this is just," it might be false to conclude and to assert "this is just" by itself, since there might be no justice except so far as the word of God was present. The replacing of the premiss by the conclusion would yield a detached conclusion where only a dependent one was warranted.

An inference is an adventure. It starts with what was supposed to be satisfactory in some way, moves on as far as possible into the realm of what had not yet been so certified, and ends by certifying something to be satisfactory in the light of what had been taken for granted. Precisely because it serves to certify what, apart from it, is not satisfactory, it involves a risk.

3.35 Processes add to what is materially implied.
(See 1.87, 3.31–33)

A BEING has a potentiality to the degree that it materially implicates the future, dictates the area in which what will actually ensue must take place. The material implication has the structure of time, relating the present to the (abstract) future, in an order of *before and after*. An actual process takes time; it occurs only in a sequence of present moments, relating them as *earlier and later*. This difference between material implication and the process which quickens it is analogous to the difference between the laws of nature and occurrences as exhibiting those laws, between theoretical and applied physics, and between formal implication and inference.

There are invalid inferences, but no invalid processes. Nevertheless there is a parallel between formal implications with their corresponding inferences, and material implications with their corresponding processes, even to the extent of permitting a distinction between acceptable and nonacceptable vivifications of implications in both cases. A process, though framed inside the area of a material implication, can subject that implication to considerable intensification by involving it in a nest of alien relations. But more, the process can end in a rather radical alteration in the nature of objects. Such alterations are the analogues of invalid inferences. Aristotle (in his account of monsters) seems to have been the first to be aware of this truth.

3.36 Formal implications and processes are not necessarily in accord.
(See 3.31–35)

SINCE a formal implication may not do justice to the richness of a material implication and the conclusion which this promises to bring about in fact, and since the process which does occur adds to what is materially implied, the conclusion of a formal implication may diverge considerably from what is produced in fact. And even where a formal implication answers quite closely to a material implication, and is used in an inference which closely parallels a process, the formal implication, precisely because the inferential process vivifies it and makes a difference to its terms, may not be in accord with that process. Processes take time to bring about both what is formally and what is materially implied. They also give a context to this which they bring about, and thus subject it to adventures not accounted for by either type of implication.

Every formal discipline must decide for itself how long it will wait for a formally implicated outcome to ensue, and how many additional and perhaps distortive features it will allow before it decides that the formal implication is irrelevant or, alternatively, that the process is irrational. Different disciplines and civilizations can be distinguished in terms of the manner in which they decide this question. A gambler lives in terms of the expectation that theoretical calculations of probalility will be fully realized in a very limited time. Should the implicated result not ensue within that time, he supposes that there are malevolent forces at work in the universe or in men. An historian not only allows for a longer run, but usually holds that what is not formally implicated by what he knows is not relevant to the course of the world. When the social sciences insist on the use of mathematics, and suppose that there must be causes for what in their results does not accord with what is implicated in a mathematical theory of statistics, they approximate the gambler. So far as they insist on observing the course of the world, and stand ready to abandon their theories when these fail to be in accord with that world, they approximate the historian. Experimental and observational sciences lean sometimes in one direction and sometimes in the other. Though often described as completely on the side of those who are always ready to abandon their theories and what they formally imply, they quite often take the opposite tack and suppose that there are unknown causes at work which account for the fact that their theories do not seem to hold.

The distinctions in 3.27–36 have been made primarily in the light of the difference in the natures of Ideality and Existence. Each of these modes governs a different set of logical constants. An analogous set of constants is grounded in the nature of God, and another in the nature of Actualities. The primary logic of God would seem, according to Plotinus, to be the production of subordinate proof upon subordinate proof, without ever reaching the stage where something is in fact inferred, treated as a conclusion over against God and his implicative mode of derivation. The primary logic of Actuality would seem, according to Kierkegaard, to be an adjunction in which there is a primary *P* to which other terms, q, r, s, can be adjoined and thereby qualified without their having a similar effect on it. In both of these modes there are analogues not only for implication and inference but for other constants and their counterparts as well.

Each mode of being provides a "semantics," a way of relating the constants and expressions in a second mode to that of a third mode. Thus, e.g., both God and Actualities offer relations connecting the two basic types of conjunction in 3.29, conjunctions which are representative of Existence and the Ideal. There are four basic types of logic, corresponding to the four modes which together exhaust the nature of being and meaning, and thus logic itself. Over-arching these four is a togetherness which never gets to be irreducibly real.

III   THE PAST

3.37   Each Actuality has its own Existence.
(See *1.22, 3.08, 3.09*)

SOME, with Aquinas and Descartes, hold that God endows Actualities with whatever Existence they have. Were God to turn his attention away from Actualities they would, it is supposed, immediately vanish into nothingness. The normal center of gravity of the Actualities is thought to be zero. Nothing less than omnipotence is able to raise them and keep them out of their nothingness; only so long as God attends to them have they some semblance of being. Such a view does less than justice to the idea of creation or of Existence. If God really creates something he makes it be. It then has an Existence of its own, over against God and everything else.

Created or not, each Actuality encloses a fragment of Existence and structures it in ways other Actualities do not. It acts in ways peculiar to it; it moves and changes, and in the case of man, can sin and defy God. The Existence it encloses is the source of the Actuality's vitality; it is what makes the Actuality effective, dynamic, able to act and interact.

3.38   Existence makes Actualities concordantly effective.
(See *1.27, 3.09, 3.37*)

THE EXISTENCE which Actualities have is part of the whole Existence. While remaining over against, it is continuous with the Existence which is resident in and peculiar to every other Actuality (as well as to Ideality and God). By virtue of the continuity of the Existence in the Actualities with the Existence which lies between them, the Actualities are related to one another across an extended space. As the whole of Existence moves on, it implicates those Actualities; these, so long as they maintain a hold on their Existence, will move into the future concordantly. Despite the fact that every Actuality exists in itself, it is, by virtue of the continuity of its Existence with the rest of Existence, not only a being which keeps abreast in time with independent contemporaries, but which interplays with them, interacts with them to constitute a single slab of present cosmic time.

3.39   Existence makes Actualities determinate.
(See *1.08, 3.09, 3.38*)

PRIMARY ACTUALITIES have Existence ingredient in them; it makes them present and effective. There are no nonexistent primary Actualities, no nonpresent ones. They cannot be separated from their Existence without altogether ceasing to be Actual. To be a primary Actuality is to be present, existent, and therefore determinate. When it is said then that Existence makes Actualities determinate this must not be understood to mean that there were indeterminate Actualities which were then made determinate. But one can speak anticipatorily of an Actuality as a possibility. Such a "possible Actuality" is made into a primary Actuality through the utilization of Existence by some present primary Actuality.

Existence makes Actualities into contemporaries. It does this, how-ever, only from the standpoint of Actualities; the Actualities confront Existence as a power which gives them a feature they otherwise would not have. Existence also makes Actualities concordantly effec-tive. Existence can do this because it is both an ingredient part of Actualities and a domain in which Actualities are imbedded. Con-temporaneity expresses a feature shared; effective concordance ex-presses a shared power and outcome. The former is a consequence of the latter. Both facts force us to look outside the confines of Actual-ities to an independent Existence, which is continuous with the Existence inside the Actualities.

Each Actuality has an essence. That essence is throughout the Actuality as surely as is its Existence. It makes every region of the Actuality part of one being. Still, when put over against the Actu-ality's Existence, the essence, no matter how specific and detailed, will be found to lack determinateness; only the Existence can give this to it. And conversely, the Actuality's Existence needs a boundary, a structure; only the essence can give these to it.

3.40   Actualities can lose their Existence.
(See 3.37)

THE EXISTENCE in an Actuality is continuous with Existence be-yond that Actuality. The continuance of the Actuality is thereby jeopardized. As Existence sweeps forward, it pulls on the Existence in the Actuality. The Actuality must use its Existence to overcome that pull—or better, to avoid a false contrasting of the Actuality with its own Existence, the Actuality must constantly assert itself with respect to the Existence which lies outside it, and endeavor to lay hold again and again of a portion of it (and the possibility in which this portion terminates) and make this its own. Should it fail to lay hold of Existence at any moment, it ceases to be. To pass away is one with losing its Existence, its dynamic power.

To persist an Actuality must re-exist. This does not mean that it perishes at each moment only to be reproduced somehow in a similar or different form. It is an existent Actuality which re-exists, which lays hold of a portion of the Existence now moving into the future and makes this its own—an effort which does not require the Actuality to give up the Existence it has and which may result in the repossession of just the portion of Existence it previously had.

3.41   Facts are realities de-existentialized.
(*See 1.10, 3.39, 3.40*)

AN ACTUAL fact is a residual Actuality, a primary Actuality shorn of its Existence and thus of its vitality—no longer primary. The fact has no power, no potentiality; it is just what it is, a brute determinate particular which owes its being to an Existence it does not contain. The fact is what Existence has made be by passing out of an Actuality. Like the Actuality, of which it is a residual derivative, the fact owes its determinateness to the operation of Existence on the possible. But the fact is even more determinate than the Actuality, since this has potentialities and is in process, whereas the fact is impotent, static.

To ask how facts come to be is to begin a quest for Existence. It is interesting to note in this regard how Berkeley, to account for the occurrence of the phenomena which he sought at first to say alone were real, was forced in invoke an effective God, and thus came out in the end merely with the substitution of a spiritual mode of Existence for the material form of it which he thought was held by other philosophers. Somewhat similarly Kant, who tried to acknowledge only a spatiotemporal manifold, was soon forced, in order to account for its presence, to acknowledge existing things-in-themselves which subtended the manifold. And in recent times Husserl's phenomenology has been undergoing a similar emendation; the outside Existence which he sought to bracket out has become a matter of primary concern for some of his followers, since only by attending to it can an explanation be found for the phenomena with which Husserl's philosophy starts.

At times we say that it is a fact that there are nonprimary Actualities, such as space, or color, or wood; we sometimes say, too, that it is a fact that something, such as a hope or idea, is indeterminate, or that something, say a possibility, has been made determinate. Such expressions involve secondary usages of the term "fact," referring to the products of Existence in derivative Actualities and in other modes of being. Their acknowledgment involves no change in principle in the use of the term "fact," since this designates any entity in abstraction from the Existence which enabled the entity to become or to have certain features.

3.42   Passing away is the conversion of an Actuality into a fact.
(See 3.41)

WHEN the present becomes past, an Actuality as in the present moment becomes past as well. But it cannot become past without losing its Existence, for its Existence has being only in the present. The Actuality may continue to exist; it may maintain itself by laying hold of present Existence once again. But as at a past moment t, the Actuality no longer has Existence in it, and cannot, as at that moment, be an Actuality. It is then only a fact.

What is true of an Actuality at moment t, is true of that Actuality forever, as at that moment. Since a fact is an abstractable component of a present Actuality, what was true of the Actuality at t is true of the fact always; the fact is wholly determinate, confined forever inside the moment t (whether this be present or past).

Actualities stand between the future and the past. In the future there are only possibilities for them; in the past there are only their derivative facts. An Actuality contains possibilities made determinate by Existence in the shape of facts, and when the Actuality moves on into the future by virtue of its grip on Existence, the shell of it in the shape of fact is all that remains of it to be past. One can then with considerable justice speak of an Actuality as a kind of transition point at which indeterminate possibilities achieve a determinateness which they never thereafter lose.

3.43   The past is a tissue of facts.
(See 2.13, 3.41, 3.42)

A FACT is what is left of an Actuality when this has been deprived of its Existence. The very passage of time, the movement of Existence, is productive of facts—a process we imitate when we abstract facts from present Actualities. Since the past is that which had once been present, it is that which once contained Existence, and now contains all that was present except that Existence.

It is true, however, that an Actuality confronts a relevant future possibility, which it has the potentiality to realize. When the Actuality passes away, must it not pass away as confronting that possibility? Must it not be true then that there are possibilities in the past, and moreover, that these possibilities remain there forever, incapable of being realized? To say that some Actuality did not pass away as a being confronting a possibility which was realizable in alternative ways, is to seem to say that there is something germane to the very being of an Actuality which does not become past. Yet to say that an Actuality became past with its potentialities and their answering realizable possibilities is to say that the past is more than a tissue of facts. It would in fact be tantamount to claiming that the past contained full-bodied Actualities. But then the past would be present.

The dilemma is overcome by noting that quite different things are future to a fact and to an Actuality. Facts do not confront possibilities; they are followed solely by facts which are followed by other facts until we come to those facts which are ingredient in present Actualities. From each subsequent fact a possibility, germane to the previous fact, can be extracted, enabling one to see what it was that had been made determinate in that subsequent fact. When we come to the present moment, we find a fact there, related to a pertinent possibility which has not yet been made determinate in the guise of some further fact; this is because the present fact is carried by an Actuality. It is only an Actuality, never a fact, that has the power to face possibilities, to confront that which has not yet been realized.

3.44 Nothing occurs in the past.
(See *3.38*, *3.41*, *3.43*)

THE PAST is a tissue of exhausted, dead, desiccated Actualities, without vitality because no longer possessing Existence. It is a realm of facts, sheer phenomena, without power or energy or movement. This point is overlooked in such plays as *Berkeley Square*, in such fancies as Wells's *Time Machine*, and in science fiction generally. If one could enter into the past, one would make that past different from what it had been, for it had been that which had not yet been entered by someone coming from a later time. He who entered the past would, paradoxically, change it, make it not 'a past which was *to be* entered.' Even more important, he who could get into the past, would not be able to see anything happening. For something to happen energy must be expended, Existence must be utilized, time must be traversed. If an act which occurred at moment t_0 continues to occur in moment t_0, when t_0 becomes past, then that act must forever involve the expenditure of energy at that moment t_0, despite the fact that new energy must be provided in order to have something occur at the next moment t_1. Not only would we then have to say that Julius Caesar is being perpetually stabbed, forever and ever, in a given moment, and that he therefore dies an infinitude of deaths, but that the energy required for this activity is forever caught within that moment, and perpetually takes Caesar from life to death.

Things spend energy only in the present; they move and change there and nowhere else. If the past were the present all over again, we would be forever doing what we once did; the present moment would be perpetually re-enacted, and whatever once existed would persist forever as substantial as it had been. Power and beings would be multiplied endlessly by the passage of time.

The past is a series of desiccated moments, mere stadia, positions, all explicit and phenomenal. The vitality of Existence, which a past thing or event had when present, has moved away from it to sustain and charge some successor, and to make possible a genuine focusing on and effort at realizing some possibility.

The past contains nothing but facts; each is just what it is, and in an unalterable relation to whatever facts may follow. The men who died in the first world war, died only once. The fact of their death is brute and final. The first world war and their deaths was followed by a second world war and the deaths of others. There are now no alternative paths possible from one to the other. Before the second world war eventuated, alternative paths were possible, but they are possible no longer except as abstractable aspects of the facts that succeeded the first world war and which had their terminus in the fact of the second world war.

It is not the nature of the past that requires historians to be hesitant and tentative, but only their ignorance. For scientists, and with respect to the future, the reverse is the case. Their predictions can be sure. But the presents that will be are yet to be freely made, and are thus ontologically outside the reach of any of their predicting.

Because the past contains nothing but facts, it is a world where determinism holds full sway. If one attends to the past or to the factuality of Actualities one is therefore not only tempted to adopt the

position of determinism but to suppose that there is a strict iso-
morphism between time and space. Past time and space have equiv-
alent properties, but this is only because facts, like things merely
occupying space, have only positions and no powers. There is a direction to present time because Existence terminates in a Future; there
is no direction to past time, in and of itself—unless we attend to the
possibilities derivable from the facts it contains.

3.45 Remembering is a present act.
(*See 1.76, 3.44*)

THE PAST cannot be re-entered without being altered. To enter
it, one would be required not only to bring into it a new element and
thereby alter it, but to introduce one's own Existence into it and
thereby make it present. When we remember we then evidently do
not make direct contact with the past. Instead, we have an idea
which claims to confront a world more determinate than one which
can be confronted in expectation; this remembered idea is had at the
same time that we confront the determinate facts about, and we, by
virtue of the rejection of the idea by these present determinate facts,
are led to refer that idea to another time, to the past, where its needed
determinate counterparts could be.

I can remember only that which I have myself encountered. This
which I encountered I can never encounter again; it is forever beyond
my reach, caught within an entirely closed past time. But I can have
an image or idea of the fact which is in the past, and can know, because of its determinateness or what it claims, that this image or idea
must be referred to a past time, and thus to one which had once been
present. Remembering is the representing of something, excluded by
what is now being experienced, as that which belongs in a past that
had been experienced.

3.46 Subsequent occurrences provide the past with new settings.
(*See 3.44*)

THERE IS one meaning to the first world war and to the deaths
it involved when one considers it by itself, and another meaning
when one considers it as having been followed by a second world
war. The theory of relativity in history which holds that there are

no steady facts and that they change with a change in perspectives, finds much support from this truth. It is one thing though to embed a fact in a new situation and see it there as having new significance, and another to suppose that it has thereby been altered. George H. Mead went so far as to claim that the "novelty of every future demands a novel past," but since he did speak of recalling his "boyhood days," he evidently did distinguish between the boyhood that he in fact had and the boyhood that he later could understand. Could the past be altered by virtue of what happened after it, causation would have to run backwards and undo what had already been done.

The past is ontologically settled, but epistemologically open, both because we do not know it entirely and because our knowledge of it can provide it with new settings which make it have consequences it otherwise would not have.

3.47   The past is necessarily related to the present.
(See 3.42, 3.46, 4.17)

THE PAST is what it is because the Existence in Actualities once made facts out of possibilities. It is the effect of that Existence, lacking the substantiality, the vitality, the finality of existent Actualities. Existence is what enables facts to be at all, both in the sense of providing the facts with their determinateness, and in the sense that its departure from them enables them to become more than present facets of Actualities. To have a position in time, the facts must be related to the Existence on which they depend for their being. Past facts are necessarily related to Existence, and thus to the present where that Existence is. Since the present is forever moving on, leaving new facts in its wake, the length of the chain of intermediary facts between any given past fact and the present constantly lengthens.

3.48   To say "x existed" is to say that the Existence which x's fact had co-ordinate with it is co-ordinate with a present fact.
(See 3.37, 3.47)

TO SAY "x exists" is to say that it is present, that its fact has an Existence co-ordinate with it. To say that "x existed" is to say that there was a present time when x had Existence, but that it has it no longer, and is therefore only a fact. If the Existence now present is not one with the Existence which was once integral to a past x, there would be no connection between the past occurrence and the present. The past would then have no relation to what followed it, or would be connected with an irrelevant present through the agency of a transcendent power. It would not be a past for a present.

It is of course the case that the Existence in an Actuality is subjugated by it to some degree. It is also true that the whole of Existence is constantly changing. Were the Existence unaltered over the course of time, it would be an Existence which was not integral to unique beings; it would be an Existence too which had no genuine duration, no real career. The identity of Existence which is present with Existence as that which had once quickened the past is an identity only of being, not of function, structure, or feature.

IV   THE CREATIVE ENTERPRISE

3.49   To reach Actualities as they are in themselves, they must be freed from the qualifications produced by Existence and other modes of being.
(*See 1.19, 1.25, 2.02, 3.10, 3.38*)

ACTUALITIES are caught up in adventures, subject to conditions, qualified in multiple ways. Each bears the marks of its encounters with other Actualities; each is affected by other modes of being. But although what other Actualities do to a given one is often something unexpected and sometimes undesirable and unwanted, the Actuality is in part what it is because of what they have done to it. The operations of other Actualities make a real, essential difference. An Actuality is what it has worked itself out to be in the face of the insistences and resistances of other Actualities. All of the Actualities together, as a result, constitute a single realm of Actuality in which the nature of each answers, as Leibniz saw, to the natures of the rest. Still, it is a fact that there are contingencies, irrelevancies. Although the effect of one Actuality on a second may be reckoned to the essence of that second, it is nevertheless true that the effect is what it is only because the Actualities happen to be in this rather than in that relation to one another.

Because Actualities are caught inside the frame of other modes of being they are affected in nonessential ways and bear the marks of the presence and action of those other modes. Thus, it is because they are sustained and interrelated by Existence that Actualities are open to experience. If, then, we wish to take our start with experience we will come to an Actuality as it essentially is, only if we can dislocate it from the thrall to which Existence subjects it. It must be freed from the particular space or time and from the spatial-temporal relations in which it happens to be. The dislocation may be physical or mental. Physically we dislocate an Actuality by holding it away from the others in space or by enabling it to persist in time. Mentally we dislocate it from space and time by attending to it, and thus offering it a role in thought, fancy or language.

3.50 The prescinding of qualities is a desirable dislocation.
(*See 3.10, 3.22, 3.49*)

ACTUALITIES subject their attributes to limitative conditions. The blue of this tie is near the brown of that desk; the blue goes wherever the tie does. The blue is subjected to irrelevant adventures by the tie, due to the fact that the tie infects the blue with an Existence not germane to it.

Distinguished qualities are derivative Actualities achieved by dislocating attributes from the Actualities in which they are resident. The simple act of sensing the blue is an act by which it is freed from the irrelevant career to which the tie subjects it. The sensing in fact frees it not only from irrelevancies, but from a subjugation by what in fact is inappropriate to its nature. If blue is anything like what it is sensed to be, nothing less than a sensing being is qualified to carry it. A dumb, unsensing tie cannot do justice to a sensed blue. Peirce, Whitehead, and Hartshorne, aware of this fact, and following in the tradition of Plotinus, Berkeley, and Kant, have gone on to suppose not that the tie is in fact insensitive, but that, as it were, it senses the blue from its own tie side. A simpler, more obvious and more adequate conclusion to draw is that which is often drawn by other thinkers and by most artists: the objects in the world are not the

best vehicles for the qualities they exhibit. To know what qualities
are we must dislocate them, hold them apart from the Actualities in
which they are attributes. Such a holding apart is achieved by virtue
of a concentration on the qualities, and an enjoyment of them without reference to the objects which sustain them.

Our very first perception requires a holding of a quality, if only
for a moment, apart from the object which happens to have it as
attribute. For that quality the reflective mind substitutes a predicate
or a universal, the idea of the quality freed from any particular
object, place, or time. The artist prefers to substitute a purer form
of the quality, in the shape of paint, sound, movement. The common
willingness of both to let qualities be freed from irrelevancies provides
a good meeting ground for the intellectual and the artist.

There is a sense, as conventionalists insist, in which any quality or
feature, any meaning or nature can be carried by any object. On this
view any sound, word, grammatical structure—stuff of any sort—
might provide an adequate support for an isolated feature or meaning.
And the very idea of "difficult beauty" substantiates this judgment.
No matter how ugly a thing may be, it is possible for an artist to so
embed it in something else as to make the product attractive and
even beautiful, and this without making us lose the ugly thing. But
it is also true that though any feature might be carried by any object,
some objects are more suited to carry some features than are others;
to make the least suited do the job that the more suited does may
require a radical change in the object, or involve the mastery of a
new way of rooting the feature in a new medium. In either case there
will be a recognition of the fact that features are not put into indifferent matters, but only into those which are receptive to those features,
either directly and simply, or via some basic reordering and making.

Strictly speaking, there are at least three kinds of blue: the blue in
the tie, the blue held away from the tie and everything else, and the
blue embedded in something other than that where it was first encountered. The pragmatist takes the first to be the true blue, the
phenomenologist takes the second, the Aristotelian and the panpsychist
take the third. The second isolates what is nuclear in the other two,
and in this sense does more justice than they do to the nature of the
color. What is hard to decide is whether or not the other two are
on a footing with respect to the color. The answer requires us to

know the nature of the isolated nucleus and to know to what degree this nucleus is hidden, blurred, distorted, inhibited by the different media. Sometimes, as in the case of shapes and numbers, the mind seems to provide a better carrier than things do; sometimes as in the case of action, Existence provides a better carrier than mind. In the case of mere qualities, such as blue, sometimes one medium and sometimes another allows the quality to function with the least distortion.

3.51   A dislocation of the natures of Actualities is desirable.
(See *1.07, 3.49, 3.50*)

ALTHOUGH the nature of an Actuality is integral to it, not in any way adventitious, exterior, or irrelevant, it is a nature which in itself has an intrinsic generality and purity that it does not have as infected by the Actuality. The Aristotelian judgment and the Husserlian phenomenological 'bracketing' offer different ways in which the natures of Actualities are freed, on the one side from the Actualities and the world in which they were encountered, and on the other side from the beliefs, hopes, suppositions, and usages to which knowers normally subject them. Aristotle and Husserl rightly and subtly exploit the process, begun in perception, to let the natures of Actualities find their own proper center of gravity, to let them be seen for what they really are in themselves apart from what the substantial interplaying Actualities reduce them to. These are great achievements.

3.52   The Ideal component in an Actuality should be dislocated, and conversely.
(See *1.21, 2.95, 3.49, 3.50*)

THERE IS a purposiveness to an Actuality because the Ideal terminates in it, affects it, and is partly inside it. As a consequence, every Actuality contains within it a universal which it has not altogether reduced to the status of bare fact.

The Platonic dialectic and the Schelerian and Hartmanian analyses offer different ways in which the Ideals in Actualities are freed, on the one side from their external Existential setting in Actualities and their world, and on the other side from the subjective judgments and interests of men. The converse effort, the freeing of Actuality from Ideality is characteristic of empiricism and positivism, the one em-

phasizing the limitations of the objective Ideal, the other the limitations of it as subjectively enjoyed. Kant's world of experience in his
first *Critique* exhibits both emphases.

No Actuality of course can be completely sundered from the Ideal
—or conversely. Indeed, every mode of being not only requires the
others to be, but must have those others as components in itself. When
then a mode of being or some facet of it is isolated or relocated, we
in effect do nothing more than discriminate a nucleal element in it,
and then try to have this element exhibited and eventually carried by
other modes in such a way as to enable it to express its native powers
and capacities with minimum distortion and maximum effect.

3.53 The divine component in an Actuality should be dislocated, and conversely.
(*See 1.23, 3.49, 3.50, 4.95*)

THE MYTH of Prometheus is a dramatic expression of man's awareness of the constraining effect that Actualities and their world have
on the divine. The life of Christ is another expression of the same
truth. The unchaining of Prometheus and the resurrection are modes
of dislocating the divine, of freeing it from the irrelevancies to which
Existence, particularly as evidenced in some Actuality, imposes on it.
The practices of the Yogi are designed primarily to promote this dislocation.

In the West the tendency is to think of God as over against the
individual, so that the freeing of the divine is a departure of it to
some other realm; in the East the tendency is to think of the self as
itself divine, so that the freeing of the divine is one with the freeing
of the self from the limitative, irrelevant adventures to which the
existing body subjects it. The converse dislocation of the Actual from
the divine is of course the act of creation, when viewed from the side
of God, and the act of commitment to nature, when viewed from the
side of the Actual.

3.54 Knowledge and art provide new carriers for freed Actualities, their qualities and natures.
(*See 1.64, 1.88, 1.94, 3.49–51*)

KNOWLEDGE involves judgment, the dislocation of features of objects and their unification in the mind under the aegis of a category

which the objects exhibit in limitative guises. The mind offers a new medium for the features, one which is superior to that which they had before, as is evident from the fact that their logical consequences can now be unfolded without hindrance or qualification. This new medium is related to the old; both are parts of one Existence, making possible a significant relating of them with the consequent accretion of the value 'truth' to what is judged.

Traditional, in contrast with the free art so characteristic of the present epoch, is dominated by a tendency to treat the new media, in which the artist embeds freed beings, qualities, and natures, as representing the very Existence in which those items had been orginially encountered. Items for it are freed, not for their own sake, but for the sake of exhibiting the world with more accuracy. The traditional master of painting does no less justice to qualities than others do today. But his concern is not with those qualities, with color and shape and relation, but with the outcome of these as in the new medium, and for the sake of showing what it is that the world, had it had such muscular colors, shapes, and relations to deal with, would have been able to exhibit. Existence in and apart from Actualities is viewed, not as that which arbitrarily limits those items, but as that which had unsatisfactory forms of those items to begin with. The embedding of the freed items inside media which are appropriate to them is thus, for the traditional artist, a way of symbolizing the nature of a purified existing world.

The attitude of the free artist is somewhat different. He concentrates on embedding the freed items, and particularly freed qualities, in media where they can be themselves, without regard for the limitative usages and meanings they have in experience. The more advanced of our modern painters, dancers, poets, and musicians offer so many different ways of giving freed qualities opportunities to exhibit themselves without regard for the way in which the outcome is related to the original encounter (as common sense tends to do) or to a purged version of it (as traditionalists tend to do). That we are still at the beginning of this venture is evident from the fact that what has now been attained in relation to some qualities has yet to be done with respect to freed Actualities and their natures, and this not only in painting but also in sculpture, architecture, drama, and fiction.

3.55   Myth provides a new carrier for freed Ideals.
(*See 3.50, 3.52, 3.54*)

THE IDEAL is encountered in Actualities in the guise of a meaning, value, or purpose. To dislocate that Ideal is to achieve something so tenuous that its presence is often denied. The medium of thought, though allowing freer play to the Ideal than that which was accorded it by the Actual, lacks substantiality even for those who have boldly affirmed the reality of meanings, standing over all else, and filling the purified mind. Almost at once one tends to turn the dislocated Ideal into a substance, to orient it in some more satisfactory being such as God. But these are precipitate treatments. Before the Ideal is treated as a substance or rooted in some other being, it should be given an appropriate mode of expression. This is one of the functions of myth. Here the Ideal is freed from the items in which it is encountered, given the cosmic dignity it deserves, allowed to express something of the dramatic and compulsive power it in fact has.

Ideologies, cosmogonies, popular religions are qualified myths having special relations to a people or society or culture. William Blake tried valiantly to forge a new mythology single-handed, but failed dismally; Wagner's and Yeats' failures in this regard were not as great but were nevertheless quite complete. Pure or qualified, the myth does not seem capable of being forged by a single individual, but to require an entire community.

3.56   Sacraments provide new carriers for a freed divine component.
(*See 3.50, 3.53, 3.54*)

SOLEMN CEREMONIES, festivals, dedicated communal activities are so many different media in which the divine, when freed from Actualities, obtains a more adequate, less distortive expression. To the degree they are successful they are sacraments, ways of enabling God to be immanent without being subjected to the arbitrary limitations to which the contingencies of the universe otherwise subject him.

Although the Jews have no doctrine of resurrection and reincarnation, they, with other religions, perpetually seek to isolate the divine component in things—particularly in various sacred books and objects

—and to provide him with his proper medium, themselves the chosen people. Apart from such reincarnations, God, when isolated as a factor in Actualities, takes on the guise of an absconding being, a Yahweh or Nirvana.

3.57 Criticism is the establishment of the import of freed items as carried by new media.

(*See 3.54-56*)

CRITICISM relates to human production. Its primary task is to make evident the extent to which the items have been freed from arbitrary governance, the appropriateness of the new media in which they are to be embedded, and the degree to which the items and the media do justice to one another. An awareness of the manner in which the freshest of artists and the boldest of speculative thinkers have read private prejudices and conventional limitative suppositions into the new carriers of freed items, provides for the recognition of styles, characteristics, modes, fashions, which qualify the new media and consequently the outcome of an embedding of freed items within those media. The charges of barbarism in ideology and of magic in sacramental practices have their counterpart in charges of perversion in the arts.

The drip painting method of Hofmann and Pollock is an attempt to provide freed qualities with a medium in no way affected by human prejudgment or bias. But this method overlooks the fact that an individual and a paint brush which move at "random" are actually moving under rather restrictive conditions and habits, with the result that in place of the limitations imposed by human prejudgment we get the limitations imposed by the conditions which happen to be operative in fact. By an irregular route one thus returns to the very type of conditioning from which one had originally sought to escape. A similar attempt at avoiding bias in mythology and sacramental activities—and subject to similar criticisms—is to be found in the frenzies of rhapsodes and in the religious use of auguries, omens, signs, portents, and tongues.

A comparison of the creative embodiments of freed entities with one another offers more hope of making us aware of the arbitrary limitations to which those items are put, even by the most creative of men, than 'randomness' can. Such comparison can cut across time or across space, the one yielding the data for comparative historical judgments, the other for comparative sociological judgments. It is because we know what a purified object is like that we can recognize that the new medium does not distort as much as the old. But in the end the giving to freed items a less distortive carrier than they had also proves inadequate, precisely because it places the item alongside other types of freed phenomena, and allows it to be affected by them. We must make use of another method, that of epitomization, if we are to know just what are (and are to free ourselves and objects from) arbitrary limitations.

3.58 Maximal freedom from nonessential qualifications by Existence, objective and human, is achieved through epitomization.
(*See 3.49, 3.54–57*)

THE AWARENESS of the limitations of the media provided in creative enterprises has led some of the most daring minds to embrace a Pythagoreanism, the use of mathematics as the frame in which to place various dislocated items. Numerology and astrology carry the practice out with respect to the divine component; theories of the grand cycle and of rhythms in history have a similar purpose in relation to the Ideal component; the 'golden section' and physiological typologies make an analogous attempt with respect to Actualities. The freed items, in these various cases, it is thought, can have no more appropriate medium than that provided by mathematics. But when one turns to the mathematician to determine how he ascertains just what determines the length, punctuation, structure of the continuum in which he seeks to embed his own ideas, we find that he looks to aesthetics, or occasionally, as with Newton, to theology, and sometimes even, as the Russians apparently do, to sociology. The most appropriate media for freed items evidently go beyond the limitations even of mathematics. Perhaps no one saw this so clearly as Plato, the last step of whose dialectic led him beyond mathematics to what conditions it and all else as well.

Epitomization is the creative embodiment of items which had been freed from the limitations of art, mythology, and sacrament, in ways that permit the items to have others in the form of special subordinate cases. The epitomization of qualities leads to the 'grand style,' where this or that quality is taken to be central and to govern an entire set of occurrences. It is this which the great actor perpetually seeks to and sometimes does attain. But no quality is rich enough to encompass all that needs to be said; in the end, as in the beginning, a quality is a derivative phenomenon and must be sustained by something more substantial than itself. Each great actor ends a period; to repeat his grand characteristic gesture is but to imitate him, and thus trap a fresh movement inside an arbitrarily restricted frame; to make a similar attempt with respect to some other gesture is to belong to his school, and exhibit a variant of what he epitomized. Nothing less than a return to experience for a fresh encounter with qualities, a new creative use of them, and a consequent epitomization will provide those who are occupied with qualities the opportunity to have a grand style themselves.

The case is different with Actuality, Ideality, and God—and the residual Existence which remains when they are maximally freed from it. Epitomization of these, in the limitative guise of great men, great ethical ideals, great religions, and great civilizations, or more adequately but abstractly in the guise of categoreal characterizations of the modes of being, alone permits of the proper subordination, clarification, and evaluation of all else.

The purified entities and epitomizations which we have so far considered take their rise with modes of being which have been subjected to limitations imposed by Existence. Analogous epitomizations can be achieved with divinized, actualized, and idealized modes. Thus, one who starts with an idealized Actuality can through acts of specification, limitation, inference, and so on, isolate the meaning of the Actuality contained within the Ideal. This which is isolated is still affected by and bears the marks of the Ideal. To know what Actuality is apart from the Ideal, one would have to operate on the outcome by means of speculation, dialectic, proof, and direct encounter. Only if we go on to make use of these will we be able to know, starting with an idealized Actuality, what Actuality is by itself, what it is for it to be an irreducible mode of being. Similar observations are to be made with respect to the derivation and cognition of the other modes of being.

V   HISTORY

3.59   Existence is made integral to and thus specified by
Actualities when and as they change in state and position.
(See 1.31, 1.32, 3.37, 3.39, 3.48)

THE EXISTENCE of an Actuality is qualified by the nature of that
Actuality. In turn, the Existence makes a difference to that nature,
involving it in adventures and serving to ground a relation which connects the Actuality with other Actualities and other beings. As a single
being, Existence pulls on every part of itself to be together with the
rest, though in oppositional ways. This pull, exerted on the Existence
in an Actuality, compels the Actuality to make an effort to keep and
renew its hold on Existence. What it has of Existence two moments
together cannot, strictly speaking, be described as having the same or
different nature in itself, for it is the Actuality which gives that portion of Existence whatever nature it has. Subsequent Actualities cannot therefore be said to possess an Existence which once belonged to
some previous Actuality, though it is the case that the Existence present today is the very Existence which had been before, and which had
been divided in various ways by the Actualities that existed before.

Actualities exist, the Ideal exists, God exists, and even Existence
exists. Ideas exist, space exists, attributes exist—anything indeed that
is in any sense. But none of the others exists in the very way in which
Actualities do. When Descartes said that he thinks and therefore exists,
he supposed that the Existence which was integral to his ideas had
the very same nature at that part of Existence which was integral to
his self or mind. But he had no right to that inference.

Hume was more precise. He rightly affirmed that every impression
had a distinct existence. It is of the essence of Hume's position, in
fact, to hold that the ontological argument is valid for every single
item of experience whatsoever. Everything had its own existence,
thought he, and that was the end of the matter. "The idea of existence
is nothing different from the idea of any object." That was his warrant
for the supposition that the Existence and the impression in which it is
integral need not or cannot be explained. But it is important to note

that Humean impressions can neither move nor change. They need not and in fact cannot struggle to retain a hold on Existence and thereby keep apace with that Existence as it surges forward into the uncharted future. But this is what Actualities try to and sometimes can do. They and Existence do not make the kind of unity which Hume recognized to hold of impressions.

3.60   Existence imposes a limit on what Actualities and other realities can do, and do with it.
(See 1.06, 3.01, 3.06–8, 3.59)

EXISTENCE has its own nature, its own rhythm, its own way of working out its destiny. It grounds space and time, and exhibits cosmic laws; it dictates to Actualities and other beings the need to struggle if they are to maintain themselves in time. These others have their effect on it as well. No untouchable, rigid domain, it is infected by Actualities, Ideals, and God who, through their integration of portions of Existence with themselves, inevitably impose limitations on the rest of it. But precisely because Existence is in each in a different way, because it is a single domain, enjoying an ultimacy of being of its own, it has a greater effect on the Existence in them than they have on it.

3.61   At any moment beings are at different stages of typical careers.
(See 3.59)

ACTUALITIES persist, and because they do, they can be correctly said to be younger than they will be at some later time, and older than they had been at some earlier time. Philosophers such as Descartes, Hume, Whitehead, and perhaps even Kant, who tend to suppose that there are no persistent Actualities, ought also to say that no Actuality is older than any other. Each is new born, and lives but a moment. Descartes and Whitehead make provision for some kind of repetition and continuity, and can speak of older and younger, not with reference to the Actualities they might encounter at any one moment, but with reference to the number of times these Actualities had been resurrected, or with respect to the length of a temporal "society" in which they might be included. But if at a given moment the Actualities do not bear the marks of having been in existence at some previous time, those Actualities cannot ground a characterization of themselves as younger or older in relation to themselves as at other times, or in comparison with other contemporary Actualities.

To say that one thing is older than another is to say that it had been in existence for some time. This we have warrant for saying only if (a) we had encountered it for a period of time, (b) it bears the marks of having been in existence for a while, or (c) it has a nature which required maturation, so that it must be somewhat along in a career. Whereas the first is consistent with an object remaining wholly unaltered for a period, and the second with its retaining the same type of features for a while, the third requires a recognition of directed changes in some of its features. The first gives us the material for memory, the second our evidence for dating, and the third provides us with data for a grounded knowledge of the past. The first tells us that it has occupied our attention, the second that it has endured, and the third that it has a history. The third depends on the second, and the second on the first.

3.62   Attention has a temporal span.
(See 3.59)

IF NOTHING can occupy our attention for a while, we could have only momentary contents; if nothing has occupied our attention for a while we could have had only momentary contents. But if we are presented with any evidence, that evidence could not be known without our holding it before us for a while, so that the very presentation of the evidence designed to show that nothing occupies our attention for a span of time would be evidence to show that something does. It might of course be urged that we might have evidence given us in a flash; but such evidence as occupying just the present moment would not be known, and if it could be known would be in no position to tell us whether or not there is a longer time span, and whether or not we had occupied it while we were noting the evidence.

3.63   No evidence can be provided to show that nothing endures.
(See 3.59, 3.62)

FOR SOMETHING to be had as evidence it must be attended to for a time. To attend to it we must continue to be. As soon as we confront any evidence, therefore, no matter what it claims to support, we know that it will support the truth that something endures. It is conceivable of course that we could have been just created with all the ideals we now have and with the belief that some of them had been attended to for a while. But we could provide no evidence in support of this contention, and if we go so far as to consider it, we will thereby demonstrate that at least we ourselves endure for a while.

3.64   Evidence that beings are of different ages can be judged untrustworthy only if there is a truth more basic than that some beings are older than others.
(*See 3.61, 3.63*)

THE PRESENT chicken is no more and no less present than the present chick; the present dusty, torn, yellowed document dated 1700 is now no more and no less present than the clean sheet alongside it. The yellowed document is here, fully, totally, exactly on a footing with the clean sheet of paper alongside. To look at it is to see nothing but what is in the present. It is yellow now, torn now, dusty now. That it was made in just that way at the same time that the clean sheet was made is conceivable; if so, both will have endured for the same length of time. It is conceivable even that both had been produced just an instant ago; if so we will have attended to them for a short period of time, through which they too will have endured. It is also conceivable that the yellowed paper was made as a yellowed paper a while ago. It will then be a yellowed enduring paper. In none of these cases ought we to say of the yellow paper (in contrast with what we can rightly say of a clean sheet which yellowed in the course of time) that it is *older* than the clean sheet. (New elements today being produced by fission are apparently somewhat like a yellowed sheet which had been made yellowed from the start; unaffected by the passage of time, each has an appropriate "life-span," at the end of which we can truly say of it, not that it had such and such an age, but that it had endured for such and such a period.)

We begin to move to history only when we have a warrant for ordering phenomena as punctuating different stages of a career. The historic consciousness begins with some such acknowledgment as that a chicken is an older chick. When Adam opened his eyes he presumably saw chicks and chickens, saplings and full grown trees. If he had an historical consciousness he would have been aware that some of the beings were older than others, and originated therefore at an earlier time than those others. If God had just created that world, he must either have denied Adam the power to relate the different objects as being at different stages in typical careers, or he tempted him to infer wrongly that the world had been in existence for some time. Accordingly we must say that if God created the universe just a moment ago, with dusty yellow paper and clean sheets, with chicks and chickens, saplings and oaks, God, for the historical consciousness, is one who lures man to err. For the historical consciousness the world always offers evidence that it was not created.

3.65 Knowledge of the past is inferentially derived from present evidence that some Actualities have different ages, and thus had origins at different dates.
(*See 1.76, 3.44, 3.46, 3.64*)

THE PAST is not directly experienced; we cannot enter into it without making it cease to be that past. Nor could it have been constructed by us without ceasing to be that out of which the present issued. Still, we can *know* it. Our knowledge of it is a consequence of our experience and understanding of present Actualities, supported by inference and reconstruction.

Confronted with a yellowed torn document covered with dust, the historian acknowledges it to have attained this state gradually over the years. He assumes that the document was first a white clean sheet and that it gradually became yellow, torn, and dusty—that is to say, he assumes that it has a different age from that of other present objects, and that the date of its origin therefore is distinct from theirs. It is not his endeavor to see the document freed from its accumulations—he does not want to tamper with it at all. Instead he seeks to interpret it by treating its present features as outcomes which can be traced back to their origins by means of plausible transformational rules, which presumably reverse the laws governing the process of Existence by which the document became what it now is.

3.66 A history is reconstructive.
(*See 3.65*)

AN HISTORIAN does not report the past; to report something one must first have some acquaintanceship. Nor does he rethink the thoughts of the past, as Collingwood supposed, for he is concerned not with thoughts but with facts, some of which are outside the area of thought. If he were concerned with thoughts he could not get to those that were past; and if he could get to them he could not really rethink them.

Taking advantage of what he knows of the laws of nature, man, and society, the historian attempts to retrace in his mind the steps by which the present came to be. A number of such retracements gives him pivotal past facts around which he reconstructs the nature of a situation which he supposes once existed. This reconstruction he tests by seeing whether or not, following out the laws of man, society, and nature as terminating in those facts, he can pass necessarily from that past nexus to subsequent facts, and eventually arrive at those facts which constitute some signal state of affairs, or at those which are in the present. It is the evidences of today that tell him that there was once a first world war, whose nature he now reconstructs to portray a situation which no one then living could have known, since none could have had the perspective and the information he now has. But this reconstruction he cannot distinguish from a fiction until he can arrive, in an intelligible plausible way over the course of an inter-connected set of facts at, say, the second world war.

What the historian produces is an account, an epistemic history. So far as he is accurate this answers to a history that has in fact taken place, an ontologic history. This ontologic history is part of a larger past, containing such nonhistoric items as the vibrations of subatomic particles, the feelings of uninfluential individuals, the shifts in sand and the waves of the sea. It is this ontologic history which the historian, with some dramatic license, and with the punctuation required by discourse and judgment, reconstructs.

3.67   Historic occurrences have significant beginnings and endings.
(See 1.43, 3.04)

THERE is nothing which suddenly begins, without preliminary or antecedent condition; there are no absolute endings. Each moment melts into the next, and what is in one is continuous with what is another. Still, there are significant beginnings and significant endings. There is a climactic character to events; they do have origins and termini, even though it be the case that those origins are but the outcome of some antecedent activity, and those termini but lead on to still others.

Historic occurrences are events with natures which provide a link between the nature of a beginning and the nature of an ending. A charge in a battle, the signing of a document, the abdication of a king are historic occurrences whose natures relate characteristic beginnings and endings. Were there no such natures, history would be the outcome of arbitrary divisions in a continuum, having no reality apart from the arbitrary decisions of men to divide it this way or that, and to characterize it in one set of terms rather than another.

3.68   The beginning of an historic occurrence is relevant to its end.
(*See 1.37, 3.67*)

ONE ITEM is relevant to another if its nature affects the nature of that other. The affecting is an occurrence having a nature of its own. One item is relevant to another therefore in a context defined by a connecting nature. The beginning of an historic occurrence accordingly, has a nature which determines the nature of the end through the mediation of a third nature, that of the occurrence. The acknowledgment of a beginning of an historic occurrence thus requires an antecedent identification of the end and of the nature of the occurrence which can mediate this with the beginning.

Because the captain was not given the aid promised him, his charge failed. The beginning of the historic occurrence, "an unsupported charge," as terminating in "failure of the charge" is "the failure of promised aid." The failure of the promised aid to arrive at such and such a time is the terminus of a different occurrence, let us say, "the failure to organize troops and supplies." We have here two distinct historic occurrences, the second of our cases representing the immediate antecedent of the first. The two occurrences are (*a*) "the failure to organize troops and supplies," and (*b*) "an unsupported charge." The end of *a*, "the failure of promised aid" is also the beginning of *b*. The beginning of *a*, "the major's decision" is not relevant to the ending of *b*, "failure of the charge." The charge of course failed because the major made the wrong decision, but the decision is not the beginning of the historic occurrence of a charge ending in failure. Decisions do not begin charges, though they may help qualify their character. The occurrence of the unsupported charge begins with the failure of promised aid; that this beginning in turn has the role of an ending in a preceding historic occurrence makes possible a traversal back in history; it does not affect the fact that it is a part of two distinct historic occurrences.

3.69   History provides explanations of facts in terms of transformations produced by Existence.
(*See 1.76, 3.65, 3.66, 3.68*)

HISTORY seeks to explain occurrences in the light of what had previously been the case. It starts with some fact and tries to get to know some fact antecedent to this by means of transformation rules imposed on the given fact. The transformation rules by means of which it gets to the antecedent fact presumably permit of a reversal of the transformations produced by Existence in the course of its relentless movement forward, both inside and outside Actualities. Having arrived at the antecedent fact by means of these transformation rules, a history can then proceed to connect this fact with the given fact by means of the converse of those rules, and thus by means of the very transformation rules that Existence presumably exemplified. In doing this it usually discovers that there are many intermediate outcomes between an antecedent fact and the given fact; these intermediate outcomes terminate subordinate historic occurrences.

Some intermediate outcomes usually become conspicuously evident in the course of a process of moving from some past fact to an initially acknowledged subsequent fact. It is the historian's awareness of the importance of these outcomes that leads him to attend not merely to the transformation rules exemplified by Existence, in the large, but also to the limited transforming rules which Existence exhibits when it is part of subordinate historic occurrences. He is concerned, say, with learning as much as he possibly can about a crucial but unsuccessful charge. Having begun with the charge as a signal present outcome, he moves back to some antecedent fact which is at the origin of that outcome, and then moves forward so far as his sense of importance and his awareness of historic occurrences permits. The awareness of the importance of some intermediate outcome usually enables him to focus on a subsequent otherwise neglected historic occurrence; his grasp of the nature of that occurrence enables him to explain an important less remote occurrence and eventually perhaps, through the mediation of a number of historic occurrences, the signal fact with which he began.

3.70 Historic occurrences have different temporal spans.
(*See 3.67, 3.68*)

USUALLY a battle takes less time to be won or lost than a war does. Both are occurrences. Both are real. Taken as units, each defines a history in which the unit of the other is either a part that must, because shorter, be abstract, or must, because longer, be at least partly inclusive of and perhaps in part a product of the smaller.

A history of battles is quite a different thing from a history of a war. The former must articulate a war, the latter must be periodized in battles. The one will deal neither with the beginning nor the ending of the war, though of course it will have a first and a last battle. The other will deal neither with the beginning nor the ending of battles, though of course whatever battles it notes will be recognized to have limited spans, even when they merge one into another.

3.71 There are unit measures for the historic past.
(*See 3.43, 3.70*)

WHILE the battle is fought, the battle is not yet determinate in nature. When the battle is over, the war usually is not yet determinate; as a rule it takes a longer time for the nature of the war to come to be than it does for a battle's. But as past the battle is just as determinate as the war. Both are over and done with, differing only in the length of the series of facts which they comprise. To use the shorter as a unit is to define the longer to be that which can be measured by the shorter; to use the longer as a unit is to define the shorter to be a distinct subdivision of the longer.

In the past the battles completely articulate the war and the war completely divides into battles. A history which is to do justice to the past recognizes this. It therefore presents the war as divided into battles, and the battles as summing up to the war—leaving out of course, for the sake of illustration, all the other elements which go to make up a war, such as preparations and alliances, general staff, and so on.

3.72   There are no determinate historic occurrences in the present.
(*See 3.70, 3.71*)

A WAR has no determinate nature until it is fought—and the fighting usually takes years. But we live by moments. The war has a determinate nature only after it is over. As a war it has full being only in the past. And what is true of the war is true of the battles, and what is true of the battles is true of the charge. We come to the end of such a process of subdivision when we arrive at unit historic occurrences, taking up only unit historic times. These can be subdivided too, until at last we arrive at final unit events and extended units of time. Were there no such final extended units of time, there would be no temporal spread at all, for out of nonextendeds no extension can be achieved. Those units cannot be divided into an *earlier* and *later* part without losing their meaning and being. They can of course be divided in thought into a part which comes *before* and another which comes *after*, but these must not be separated out to constitute distinct events at different times.

Times comes in gulps, in atomic moments, but these moments or gulps are too short for history. We live successively in and through nonhistoric moments, but thereby bring about a sequence of moments which have a nature that can be exhibited only so far as that sequence is past. What is now taking place is not history until it is over.

In the present only nonhistoric units are real; they alone constitute the present. They alone are neither too short not too long to encompass what is now taking place. But as in the past, the nonhistoric unit is a subdivision of an historic occurrence, no more, but also no less real than those occurrences.

3.73   Incompleted historic occurrences are grounded in the present.
(*See 3.72*)

WHEN the battle achieves a determinate nature as an historic occurrence, the war may not yet be over. Still the battle is a battle in that war. The nature or essence of the war affects that of the battle, as surely as the nature of the battle determines the nature of the war.

The war, while the battle is being fought, is a possibility which the battle is actualizing; it is an essential connection relating the battle to other possible battles and occurrences, a unity of meaning which gives structure to the sequence of incidents in the battle and what will follow on it. And what is true of the war in relation to the battle is true of the battle in relation to smaller historic occurrences, and so on until we reach a limit in that unit nonhistoric occurrence which alone can be present.

An atomic moment has too short a span to accommodate an historic occurrence. But were the historic occurrence not in some way involved in the atomic moment, an acknowledgment of an historic occurrence in the past would then be an acknowledgment of something alien to what actually took place. The smallest historic occurrence is an effective mode of relating a unit present occurrence to what is concurrent and to what in fact follows. Within that historic occurrence there are more and more attenuated, indeterminate patterns of occurrences demanding longer and longer temporal spans in order to be exhibited as the natures of historic occurrences. The longest possible historic occurrence terminates in the Ideal or abstract Future; like every other historic occurrence, it is rooted in an atomic nonhistoric occurrence.

Because there are more limited possibilities than that of the mere Future, there are possible historic occurrences of varying lengths. A present nonhistoric occurrence grounds a plurality of indeterminate historic patterns of occurrences of different lengths, because it is related to a plurality of possibilities more and more indeterminate, and more and more remote, of which the furthest is the all-inclusive Future.

3.74 Every historic occurrence must be at least two moments long.
(*See 3.67, 3.71, 3.72*)

A UNIT historic occurrence has a longer span than a unit physical occurrence. It has a nature which relates the nature of something earlier with the nature of something later. Since those natures are not fully realized until the occurrences which they terminate have in fact occurred, the historic occurrence which links them must be at least two moments long. The longer an historic occurrence, the longer is the sequence and the greater is the number of moments of nonhistoric occurrences which it includes.

A war comprises all the incidents that occur from its beginning to its end, but it is better analyzed as a sequence of battles than as a sequence of charges. Each type of historic occurrence has its own type of unit. The natures of those units require spans less than that of the given historic occurrence, but greater than that of any other type of event contained within that occurrence.

Physical occurrences such as a combining of chemicals, a waning of the moon, and so on, which take more than a unit of time to be realized, are to be understood in ways similar to that in which historic occurrences are to be understood. But there are differences. The difference between physical occurrences of more than unit length and historical occurrences is a difference between two equally real and significant modes of linking unit physical occurrences. The shooting of Lincoln is at once nonhistoric and historic. As nonhistoric it relates to a bullet in its flight and the piercing of a man's flesh, and so on, with its inevitable, predictable outcome. As historic it relates to an assassination as a way of connecting the bullet with the contingent tempers, proximity, etc., of Booth and Lincoln.

There are some who hold all nature to be a special case of history, others who take all history to be a special case of nature, still others who think that the two of them are equally real but distinct and perhaps even wholly independent. But only the view that they are equally real, equally immersed in Existence, relating what are sometimes the very same events in different patterns, thus giving them different successors and therefore meanings, allows us to say that the assassination of a president is the killing of a man, i.e., is at once a social, an historical, and a physical occurrence.

3.75   An historic field contains a number of occurrences not related in sequence.
(See 3.74)

A HISTORY embraces a number of sequences of historic occurrences. It spreads over space as well as over time. As spreading in both these ways it constitutes an historic field. Within that field there may be an occurrence which occupies its entire temporal length. But whether

there be such an occurrence or not, there must also be other occurrences in it which take place within the time span of that field. A
war comprises many battles, some of them fought at the same time.
Some of those battles may have begun just as others are ending; other
battles will overlap more completely. But all the battles are contained
within the field of the war.

3.76   An epoch is a field of works of art, structured by myth, and sacramentally unified.
(See 3.54-56)

WORKS OF ART are the outcome of the embodiment of freed qualities, Actualities and their natures; sacraments are the outcome of the
embodiment of a freed divine element; myths are the outcome of the
embodiment of a freed ideal component. Taken in their spatial and
temporal spread they constitute a field inside of which multiple occurrences take place, occurrences which exemplify these three types
of embodiment, or some mixture of them. As a rule it is the myth
which defines an *epoch,* the others serving to qualify and punctuate it.
But an epoch can have as its dominant note either sacraments or works
of art. It may thus be primarily cultural, religious, or aesthetic.

3.77   A civilization is a field containing great men, given direction by an ethical norm, and unified by a religion.
(See 3.58)

THE LIMITATIONS to which an epoch subjects Actualities and their
features, the Ideal and God, should be overcome. The overcoming of
these limitations involves a further freeing of Actualities, the Ideal,
and God, so as to make them fundamental to the understanding and
the being of all else. When these elements are rooted in a freed Existence, they respectively appear in the guise of works of art, i.e., as
great men; in the guise of an effective historic ideal, i.e., as an ethical
norm; and in the guise of the divine in history, i.e., as a dominant
religion.

A great man—Hebrew prophet, Greek hero, Christian saint—is an
Actuality, freed, maximized, given locus in a civilization. An ethical
norm, say of public welfare, whether consciously entertained or not,
and expressed in terms of material goods, pleasures, virtue, or activity,
is the Ideal component in Existence, freed, maximized, and made his-

torically relevant. A religion, institutionalized or not, expressed in rituals, beliefs, creeds, or works, is the divine component in Existence, freed, maximized, and reintroduced into the purged Existence. All three are as close to the being of Actuality, Ideality, and God as it is possible for one to get who starts from and remains within the area of Existence.

A civilization is a spatiotemporal historic field, carrying all three epitomizations as qualitative modifications of an epitomized Existence. Each can serve as the medium for the others. A great religion sustains great men, ethics, and civilizations; e.g., Christianity offers a medium for the production of saints, summas, and states. A great man, e.g., a Mohammed, serves as the medium for a great religion, civilization, and ethics. A great civilization, e.g., the Greek, sustains heroes, philosophies, and mysteries. One or the other of these epitomizations may be dominant, and mixtures of them may occur at any time. But in any case, within the civilization, an epoch—not necessarily of shorter duration—can be found which specializes and delimits the epitomized elements. And within the epoch there are smaller historic fields, with shorter temporal spans and smaller spatial spreads.

3.78   The men of a given civilization constitute a people.
(See 3.77)

THE NATURE of a civilization is constituted by men, a religion, and an ethical norm. The men are affected by and affect the religion and norm.

A *people* includes all the men in the civilization. Only a few of those men may be definitory of that civilization, but all of them express it in various degrees. Great men, by virtue of their excellence as Actualities, help define the nature of the civilization; but as individual beings, as finite, unit beings, they are, as are all the other men in that civilization, part of the people in which that civilization is expressed and carried.

There are of course many things that men do which have no ostensible reference to their greatness, their religion, or their ideals. These things can be understood to constitute a kind of civilization when this is treated as the outcome of delimited versions of men, religion, and ideals. Just as a war has its heroes, its faith, and its dedication, industry can be said to have men of magnitude, a more or less explicit unity reflecting the meaning of the dominant religion in that context, and an objective which is in some accord with other objectives in that society. Together these express in a specialized form the characteristics of a civilization.

3.79   A guided people make up the body of a civilization whose nature is defined primarily by great men.
(*See 3.77*)

IN SOME civilizations, great men are at the center; it is what they say and do and think which dictates the nature of the religion and the kind of ideal that all will pursue, and thereby determine what the nature of that civilization will be. The Golden Age of Greece seems to be one such civilization, the time of the Hebraic prophets another, early Christianity a third, the Reformation a fourth. At the present time, India is a civilization with a major focus on Gandhi and the men he inspired. In all these, the religions and ethics take much of their color from great men, the primary source of the character of the civilization.

In historic fields of smaller compass than a civilization a similar dominance by men, great not as men but in some enterprise such as art, can often be discerned. Bach defines a world of music and gives a new meaning to religion and the ideals carried by it; Shakespeare has the same effect in drama; Napoleon has a similar role in the art of war, and so on.

There is no steady relation which great dominant men have to religion and ethical norms, since the men are remade by the very items that they qualify. An Augustine is changed by the very religion and ethics he helps define, as is a Schweitzer or a Gandhi. Yet it is these men who constitute the nature of their civilizations; the religions and ethics qualify, enrich, and extend that nature rather than the reverse. The people in such civilizations is a *guided* people, a people led or inspired primarily by humans who are works of art, i.e., great men.

3.80   A religious people make up the body of a civilization whose nature is defined primarily by a religion.
(*See 2.86, 3.77*)

RELIGION as public, social activity is expressed in institutions, ceremonies, rituals, and sacramental objects. It need make no reference to any supernatural or personal being, though it must make a reference to something permanent and of value.

An entire people might share a religion and yet may have no genuine faith. Their activities may be routine, conventional, habitual, unreflecting. Nevertheless, even their religion cannot be wholly confined inside a state. The range of a state's interests, ideals, and time span leave out too much to make possible the exhaustion of a religion inside its limits. But the religion could be encompassed in a civilization, for what a religion takes to be permanent might exhaust its being or its functions over the whole of the time in which the civilization exists. There are, however, religions which cannot be kept inside the confines of a civilization since they judge, oppose, criticize all civilizations, insisting on values no civilization could encompass.

It seems quite evident that there was a time when the Hebrews had a religiously dominated civilization. The Middle Ages offers a different civilization, but one which was also religiously dominated. Islam (and, before the English domination, India) seems also to be properly characterizable in this way. In these civilizations there are great men. These men presuppose the religion, even when they contribute to it and reconstitute it. The prevailing ethics, too, clearly presupposes the dominant religion.

Different virtues, objectives, and values are stressed in different religious civilizations. The Hebrews emphasize an adherence to the law, the Christians the act of love, Islam the virtue of obedience, the Hindu renunciation, and the Buddhist compassion. No one of these stresses, of course, is ever pure or unrelated to the others, and no one of them means in the context of its civilization what it means for those who view it from without. Each civilization expresses its own virtues and the virtues of the others in quite different ways.

3.81   An ethical people make up the body of civilization whose nature is defined primarily by an ethical ideal.
(See 3.55, 3.77)

AN ETHICAL PEOPLE is one which has isolated the Ideal as it is found in experience, and has overcome the limitations which myth imposes. For generations the Chinese and perhaps also the Japanese have been under the domination of an ethical civilization, to which their religions and great men were also subject. The great Chinese is not a saint and not a hero but a good man; the religion of a Confucian is a qualifying note in an ethical life.

It is somewhat common practice to speak of the Hebrews as though they also had an ethical civilization, and sometimes it is said that the Romans had one. But it is hard to escape from the religious temper of the Hebrews; the brooding presence of God perpetually pervades their civilization. And the Romans seem to have stressed great men more than any ideal, though their great men, to be sure, were acknowledged to be men supreme in virtue. Much however could be said in defense of the view that it is our own current civilization which is essentially ethical, with a dominant ideal qualified by Christianity on the one side, and by outstanding men, of quite different types, on the other. Evidence for this opinion is to be found in the fact that the hero, the prophet, and the saint are not now, as they once were, thought to be superior to or different from ethical men, but are instead taken to be just ethical men who are more daring or gifted or religious than the rest.

3.82 There are three types of civilization.
(See 3.79–81)

A CIVILIZATION is Existence epitomized and serving to characterize an historic occurrence encompassing a people. Civilizations have cross-currents, and their various parts move at different paces; it is doubtful whether there ever was a civilization in which the people were purely of one type. Not only do civilizations gradually pass into one another, not only are they subject to various contingencies, but each has strands which stress features of other types as well. A Christian world does not altogether exclude the existence of heroes of the Greek sort; nor does it exclude the merely ethical man, alert to obligation and negligent of his own perfection as a human being. The civilizations which have dotted the course of history mix great men, religion, and ethics in various degrees and ways. But this does not preclude a fairly accurate characterization of many of them as stressing one of these and thus as being primarily of one type rather than another.

A confusion between types of civilizations and actual civilizations seems to be behind the transition some historians make from a *philosophy of history* to a *philosophical history*. A philosophy of history dissects and analyzes, compares and categorizes; it attempts to isolate the main features of an historic occurrence, to characterize the nature of civilizations, and to indicate their basic varieties. A philosophical history tries to show that history has a definite pattern and outcome. Such philosophical historians as Hegel, Marx, Spengler, and Toynbee suppose that civilizations have inevitable termini, and give way to others in a definite predictable way. But there is no need to suppose that civilizations necessarily succeed one another in any particular order, or that the whole of history has a predesignatable structure and terminus.

3.83   A people exhausts its being and meaning in a civilization.
(See 3.78)

A PEOPLE is the body of a civilization. When that civilization passes the people passes as well. It has no other nature, no other life than that which it had within that civilization. It is foolish to say that the historic Greeks should not have had slaves. To take away the slaves from them, even in thought, is to take them out of their civilization. As an historic people they are no more or less or other, and could not be more or less or other than they in fact were. If we limit our historic field or concentrate on even a short occurrence, a similar consequence must be drawn. We cannot say of the historic Plato that he could have written another dialogue additional to those he had written; we could not rightly say that he could have written even another syllable, if by the historic Plato we mean the man who, at the time such a dialogue or syllable would have to be written, was in fact doing something quite different. The Plato who was sleeping or walking or trying to govern was at those times in no position to write anything; but that Plato is the historic Plato. Just so, the Greeks are the people who did whatever they did do during the period of their civilization; to say of them that they might have or should have done this or that is to tear them out of the world where they in fact were Greeks, and to view them as something distinct from the actual historic people that they were.

3.84   A people's potentialities are not exhausted in a civilization.
(See 3.43, 3.78, 3.83)

EVERY BEING that persists through time has potentialities. To say that it is exhausted in the occurrence where it has a beginning and an end is in effect to say that it perishes without any unused potentialities.

Every being, it would then have to be said, inescapably fulfills itself. This is absurd, flying in the face of our awareness that a baby dies with a life unlived, and that the most aged of men still has potentialities unrealized. Yet it seems equally absurd to suppose that there are genuine potentialities in the dead, factual past. There is nothing that the dead *can* do, and this is one with saying that they have no potentialities.

When we view a people in the past as the predecessor of another, we see the people as not yet having fulfilled itself. When we view a people as in the civilization where alone it has its historic full being, we see it as a people whose potentialities are wholly expressed and fulfilled there. In the one case the people is thought of as demanding a successor, as having potentialities which cannot be actualized by itself as contained within that civilization; in the other case the people is thought of as apart from every successor, and as being just what it in fact is. Its "unrealized potentialities" then but express the fact that its Existence has moved on to a successor.

A potentiality must be realized. If it remained unrealized it would in effect be that which the universe precluded from being realized. But what could not possibly be realized is not a potentiality at all. What realizes such a potentiality is the process by which other beings and people come about. The being and the people are not thereby ennobled. They pass away, and that passing away may be regrettable, tragic. The historic occurrence that they define or constitute might conceivably have been richer had they continued to be.

In one sense then every being and every people passes away with itself fulfilled as just that being and people, no more, no less, no other. In another sense a being or people passes away unfulfilled, less than it could have been. And in a third sense, every being and people is inevitably fulfilled in that it is followed by other beings and people. In the first case we stress the determinate nature, in the second the promise, and in the third the role which the beings and people play in history.

3.85 A people has a nature not exhausted in a civilization.
(*See 3.73, 3.83, 3.84*)

JUST as a man can be a swimmer even when he is not in the water, just as a child is a genuine human though it has not yet exhibited fully the human nature that it has, so a people can have a nature which it has not yet made fully manifest. In addition to the *ingredient* part of the nature that a being then and there possesses, concrete, individualized, exhausted, there is a *relational* part which links it with others, with what will be. The nature of a being in history is partly ingredient and partly relational.

A people's nature has an ingredient and a relational part. The latter is fully expressed and exhausted not in the civilization of that people but in the way in which that people becomes transformed into its successor. The manner in which the Greek civilization gave way to the Roman embodied that residuum which the Greeks did not exhaust in their civilization.

3.86   A people has an organic unity not exhausted in a civilization.
(*See 3.83, 3.84, 3.85*)

IN ITS CONCRETENESS a people is no simple unity; it is beset by conflicts, oppositions, whirlpools, crosscurrents. Only by abstracting from all these is one able to characterize it as a single people. It is then seen to have two kinds of unity. It is a people which, despite all conflicts, has a unity determined by the civilization. That unity is descriptive of the people, not prescriptive, not holding them together, unifying them in fact. Such a descriptive unity fails to do full justice to an organic unity in which part sustains part. That organic unity is historically exhausted not in the civilization, but between the civilization and a successor. It is to be accredited to a people when that people is set over against its successor. This is but to say that an organic unity is an ingredient unity set in contrast with, i.e., related to, a subsequent unity ingredient in another people, and that only when it is so related does the people become organically one. In history, to be organically one is to be past, dead; it is to be unified only in reaction or opposition to what follows it in time.

3.87   A people faces a standard not exhausted in a civilization.
(*See 3.81, 3.83*)

EACH PEOPLE has an ethical norm it more or less realizes throughout every stage of its career, and which offers it a standard in terms of which it can judge itself. No people does full justice to the demands of that norm; in terms of its own standard it is deficient, criticizable.

As an historic phenomenon the standard is an abstract prescriptive future relevant to a people. The concrete future which actually ensues realizes that abstract future; consequently the prescriptive future for one people becomes the descriptive present of its successor. Although no people succeeds in realizing it fully, so that it always remains outside the people as a standard, the ethical norm thus achieves realization in the shape of the people who succeed. To be sure, the succeeding people does not realize it as an ideal, as that to which it should conform, but only as a possibility which it makes determinate unawares, and thereby inevitably realizes. The succeeding people thus does not satisfy the demands of a previous people's ethical norm; these demands are made solely on the preceding people. But the succeeding people does satisfy the demands of the possibility to which that ethical norm reduces when held apart from the preceding people.

There is then this much truth in the idea of inevitable progress: a succeeding people by its very existence fulfills the residuum of the norm which the preceding people failed to fulfill. However, instead of yielding to that norm, exemplifying it, the succeeding people embody it, subjugate it, make it a facet of themselves. It has a prescriptive character only for the preceding people. It therefore does not express that Ideal in terms of which all peoples are to be judged.

It is to be noted that whereas the being and meaning of a people is exhausted in a civilization (3.83), the people's potentialities, nature, unity, and standard (3.84-87) are exhausted in the coming to be of a successor to the civilization.

VI   BEYOND HISTORY

3.88   Civilizations are comparable because there are principles which apply to all.
(*See 3.84-87*)

THE POTENTIALITY, nature, unity, and norms of a people and its civilization require some reference to a succeeding people and civilization. They express what the Actual, Ideal, Existential, and Divine, in time and as germane to two connected peoples and civilizations, can be. But *any* people and civilization can be compared. There is comparison possible betwen ourselves and the Greeks, even though they were directly succeeded not by us but by the Romans. Such comparison must make use of principles which are not exhausted at any one time; they must be principles which transcend any number of peoples and civilizations. If those principles are exhausted in the totality of peoples and civilizations, they are *universal principles* of history. If not necessarily exhausted by the totality of peoples and civilizations, they are *normative principles* for history.

A universal principle is an epitomized abstraction from Existence used to measure a civilization and a people; a normative principle is a mode of being, viewed as imposing conditions on history. The former is a derivative from Existence and enables one to compare different parts of history; the latter is derived from what is outside the realm of Existence and enables one to assess the whole as well as the parts of history. If we had neither measure, comparisons of a number of peoples and civilizations would be arbitrary, made in terms of standards which none exhibits, or in terms of some one chosen people or civilization, no more fitted than any other to measure all the rest. If we did not have them it would be impossible to criticize the entire course of history as deficient, bad, less good than it could have been and perhaps less good than some other form of being. We can objectively judge any civilization in relation to ours or to any other, only because there are principles which transcend our own and the others, and in terms of which all can be compared.

3.89   Great men provide universal principles measuring the creative energies of a people and a civilization.
(See 3.58, 3.76, 3.79, 3.88)

GREAT MEN are epitomizations of Actualities. They are works of art of the greatest magnitude. In each civilization there is a different type of great man. To say this is to subordinate the men to the civilization. That need not be done. Great men can, instead, be viewed apart from a civilization, as in root alike, as so many instances of "the great man." It will then be possible to compare different civilizations with respect to the number, magnitude, and nature of the great men they include. The civilizations with the least number of such men, or whose great men have only some partial human virtues carried to an extreme, can then be judged as inferior to others, as civilizations with less creative energy, i.e., with less flexibility combined with power, than those others.

From the point of view of the idea of "the great man," history is a laboratory for the production of perfected Actualities. Each civilization can be dealt with as occupying a limited part of that laboratory and as experimenting with different men and agencies in order to bring about the best of men. The idea of the great man which these different civilizations are to realize is exhausted by the totality of whatever great men are in fact produced in the course of history. History with its civilizations is from this perspective but an epitomization of Existence, which has found perfect lodgment in the totality of great men, the epitomization of the Actual.

3.90 A religion provides a measure of the purity of a people and a civilization.
(*See 3.80, 3.88*)

EACH CIVILIZATION has a religion peculiar to it, a 'civilized' religion. To say this, however, is not to take the position of the religion itself since, from the standpoint of the religion, a civilization is only a more or less adequate expression of it. For each religion there is a "city of God," which the different cities of men exhibit with more or less adequacy or purity.

Each religion provides a means for comparing different civilizations and peoples, and thereby enables one to escape from the relativity which judges one civilization in terms provided by another. But, precisely because there are many civilized and also other-worldly religions, a religious test of civilizations introduces a relativity of its own, unless one can isolate a single true or perfect religion, or the "idea of a civilized religion" which the different civilized religions more or less exemplify.

The "idea of a civilized religion," which all civilized religions exemplify, is an epitomization of a derived divine element. Such an idea may of course be perfectly exemplified in some extant religion. All civilized religions make the claim that at least they exemplify the "idea of a civilized religion" better than other religions can or do. Since religions conflict and deny one another, their oppositional claims require an antecedent determination of what the perfect epitomization of the divine is like, and a testing of each in terms of this. So far as they fall short of the test they must be acknowledged to be so many different cases where a divine component has been freed but rather arbitrarily and limitatively embodied in some medium not altogether appropriate to the exhibition of that divine component in its purity. But whether or not there is a perfect realization of the "idea of a civilized religion," that idea enables one to compare different civilizations and peoples as more or less pure, as more or less divinely sanctioned or disdained. And that idea will be exhausted in the totality of civilizations and peoples, since it is only in an epitomization of a derived divine component that the whole of history can be at once contained and measured.

3.91   Ethical ideals provide a measure of the moral worth of a people and a civilization.
(See 3.81, 3.88)

EACH CIVILIZATION has its own peculiar ethical demands. Each can be measured in terms of the civilization which in fact ensues on it. But these different ethical ideals and the civilizations to which they are relevant can themselves be compared. This requires that there be some criterion applicable to them all. Such a universally applicable criterion offers an epitomization of the Ideal component in Existence in the shape of ethical ideals which measure the worth of a civilization, and which must be expressed and exhausted over the whole of time. It will enable one to say that a civilization may fail to do all that ought to be done, even when it lives up to its own norms.

The philosophy of history of a Hegel, Marx, or Dewey makes use of such measuring ethical ideals. The view has the merit of affirming that there is a way of evaluating all civilizations, which requires no recourse to a transcendent or nonhistorical phenomenon, and which in fact spends itself over the entire course of history. Each civilization, on this view, illustrates with more or less adequacy that value which, initially derivable from any civilization, is epitomized in the guise of a universal, final ethical ideal of excellence.

Great men, religion, and ethics provide measures for any part of history. They are to be contrasted with the nature, unity, and standard that are exhausted by the arrival of a subsequent civilization. But they are also to be contrasted with the natures, unities, and values which transcend any stretch of history. Though we should judge all civilizations and peoples by the standards set by great men, religions, and ethical ideals, we must judge the whole of history by other and higher principles.

3.92 Peoples and civilizations have hovering natures, unities, and values, exhausted only in a longer history.
(See 3.46, 3.73, 3.85–87, 3.89–91)

EVERY PAST ITEM has an ingredient nature, value, and unity, expressing just what it is, as that determinate fact within a bounded segment of past time. Every past item also has a relational status by virtue of which its ingredient nature, value, and unity accrete relational significance, and with respect to its successor. But every past item too is part of a history larger than itself, and even larger than itself as together with its immediate successor. When and as a past item is determinate, as this particular with this ingredient and relational significance, it must also have an indeterminate status with respect to all the other items which are to eventuate in the course of history. If there is a third world war, the first world war, without losing its determinate being as that which is just what it was, no more, no less, and no other, and as that which gave way to a second world war in just the manner it in fact did, must, when it occurred, have had the indeterminate status of being "the first of three world wars." But not until the third world war in fact occurs can that status be wholly determinate; until then "being the first of three world wars" must be a nature which only hovers over the first world war. Since the past tolerates no indeterminates to be made determinate by what follows later, the hovering nature "the first of three world wars" testifies to something external yet relevant to the past. And what is true of a nature is true of value and unity. A past item has an indeterminate hovering value and unity which it does not fully embody, and which can be exhibited only after the passing of a period longer than that required for the item and its successor.

Any fragment of history has an indeterminate hovering nature, value, and unity which will be made more and more determinate in time. It is the virtue of the naturalistic or immanentistic philosophies of history of Hegel, Marx, and Dewey to recognize that such hovering natures, values, and unities must be realized in history, and that when a part or the whole of history is over, there is nothing in them which is unfulfilled. These thinkers tend to suppose that the last stage of the history is one where the residuum of an otherwise unsatisfied possibility is satisfied. This fortunately need not be made an essential part of their theory. But it is essential to the theory to hold that what no civilization in fact ever exhibits is not relevant to any, and that any one can be related in time to any other. There is truth in what they say, but it is less than what must be said.

A hovering nature, unity, or value for any bounded segment of history, since it permits of a relating of this and distant segments, achieves realization in the guise of a pattern or relation between these segments. But once it be recognized that other modes of being also are determinative of the course of history, it is possible to do justice to history as the story of Man, the revelation of God, or the exemplification of the Ideal. This the next three theses attempt to make evident.

3.93 The whole of history, and derivatively any people, may be unfulfilled, fail to be actualized maximally.
(See *1.47, 3.85, 3.88*)

A PEOPLE has an ingredient nature only when it is wholly past; it has a relational status with reference to a succeeding people; its hovering nature is exhausted in a history longer than that of a civilization. Acknowledgement of just the ingredient part precludes any criticism or evaluation; acknowledgement of just the relational precludes criticism or evaluation except in terms of what follows immediately after; an acknowledgement of just a hovering nature precludes a criticism or evaluation except in terms actually exemplified in some instance, or in all.

The parts of history, however, may not only be evaluated in relation to others or in terms of some standard exhausted over the course of history; they can, they must be evaluated in terms of a criterion which may never be exhausted in time. It is conceivable that all the occurrences in history, *severally or together*, may fail to measure up to some standard of excellence, some normative principle for history. The whole of history would then be condemnable as defective, as failing to be as excellent as it might have been. It is this judgment that

no Hegelian can make. There are for him no temporally unexempli-
fiable universals, values, standards, possibilities, criteria; all these are
for him exhaustively realized in time.

Every Actuality has an inside, an interiority. This comes to highest
expression in the guise of the human self which, because outside
history, can provide criteria in terms of which history can be judged.
From the standpoint of Actuality, and therefore of the self, one part
of history is superior to another so far as it permits and encourages
the flourishing of free individuals. And the whole of history is to be
judged as more or less excellent depending on the degree to which it
proves to be a field allowing and encouraging the full expression of
the free individual.

3.94   The whole of history, and derivatively any people, may be incoherent, fail to be unified maximally.
(*See 2.14, 3.86, 3.90, 3.93*)

HISTORY in whole and part is a locus of conflicts, tensions, am-
biguities. In terms of the unity which is God, every part of history
and the whole of it is defective, not unified sufficiently. From the
point of view of God the whole of history is found wanting, even
when it is the case that the hovering unity which that history must
exhibit is exhibited perfectly in every segment of it. The unity which
God demands of history is not defined in terms of what that history
does or even may or can do. It prescribes to history, evaluates it,
criticizing the whole of it and every part so far as it is not perfectly
unified. Only because God provides a unity, which in being and in
demand is in complete independence of what history might produce,
is it possible to measure the worth of whatever historically occurs,
and to scale it as more or less unified, more or less pure.

3.95   The whole of history, and derivatively any people, may not be wholly good, because it fails to be idealized maximally.
(*See 2.15, 3.87, 3.91*)

FROM the standpoint of the Ideal, history is a set of occasions or
loci where the Ideal can be embodied in the form of the Good. The
Ideal by making an incursion into history provides it with a value
which the totality of historic occurrences will exhaust. But the Ideal

also stands outside history, and as outside offers a test for the whole of it.

There is evil, ugliness, tragedy, and misery throughout history. And even if there were not, the kind of value which can be exhibited only over a stretch of time falls short of the rational translucency which the Ideal demands of anything that would be excellent. Every segment of history may illustrate the value which the Ideal gives history to exhibit. But whether the value is exhibited in every part or not, from the standpoint of the Ideal itself, what occurs in history is not wholly good because not wholly ideal.

3.96 From the perspective of Actuality, the whole of Existence is only potentially excellent.
(See 3.09, 3.93)

HISTORY is but a facet of Existence, and therefore Existence too can provide a norm for judging history. In terms of Existence history is a derivative, inadequate way of encompassing what occurs in time. History will never encompass all that exists; it does not have room for every physical event or individual.

History is also criticizable from the perspective of Actuality; it cannot, we saw, meet the standards set by the self. Nothing which is not wholly individual and free can content the self. The self even finds Existence (and God and the Ideal as well) to be insufficiently free and individual. From the perspective of Actuality, Existence is only raw material for an individualization and a genuine canalized, well-directed, responsible freedom. Existence must become ingredient in and subject to Actualities if it is to share their virtues.

3.97 From the perspective of the Ideal, the whole of Existence is not wholly rational.
(See 3.10, 3.95)

FROM the perspective of the Ideal, Existence adds implications to what is logically implied. But these implications do not make Existence a rational world from the standpoint of the Ideal. The career of Existence outruns the reach and control of the Ideal. Existence, consequently, will never altogether exemplify the Ideal. Not only history, then, but the entire realm of Existence is seen to be not translucent, not excellent enough, when viewed from the perspective of the Ideal. (A similar criticism of Actuality and of God can also be made from this perspective. They too are not excellent enough in terms of the standard of rationality which the Ideal portrays. The one lacks the Ideal's universality, the other its translucency.)

3.98   From the perspective of God, the whole of Existence is incoherent.
(See 3.11, 3.94)

FROM the perspective of God, Existence is the domain of becoming. But no becoming is perfectly unified; there is always a merging and a passing away. From the perspective of God this is a defect in Existence. From the perspective of God, not only history then but the entire realm of Existence is radically defective. (A similar criticism of Actuality and the Ideal from this perspective can of course be made; they too are not sufficiently coherent in terms of the standard set by the unity which is God.)

In 3.84–87 we distinguished four facets of a people which are exhausted in the coming to be of its successor. In 3.89–91 we distinguished three universal relevant principles in terms of which any two peoples or civilizations can be compared. In 3.93–95, we distinguished three normative principles which are imposed on peoples and civilizations and which they cannot wholly realize. In 3.96–98 we distinguished three ways in which, not merely history, but Existence itself falls short of excellence.

Platonism gains strength from the truth of 3.93–98. But Aristotelians insist on 3.84–87. Both sides meet in 3.89–91.

VII   EXISTENCE   AND   THE   OTHER   MODES

3.99   Actuality, the Ideal, and God are deficient from the perspective of Existence.
(See 3.12)

FROM the perspective of Existence, an Actuality is a focal point, lacking the energy, the driving dynamics, the all-encompassing vitality of Existence itself. From the perspective of Existence, the Ideal is the universal abstract Future, lacking the plurality, the divided explicitness of Existence. From the perspective of Existence, finally, God is essence, lacking Existence's extensionality, its capacity to be in and through space and time. In terms of Existence, these are serious lacks, marking defects in their natures.

The other three modes of being incorporate some Existence in them. To some extent they must then satisfy the standards set by Existence. In terms of those standards they are to be viewed as being more or less effective at different times, depending on the degree and manner in which they make use of Existence.

Each mode of being is present in every other. It therefore to some degree does meet the standards set by the others. What it can never do is to meet those standards entirely, for they are in the end different from it in temper, being, and function.

3.100   Existence provides testimony to the reality of Actualities.
(See 1.27, 3.06, 3.12)

EXISTENCE is a mode of being with its own rhythms and laws. But it has features which cannot be accounted for without making reference to Actualities. Firstly, Existence is a locus of relations, and this requires that there be termini, beings outside and independent of it in which its relations can terminate. Secondly, the structure of Existence is variable in space and over time, a fact which can be explained by recognizing changes in the concentration of Actualities at various places. Thirdly, there is an irregularity to the rhythms of Existence; it is subject to pulls and resistances, attributable to Actualities as withstanding and opposing the whole of Existence. Yet these Actualities may not be ultimately real, so far as the testimony which Existence provides is concerned; they might from that perspective only be expressions of some other mode of being, such as God, as Spinoza seemed to have held.

Similarly Actualities testify to the reality of Existence, since they are subject to a pull by the whole of Existence, can be related as incongruous counterparts which require for their understanding a reference to a space outside them, and are real co-ordinated contemporaries, requiring a domain in which they can be separate yet together. But the testimony does not prove that Existence is a real mode of being; it may, as Spinoza supposed, be but a facet of God or, as Hegel thought, be but a facet of the Ideal.

3.101 Existence provides testimony to the reality of the Ideal.
(See 2.96, 3.12)

THIS PROPOSITION is the reciprocal of 2.96, where it was shown that the Ideal provides testimony that there is a real Existence. The Ideal, while selfsame and formal, is involved in the affairs of the cosmos in such a way as to require reference to an Existence which—so far as this testimony is concerned and as Plotinus supposed—may not have a real being of its own. Similarly, Existence offers testimony to the reality of the Ideal; it has a directionality, which as determined from without, is to be explained by reference to what is now possible to it. That presupposed possible may not, so far as the testimony of Existence goes, be a final reality. It is conceivable that it might be nothing more than one of God's expressions, as Irenaeus seems to have held; or it might conceivably express the nature or desires of an Actuality, as William James seemed to believe.

3.102 Existence provides testimony to the reality of God.
(See 3.01, 3.14, 4.21, 4.86)

THIS PROPOSITION is somewhat anticipatory. In 4.21, it will be used to ground a proof terminating in God. For the moment it suffices to observe that Existence has a unity, an essence which, though belonging to it, is nevertheless over against it. The presence of this essence testifies to a being which imposes the essence on it. A being with such a capacity is conventionally termed 'God.' He may not, so far as the testimony of Existence is concerned, be a real being; it is conceivable that he is only an idea expressing the unifying power of a judging human mind, as many humanists hold.

Similarly when account is taken of the fact that God is omnipresently effective in a world not altogether good, he will provide testimony to the reality of an independent Existence. Such an Existence could conceivably be an attenuation of an Actuality—as Existentialists hold—and not be a fundamental mode of being at all.

3.103   Existence partly satisfies the needs of Actualities.
(See 1.14, 3.12, 3.40, 3.41, 3.100)

DEPRIVED of Existence an Actuality is just a fact; with Existence it is present, vital. An Actuality needs Existence if it is to be substantial and flexible, self-maintaining and internally diverse. Could Actualities master the whole of Existence they would have within their control the entire energy, the very being of space and time that characterizes this universe. Each Actuality reaches out into an Existence not integral with it, to make this part of itself so that it can become the master of that which otherwise would move away from it and thereby reduce it to a mere fact. Reciprocally, Actualities partly satisfy the need of Existence to achieve stability, focus, a plurality of distinct vantage points from which effective action can issue.

3.104   Existence partly satisfies the needs of the Ideal.
(See 2.99, 3.07, 3.12, 3.101)

APART from Existence, the Ideal would not be an effective Ideal for this cosmos, but at best only an objective for distinct Actualities or a principle for an eternal God. The Ideal needs Existence to provide it with the status of a cosmic reality in space and time. The Ideal in turn partly satisfies the need of Existence to be purposive through and through. Without the Ideal, Existence would have no direction; it would be just a chaotic onrushing.

3.105   Existence partly satisfies the needs of God.
(See 1.15, 3.04, 3.102, 4.86)

THAT God has needs, to be satisfied by other modes of being, is evident from the fact that there are such other modes. Just what his needs are, and how these modes satisfy them, must await an account of the nature of God. But for the moment it is sufficient to observe that God to be effective everywhere, and this without compromise to his unity, needs that single field of action which is provided only by Existence—just as Existence, to be fully in and of itself, needs to be united with an organizing unity which only God can provide. Neither one satisfies the other fully. There is a recalcitrance to Existence which precludes its allowing God to be adequately effective, and there is a transcendence in the divine unity which prevents Existence from making it entirely its own. Not until the other modes of being supplement the contribution of Existence or of God, does either God or Existence achieve the opportunity or unity, respectively, which it requires. God, the Ideal, and Actuality together give Existence the unity it needs in order fully to be; and Existence, the Ideal, and Actuality together give God that opportunity for effective action which he needs in order that he be himself most excellently.

3.106   Existence supplements the contributions other modes make to one another.
(See *1.14, 1.25, 2.20, 2.104, 3.13, 3.103–5*)

ACTUALITY'S NEED to be permanent is satisfied only by God, the Ideal, and Existence together. God gives it the status of a permanent other, the Ideal gives it the status of a permanent instance of the Ideal, and Existence involves Actuality permanently in the affairs of the space-time world. So far as God and the Ideal fail to fulfill their respective tasks towards Actuality, they impose a burden on Existence. Instead of being occupied merely with making Actualities part of the space-time world, Existence must then make them, while part of such a world, into beings which stand over against all else, and serve to sustain a meaning. Similarly, the Ideal's need to be realized is satisfied only by God, Actuality, and Existence together. God gives the Ideal the status of a standard, Actuality gives it the status of the Good, and Existence gives it the status of a Future. The failure of God and Actuality to satisfy the Ideal as it faces them, makes the Future which Existence faces more determinate than it otherwise would be; it is this more determinate future, carrying part of the unfinished work of God and Actuality, which Existence struggles to realize. Finally, the Ideal, Actuality, and Existence give God effectiveness, the first in the form of a principle expressive of divine intent, the second in the form of a being of virtue qualified to exhibit God's meaning, the third in the form of a cosmic space-time frame. The failure of the Ideal and Actuality to do justice to the needs of God makes the cosmic field, which Existence offers to God as an area for his activity, to be more receptive to the divine intent and less antagonistic to his meaning than it otherwise would be.

3.107 The Ideal relates Existence and Actuality.
(See 2.101, 2.102, 3.40)

EXISTENCE has one rationale, Actualities another. By virtue of the incorporation of part of Existence within an Actuality, there is an inevitable pull exerted by that part against the whole; conversely, by virtue of the continuity of the incorporated Existence with the larger and more effective Existence beyond, there is a pull exerted by the whole against any incorporated part. Without the Ideal they would always be opposed to one another. The Ideal, by providing an objective common to both of them, enables them to be harmonized in prospect and partly in fact.

Semantic rules and rules for action are ways of using the Ideal as a mediator between Existence and Actuality. And as Plato saw the Ideal can, in the guise of the rationale of a demiurgos, also relate God and Existence. Analogously a religious ethics offers us the Ideal as a mediator between God and Actuality.

3.108 Actuality relates Existence and the Ideal.
(See 3.40, 3.107)

EXISTENCE is perpetually productive of an Ideal limit or effect; the Ideal perpetually tries to govern the process of Existence in the endeavor to turn it into an instance of itself. Actuality relates the two efforts. It provides the Ideal with a means through which it can be realized in Existence. Conversely, Actuality functions as an agency for Existence, a means by which Existence can effectively make the Future vary in consonance with the relevant needs of the present.

The Existentialists, in their theory of commitment, attempt to show how an Actuality mediates between the Ideal and Existence. Their view is analogous to that of the prophets who view themselves as mediators between God and the Ideal, and to the Kierkegaardian singular Actuality which mediates between God and Existence.

3.109 Existence relates the Ideal and Actuality.
(See 3.01, 3.107–8)

EXISTENCE is the agency by means of which what is distinct can have a common field of operation. It relates as it separates, holds together what it divides. Existence keeps all the various Actualities within the orbit of a single Future, thereby enabling them to move into the next moment concordantly; at the same time, Existence limits the independent activities of Actualities, thereby enabling the Ideal to be multiply realized in related ways. Were there no common Existence the Actualities would not share a common present, nor would there be any spatial relation between the various realizations of the Ideal.

Kant's theory of the schematism, which views an existing time as the mediator between categories and actual entities, is a brilliant illustration of the use of Existence as a mediator between the Ideal and the Actual. An analogous function is attributed to history by Augustine, for this serves to mediate the Ideal and God. Ethical commands serve a similar function for Thomas Aquinas, since for him they are moments of Existence mediating Actuality and God. (These various mediations are here being viewed as oriented towards that which is mediated. Each mode also mediates the others when they are in it, as will become most evident when we deal with God, as e.g., in 4.90.)

3.110   A "proof" of a mode of being involves the use of the other three modes.
(See 3.100–102, 3.107–9, 4.12, 4.56)

EACH MODE of being provides testimony to the reality of some other. Each is related to that other. Each can be made to give way to that other. And each can be "proved" by starting with the testimony, relating this to the desired conclusion, and then proceeding to isolate that conclusion.

Every one of the modes should have its proof. Now there have been thinkers, primarily epistemologists, who have seen the necessity of proving the reality of Actualities. Others, primarily ethicists, have seen the necessity for proving the reality of the Ideal. Still others, primarily cosmologists, have seen the necessity for proving the reality of Existence. But on the whole these proofs have not occupied the forefront of attention. Interest seems to have been concentrated almost exclusively on proofs of the reality of God. Yet, as will be evident in the next chapter, were any of the other modes not acknowledged, no proof of the reality of God would really be possible. Conversely, were there no God acknowledged, there could be no adequate proof of any other mode.

The ordering of the present chapters is in consonance with the traditional spirit of seeking a proof of God, and it is to this we will immediately proceed. But it is not to be forgotten that each mode of being provides as good a beginning, as good a relation, as good an agency, and as good a terminus of a proof as any other, and that once a proof of God's reality has been achieved one can, with the help of two more modes, provide proofs of the reality of each of the others— proofs which are no more and no less sound or revelatory than a proof of God.

CHAPTER 4

God

I   PROLOGUE

4.01   Each mode of being is ingredient in the others.
(*See 1.15, 1.25, 2.98–100, 3.60, 3.100–102*)

THERE are four co-ordinate, irreducible modes of being. Each has its own nature and integrity. An adequate knowledge of them all will require the achievement of a position of neutrality in which each can be recognized as over against all the others. But since each is being in an essential mode, no one of the modes can truly be except so far as it is one with true being and thus contains within itself something of the others. This is essentially Anaxagoras' insight, and in a way Leibniz' too. In every part of reality one can find all four modes of being, though to be sure as inside a mode the other three are and function in ways which diverge somewhat from the ways they are and function over against that mode. Over against one another the different modes stand out as pure, unaffected by the others. Ingredient in one another, the modes of being give reality to one another, but thereby suffer qualifications. The internal presence of other modes in a given mode does not change the nature of that mode as in itself or as over against the rest, but it does enable it to *be*, in itself and over against the rest.

4.02   Each mode of being needs the others.
(*See 1.14, 4.01*)

THOUGH each mode of being has subjugated forms of the other modes within it, those other modes still remain outside it. No mode of

being possesses the others in their full concreteness. All are on a footing, independent, irreducible, final. Because each lacks the reality
which the others possess, each is imperfect. And since there are four
modes of being, each is triply imperfect, imperfect from three sides.
Each expresses a three-pronged need for the others which are outside
and independent of it, defining it to be incomplete because it lacks
their reality. Each needs the others, not consciously or biologically,
but ontologically, as external conditions outside its control, determining it to have the status of a being which is not and cannot be the
whole of being.

4.03   Each mode of being seeks to adjust itself to others.
(See 1.24, 1.25, 2.98–100, 3.103–5, 4.02)

TO BE CONDITIONED by what is external is to be dependent on what
is external. It is to have one's entire being at least jeopardized, for the
external being dictates to some extent what the conditioned being is
and can do. The fact that this conditioned being may reciprocate, and
condition what conditions it, does not improve the situation. A double
jeopardy increases, it does not eliminate difficulties.

Were all the modes to make an effort to subjugate one another,
they would, were their powers equal, frustrate one another perpetually; and if their powers were unequal some one of them would
reduce at least one other to the status of a derivative or subordinate
being. If one mode wholly subjugates another it thereby shows that
that other is not a final, irreducible being.

No being succeeds in wiping out the conditions to which others
subject it. No being ever could do this without thereby becoming the
whole of being. Still, each acts independently to give the total cosmos
a kind of life (to speak the language appropriate to Actuality), something like a career (to speak the language appropriate to Existence), a
sort of structure (to speak the language appropriate to the Ideal),
and some unity (to speak the language appropriate to God). From
its own perspective, each overcomes the limitations which the others
impose. But none really does so. Each fails to deal adequately with
the others, with the consequence that each always has work to do
and even new problems to deal with.

4.04 Each mode of being partly satisfies the others.
(*See 1.118, 2.98–100, 3.103–5, 4.02, 4.03*)

THERE IS a lack to each mode of being, precisely defined by what ever reality the remaining modes possess. Each takes account of the other modes, turns them into data, thereby defining them to be nothing apart from it. But these others continue to remain outside its perspective, compelling it to take account of new data all the time. In its acceptance of the data which the others enable it to have, the being satisfies the other modes, giving them a place in its economy, allowing them to function in it, not in their full concreteness, not as substances ingredient in it, but rather as meanings or qualifications carried by it.

4.05 Each mode of being imposes a burden on every other.
(*See 1.14, 2.21, 2.104, 3.13, 3.106, 4.04*)

A MODE of being shows a different face to each of the other three modes, thereby presenting them with distinct tasks. These tasks have an immediate and a final nature. The immediate task is the mastery of the others in the guise in which they present themselves to it; the final task is the completion of a grand totality of immediate tasks, for behind every immediate task is another, expressive of the fact that the others have beings of their own. Neither task, the immediate nor the final, is ever fully completed, due to the distance and the recalcitrance of the mode. But every task ought to be completed, and what ought to be done can be done, if not by the being that ought to do it, then by some other. The failure of one mode of being to do what it ought for another leaves over material for the others to deal with when they act to complete their own respective tasks. This material changes the character of their tasks, in both its immediate and final form, making it more determinate than it had been.

Each mode of being fails to complete its task with respect to some second, leaving over to a third and fourth the need to make good the failures of the first. Only jointly do the first, third, and fourth do justice to that second. Because Actualities for example, fail to do for the Ideal all they ought, God and Existence are compelled to realize, as they inadequately engage in their own respective tasks in relation to the Ideal, all that the Actualities failed to do on behalf of that Ideal. The Actualities should have realized the Ideal in the guise of the

Good. But they do not realize it, and what they fail to do must be residually realized by God and Existence.

4.06 Each mode of being provides testimony to the reality of the others.
(See *1.11–13, 2.95–97, 3.100–102*)

A *descriptive* feature or status is one without which a being would not be what it then is. An *essential* feature or status is one which the being intrinsically possesses, one which it must have. "Being near" is descriptive of the object in my hands; it is not essential to that object, since the object could conceivably be at a distance. Descriptiveness refers to an object in its concreteness, possessing whatever features it does have; it may encompass features which owe their presence to other realities as well as features which the object possesses by itself. Essentiality, on the other hand, refers just to the object in its being, and thus only to what may relate to the being in an abstracted but still conceivable state, as torn away from the contingent situation in which as a matter of fact it happens to be. There must be some descriptive features which are nonessential, unless beings never did make a difference to one another. These descriptive nonessential features *characterize* objects, manifesting the passivity of objects to imposed factors. And some descriptive features must be essential, express *characters* of the object, for otherwise beings would have no natures of their own. Traditionally the two ideas have often been identified; what was descriptive was thought by rationalists to be essential, and what was essential was thought by empiricists to be descriptive. Distinguishing them enables us to see how one mode of being can provide testimony to the reality of another.

Testimony is evidence; it may be verbal and propositional, or silent and ontological. Most testimony is of the latter sort. It is the kind of testimony which the modes of being provide to the reality of one another. A mode of being provides such testimony if it has features which are not essential but are descriptive of it, i.e., if it has features, not implicated in the idea of it, without which it would not be a real being in this cosmos. A testifying mode behaves in ways, exercises functions, and exhibits traits which it need not have, and which one can conceive it not to have—though of course not without at the same time conceiving it to be no longer in this cosmos. Since it is the other modes which endow it with these nonessential descriptive traits, it is one and the same thing to say that each mode of being provides testimony to the reality of the other modes, and that all the modes together exhaust the whole of being, define a cosmos.

"Accidental" characters testify to a reality outside the being in which they are, for they are nonessential features descriptive of the being as it is in the world. In Aristotle's system the accidents provide testimony to the reality of matter; in other systems they testify to the reality of relations, external pressures, and so on. The fact that one "accident" can be substituted for another without affecting the essential nature of that being has led some Aristotelians to suppose mistakenly that all accidents could be sheared off to leave us with the being as possessing only essential features. But the fact that an object has nonessential features cannot be cancelled out without cancelling out the fact that the object is in the world. These features provide evidence that the object is partly determined from the outside, that there is something other than it which makes those features descriptive of it.

Each mode of being has "accidental" features, i.e., nonessential traits which are descriptive of it as a being in the cosmos, and which therefore testify to the reality of other modes of being. This truth does not affect the fact that every being has a singular, all-inclusive essence, and that every single trait of the being is an expression of that essence. What the being expresses is qualified, altered, partially transformed from without, thereby becoming descriptive of it.

4.07   Each mode of being provides both direct and indirect testimony to the reality of others.
(*See 4.06*)

DIRECT testimony of another mode of being is provided by nonessential descriptive features having natures which instance the nature and require the activity or presence of that other mode of being. *Indirect* testimony of another mode of being is provided by nonessential descriptive features which, while instancing one mode of being, require the presence or action of a different mode of being. Direct testimony refers us to a being acting in such a way as to make a feature of itself descriptive of another; indirect testimony refers us to a being acting in such a way as to make a feature belonging to something else descriptive of a third. A finger print—strictly speaking, whorls and ridges smudged on something—offers direct testimony to a finger with similar whorls and ridges; a stabbed man provides indirect testimony to the identity of the culprit who thrust in the dagger. The detective sifts the available evidence in the hope of isolating some direct testimony, as the surest and safest way of getting to know who the culprit is.

Plato thought that knowledge provided indirect testimony to the reality of a pre-existent soul, and direct testimony to the reality of the Good. Descartes thought that his errors provided direct testimony to the reality of a maladjusted will and mind, and that his finite truths provided indirect testimony of the existence of a concerned God. Those who argue to the reality of God from the supposed fact that this world has more order to it than chance could provide, think of the order as providing direct testimony of an ordering God and indirect testimony of a purposing God. The latter presumably is God in himself, the former being but a surface facet of him. In this case, the supposed indirect testimony provided by the order of the world is thought to refer us directly to a divine idea of order, and indirectly to a God who purposely imposes that order.

It is possible to treat testimony in another way. One can, for example, think of the order of the world as a consequence of a purpose; one can think of it even as being the consequence of an act of God, in no way like any feature of him. The order of the world could then be said to require the reality of a God in whom a purpose may be resident or who expresses himself purposively. Direct testimony would on this view, as before, point to a being which possesses some trait or other that the testifying feature instances, but indirect testimony would have the role of directly pointing to a being which is a source of the testifying trait. This interpretation has the advantage of not requiring, in the case of indirect testimony, that a testifying feature should instance a feature of another being. The only testifying traits, whether direct or indirect, useful in proving a mode of being, however, all instance characters of modes of being. If one forged proofs by taking account of traits which indirectly testified only to an exterior source of those traits, one would know nothing about the nature of that source. We need testimony, direct or indirect, which allows us to know the characters of other beings. Only direct testimony enables us to know the characters of the beings responsible for the presence of testifying traits. Indirect testimony can never do more than enable us to determine the characters of one being while merely directing us towards another, perhaps quite distinct from it, which is responsible for the presence of the testifying features.

4.08   Each mode of being relates two other modes of being.
(*See 3.107–9*)

THE MODES of being are existentially distinct from one another; they exhibit a meaning or Ideal in different ways; they are localized in Actualities; they are unified. Consequently there are four types of relation, four ways of connecting testifying traits to what they testify. A trait may testify to a being existentially distinct from the being in which the trait is resident: a fingerprint testifies to a finger. It may testify to a being which has a meaningful relation to the trait or its object: an act testifies to an intent. It may testify to a being which is located in a larger Actuality: kidneys testify to a heart. It may testify to a being which makes a unity with it: a husband testifies to the reality of a wife. In each case there is a different mode of being serving to relate testimony to an appropriate object.

Each mode of being has three descriptive nonessential features testifying to the reality of the other three modes. Each also has three descriptive nonessential features pointing to the other three modes in their role of relations. Only the first set of features has been stressed, however, since they are sufficient, for our purposes, to justify the acknowledgment of other modes, as able to have a relational status.

4.09   A being is related to another by a third in a primary and a secondary way.
(*See 4.07, 4.08*)

A PRIMARY RELATION connecting one mode of being with another is provided by any mode of being; a secondary relation is a qualified primary relation, expressive of the modification to which one mode of being subjects another. So far as Existence, for example, alone mediates Actuality and Ideality it provides a primary relation between them; so far as it is qualified by divinity it provides a secondary relation between them.

Both primary and secondary relations may be sustained by the very being which provides one of the terms. The Ideal may offer a primary relation connecting the Ideal with Actuality; the Ideal as qualified by Existence may offer a secondary relation connecting the Ideal with Existence. Both types of relation, to function in a proof of a mode of being, however, should have one term which begins with testimony and another which ends with what one seeks to prove. And if a secondary relation is to serve in a proof, it of course ought not to be one which is qualified by the being at which the proof is to terminate, since it would then obtrusively beg its question.

4.10   Each mode of being enables one to hold any other apart from the rest.
(*See 1.82, 4.08, 4.09*)

EACH MODE of being can be existentially distinguished from the others; each mode of being can be made to instance the Ideal in a special way; each mode of being can be referred to by Actualities and particularly by a mind; each mode of being can be made the object of a distinguishing act of unification.

To terminate in a mode of being one must relate it to a testimony in a primary or secondary way, and then in one of the above four ways traverse the route defined by the relation. The relation which one mode of being has to a second by virtue of a third is used by a fourth. The third provides the fourth with a kind of rule, a structure to be exhibited in the course of an activity. The fourth, if it follows the route of a legitimate rule connecting the testimony with its object, ends with a being "proved."

Existence and Actuality, for example, are related by the Ideal. Starting from Existence, God can in an act of unification traverse the route defined by the Ideal to terminate in Actuality; starting from Actuality he can, in an act of unification, traverse the route in an opposite direction to terminate in Existence. The illustration is perhaps unfortunate, for of all possible ways of proving, none has had so little attention as that which can be performed by God. God, as providing route or traversal or both, is usually dismissed as a mere figment of the imagination. This is arbitrary, but no more so than the other traditional restrictions various thinkers have imposed on proofs. Logicians usually recognize only a route and then only if it has an Ideal character; existentialists attend primarily to a traversal and then only if it is performed by an Actuality; cosmologists acknowledge both route and traversal, but only as facets of Existence. All infer in warranted ways, but they overlook essential features in their own proofs, unwarrantedly deny the legitimacy of one another's proofs, and fail to recognize the existence of still other types of proof.

4.11 Each mode of being permits of the detachment of a directly or indirectly originative being.
(*See 4.10*)

IF AN ACT of detachment terminates in a *directly originative* being it terminates in one which is in a primary relation to a testifying being; if it terminates in an *indirectly originative* being it terminates in one having a secondary relation to a testifying being. The former arrives at the object of direct testimony, the latter at the object of indirect testimony. The one reaches an object which intrinsically possesses the trait that the testifying being had descriptively but nonessentially; the other reaches an object which has only the power to impose such a trait on another. The one therefore reveals something of the nature of a being; the other tells us of its power, and incidentally also tells us something about the nature of some other being, which is subject to that power.

4.12 A "proof" of a mode of being begins with testimony, acknowledges a relation, and terminates in the being.
(*See 1.80–86, 3.110, 4.06–11*)

A "PROOF" begins with that which determines a possible conclusion. It follows the route which connects that beginning with that possible conclusion. And it ends with the detachment of the conclusion from the relation which united it with the beginning. Without testimony there would be no particular direction for the proof to go; without a relation connecting it with the possible conclusion, there would be no validating structure for the proof; and without a termination at the being to be proved there would be no concluding.

A proof does not necessarily begin with or end in propositions, nor does it take place only in the mind or on paper. It can begin with, traverse, and end with modes of being. It may begin with one mode of being, move through a second over the route given by some third, and end in a fourth. Such a proof has the same virtues and vices as any other type of proof. It has a certifiable structure, justifiably linking a beginning and an end, and it vitalizes the structure in a way which cannot be wholly predicted. For logicians, to be sure, a proof has a limited kind of formal structure, and an inference—where allowed to come into consideration at all as an act terminating in the conclusion along the route provided by the formal structure—is a mental act. They in effect make use of specialized versions of the Ideal and Existence. But there is no preferential status that any mode of being enjoys as premiss, rule, act of concluding, or conclusion; nor is there any need to deal only with specialized versions of the modes of being.

4.13 There are three basic and six subordinate testimonies for, relations to, and terminations in God.
(*See 4.07–12*)

EACH MODE of being provides direct testimony to the reality of God, by virtue of its possession of a descriptive but nonessential trait which is nevertheless essential to God. In addition, each mode of being has descriptive and nonessential features which are iconic with those possessed by two other modes of being but which it has acquired only through the agency of God. Also, each mode of being serves to connect two others with God, the being who possesses the testifying trait; and, as qualified by other modes, each serves to connect them with God in a secondary way. Each mode, finally, terminates in God as directly or indirectly originative of nonessential traits. These basic functions must be distinguished and clarified, if we are to make satisfactory use of them in proofs of God.

II   TELEOLOGICAL BEGINNINGS

4.14 Teleological testimony offers evidence requiring God for its explanation.
(*See 4.06, 4.07*)

TESTIMONY is offered by any descriptive feature not essential to the being in which it is. If the feature is permanent it offers testimony to the reality of a distinct mode of being. If the permanent feature is an essential feature of God, it offers direct testimony to the reality of God. If the feature is essential to some other mode of being but requires the action of God in order to be present in the testifying being, it offers indirect testimony to the reality of God. Both direct and indirect testimony is "teleological"; each is expressive of a purpose, not in the sense that it necessarily expresses some deliberate intent by God, but only in the sense that it testifies to the fact that God has made his presence and therefore something of his nature or power manifest in some other mode of being. To testify teleologically is of course not yet to prove anything. Testimony provides only the beginning of a proof of God. A teleological approach is quite distinct from a supposed teleological proof of God. The former offers a way of looking at testimony; it provides just the premiss for a proof of God. The latter moves away from such a premiss to a conclusion. The former is an indispensable part of any proof; the latter is not a proof at all. (On this see 4.24.)

One can avoid making a reference to God if one affirms that (a) the features said to offer testimony are not there at all; (b) the features are not descriptive; (c) the features are essential; (d) though non-essential the features are merely adventitious; (e) they offer testimony to a being other than God. The first alternative raises a question of fact; this question cannot be avoided by characterizing a feature as illusory or not real, for what is to the point is not the reality of the feature but whether or not it is present and what it entails. The second alternative raises a question about the features of a being as part of the cosmos; the fact that the features may be vague or be in part a function of some other beings does not affect their descriptiveness. What is relevant is that they do pertain to the being. The third alternative raises the question as to whether a feature only characterizes or is a character of a being. As part of the cosmos, as just the being it is in the setting it has, the feature characterizes, is characteristic; if it is essential to the being the feature is a character of it. Only the former can be conceivably removed without destroying the being. The fourth alternative raises the question as to whether or not removable features may as a mere matter of fact be present without any relevant cause or reason. The question is resolved by showing that the feature is not only incapable of existing on its own, but must have been imposed on the testifying being. Finally, the feature might be supposed not to instance a divine attribute and thus not to refer to him at all, or (where it is thought to instance a divine attribute) may in fact have been produced by, and thus indirectly testify to some other mode of being. The resolution of this question depends on a knowledge of what an instance of a divine attribute is, and what does and does not depend on the exercise of divine power. Before there can be a proof of God, all five difficulties must at least in principle be overcome in connection with the three primary and six secondary testimonies that Actuality, Ideality, and Existence offer regarding the reality of God.

4.15   A substantival teleology begins with primary Actualities offering direct testimony to the reality of God as their Absolute Other.

(See *1.08, 1.14, 1.16, 1.23*)

EACH PRIMARY Actuality has an inside, an inwardness, a self-substantiality, which it holds apart from all else. If it did not, it would not be a distinct individual. I, for one, am limited, exclusive. I can never meet myself coming towards me; whatever I encounter is the other of myself.

An Actuality cannot be an other unless there be something for which it is the other. To be an other requires that there be another. The otherness of an Actuality is characteristic of it but is not of its essence. The otherness depends for its being on the reality of something outside the Actuality. Its role of being an other must be imposed on it. It becomes an other only because there is some being correlate with it, at least as irreducible, as unitary, and as withdrawn as itself.

Each Actuality is a limited case of Actuality, vitalizing, delimiting, qualifying, intensifying features pertinent to all Actualities. Since to be Actual is to be "other than," and since "other than" is a reciprocal relation, requiring its terms to be equally effective, the correlate of an Actuality must be at least as real as it is. Each Actuality therefore must be other than some being which is unaffected by the fact that there might be this or that Actuality in the world. That being is the other of Actuality. As such it must continue to have being at least as long as there are any Actualities at all. It must therefore be another mode of being, as fundamental, as irreducible, as indestructible as Actuality. But it cannot be the Ideal, since this lacks the inwardness which is needed if there is to be a true other for a being with an inwardness. Nor can the true other of Actuality be Existence, since this lacks the unity which the correlate of Actuality must have. The Ideal and Existence of course are other than Actuality, but they are not its Absolute Other; this would require them to have an inwardness, a unity and a substantiality matching that of Actuality. There is no alternative left but God.

God is all inwardness as it were, requiring everything else to be distinct from him. Only that which has an inward withdrawn being of its own, as Actuality does, could directly testify to his substantial unitary inwardness. Only it directly testifies that he is the Absolute Other. (Since "other than" is a symmetrical relation, God himself must offer testimony, as we shall see in 4.67, to the reality of Actualities.) Ideality and Existence testify to God as one who imposes some other kind of status on them, enabling him to enjoy some other role than that of being their Absolute Other.

God is the Absolute Other of all Actualities, each of which is representative of Actuality. And each one of these Actualities has the role of an other with respect to other Actualities. As holding itself away from the rest, each is an other relative to them, fluctuating in content and significance; as a representative of Actuality, each holds its whole being away from, is a constant other, a correlate of God.

Arguments grounded in the fact that men have minds, consciences, feelings, secrets, are limited forms of the substantival teleological approach to God, since they start with a particular type of Actuality, to wit, man. But other kinds of Actualities have an inwardness as well; each is self-centered, excluding and being excluded by all else as surely as is man. Any one of them can therefore provide testimony to the reality of God in the guise of the Absolute Other.

4.16 A rationalistic teleology begins with universals offering indirect testimony to a God concerned with the Ideal.

(See *1.16, 1.26, 2.19, 4.07, 4.15*)

EACH PRIMARY Actuality is an individual. Every essential feature of it is submerged within its individual nature. In one sense then nothing could be more incorrect than to say of it that it is a being of a certain kind, for it is nothing but itself, absolutely unique and unduplicatable. It is wrong in a way then to say of Socrates that he is "a man." Socrates is not "a man"; he is this man, or better even, he is this individual, uncatchable within any general expression or category. "A man" does not eat, sleep, die; it is outside the area of that unique, specific, unduplicatable being, outside that deciding, willing, lonely, 'Dasein' which is man. "A man" is neither male nor female, tall or short, happy or unhappy, here or there. Since I am male, short and happy it cannot be the case that I am "a man." Ecce homo; here in me is where "a man" is; "a man" is but a submerged, subjugated, qualified, altered, a mere abstractive aspect of myself, this unique individual. As distinct from me it is a nonessential feature; I do not need it in order for me to be the living existing individual that I am.

But it is also true that "man" is a feature of each and every one of us. Socrates and Plato are equally men; there is a human nature common to them. What "man" implies applies to both of them. It is because Socrates and Plato are both men that we know that they both breathe, eat, sleep, love, die, that they have heart, head, lungs, liver, kidneys, self, mind, and will. "Man" in fact is but one of a host of universals which pertain to them, to me, to you and to other humans. These universals describe them.

All Actualities have "Actuality" as a universal, descriptive feature. This is too indeterminate to stand by itself; it cannot be imposed on every Actuality by the Ideal, for the Ideal subjugates the beings with which it is occupied, and thereby denies individuality to whatever may be Actual and under its sway. Nor can the character "Actuality" be imposed on every Actuality by Existence, for Existence too is not considerate of the individual. God alone allows universals to be sharable and individuals to be private, and provides the power making it possible for these two dimensions to be together in a single unity without loss to the integrity of either.

In themselves universals do not provide testimony to the reality of God. But as united with individuals, they do provide indirect testimony to him as a being who has the power to make those universals one with those individuals, without compromising either side. To affirm, "I am an Actuality" is to provide indirect testimony of God, the being who makes it possible for me to be both one and one of a kind.

Theologians often refer to the noble nature of man, the order in which Actualities occur and act, or to the hierarchy of excellence in which all Actualities fall, as evidences of a purposing God. It is questionable whether any one of these is more than a transient feature, and it is questionable whether, even if it offered a nonessential characteristic, it would provide direct testimony to the reality of God. Nobility, order, and hierarchy do not seem to be essential features of God; if they were permanent characteristics of Actuality they could provide only indirect testimony of him.

4.17 An historical teleology begins with facts offering indirect testimony to a God concerned with Existence.
(See *3.41, 3.47, 3.102*)

A FACT is an Actuality de-existentialized. Existence moves on perpetually, bringing about new present moments, and what had been at some previous moment is, as at that moment, a desiccated Actuality, shorn of power and substantiality. Yet what is past stands over against what is present; it has a being of some kind, making it a possible topic for an historical study, and the proper terminus of a memory. It has a kind of existence, despite the fact that all Existence has moved on to the succeeding present. Otherwise the past would be nonexistensially related to the present, be a mere adjective of the present, incapable of standing over against it. This means that there must be a being which enables it to have something like an existence. It cannot get this from Existence itself; it is past precisely because all Existence has moved away from it, without residue. Nor can it get it from the Ideal, for the Ideal equates it with the present as merely another case of the Ideal. God alone could endow the past with a nondynamic facet of Existence which, though not essential yet is descriptive of it. If then by creation one means "the giving of Existence" to some determinate essence, as the Thomists seem to hold, one ought properly to say that God created the past rather than the present.

Many men acknowledge that there is a God on the basis of testimony offered in history. The writing of the Bible, supposed miracles, fulfillments of prophecy, incarnations, resurrections, and revelations are often offered as past facts which provide adequate testimony to the reality of God. It has been seriously questioned whether these are genuine facts. If they are, they are but a selection from a larger, equally

satisfactory body of evidence. Every bit of the past offers good testimony for the reality of God. But none, including these selected items,
offers direct testimony. The fact that there is a past, or that this or that
object is in the past, points only indirectly to God, since he does not
have the kind of existence which an impotent past must have.

4.18   A moralistic teleology begins with normative possibilities, directly testifying to an evaluating God.
(See 2.13, 2.14)

SOME POSSIBILITIES are actualized in the course of time. Present
Actualities act to make them real. There are other possibilities which
may never be realized in this world—the Good and subordinate norms
that things ought to reach and exhibit.

The Good is at once relevant and exterior to Actualities. Were it
only relevant, the Good could be exhausted by any and all of them;
were it only exterior, it could be without any bearing on them. But
it is not an essential feature of the Good that it be exterior. It could
conceivably become one with Actuality. To be exterior it must be
made and kept exterior.

Actualities cannot make the Good exterior to themselves, for it is
they who face it in just that guise as their objective. Nor can it be
Existence which does this, for though it has power enough to make
the Good relevant to all Actualities, or to keep it apart from them, it
does not have the capacity to make it stand apart as a norm for them.
God alone has the power and dignity to keep exterior a relevant norm
in terms of which the worth of the universe and the things in it are
evaluatable as defective.

The Ideal in its very nature is exterior to, and has a facet relevant
to Actuality; it is only in the fact that it is exterior while and so far
as it is relevant to and yet unrealized by Actuality, it is only because
it has the role of the Good that it offers testimony to the reality of
God. Exteriority is a descriptive nonessential feature of the Good,
testifying to a power which keeps the Good over against the Actualities that might otherwise subjugate it. It is a feature which provides
direct testimony of the reality of an exterior being capable of holding
apart from Actualities the standard in terms of which they are properly judged. The view that there are measuring archetypes, laws,

principles, ideas which are the concern of an infinite being is a specialization of a moralistic teleological approach. The measures are limited forms of one absolute normative possibility, the Good.

4.19 A directional teleology begins with realizable possibilities which indirectly testify to a temporally oriented God.
(See 2.09, 2.13, 3.94, 4.18)

A NONNORMATIVE possibility for this world must eventually be realized in the course of time or be a possibility in a purely logical sense. What the world precludes is no possibility for that world. But the possibility in itself obviously does not guarantee its own realization. Nor can Actualities guarantee the realization, for they frustrate one another all the time. What they do not realize today they may not realize tomorrow, and so on through endless time. Nor can Existence guarantee the realization of a possibility, since it has no capacity to know how to alter the relations of possibility to Actuality so as to make sure that what is not realized today will be realized tomorrow. Only a God has the power to keep nonnormative possibilities realizably relevant to Actualities. Such relevance is a nonessential feature, acquired by the possibilities by virtue of the manner in which God deals with them.

Aristotelians tend to view all possibilities as not only relevant to the world and its things, but to be exhausted by them in the course of time. Actualities inevitably and on their own, they suppose, can fulfill whatever possibilities there be. For them the Actualities are final substances which, though potential or incomplete at any given time, will eventually be completed. These thinkers are not, strictly speaking, entitled to the belief that the Actualities can achieve this completeness solely through the efforts of the Actualities themselves, and in any case, the completion could conceivably be delayed indefinitely. Some of these Aristotelians, Hegel at times for example, seem to hold that the Ideal works as a leaven in things and so affects them that they learn to accommodate it more and more. In this way, it is assured that the Ideal will be realized. But his assumption seems unwarranted by the facts and unnecessary in theory.

Possibilities as not yet realized are exterior to the realizing Actualities. This exteriority the Aristotelians guarantee in the very way the Platonists guarantee their relevance—they root the possibilities in a *tertium quid*, in some other reality. As a consequence, the Aristotelian view is not as distant from the Platonic as is usually supposed.

At every moment the Platonist's forms are "participated in" in various degrees. One can even say that his normative possibilities are exhausted over the course of time in the guise of components in a substance, such as a world-soul, which has different moral weights at different times, depending on how effectively it relates the norms to Actualities. And, on the other hand, since at any time the Aristotelian forms may not be realized, one can even say that his historically significant forms, through the aid of God, stand over against Actualities and measure them. Platonism and Aristotelianism seem now to reverse their positions. Nevertheless, the positions are distinct and not interchangeable. The main differences between the two views are firstly, that the things in this universe are final substances for Aristotelians and morally qualified fragments for Platonists; secondly, that whereas the primary function of the Aristotelian *tertium quid* is to guarantee the exteriority of the forms, the primary function of the Platonic *tertium quid* is to guarantee their relevance. But more important for the present purposes is the fact that thirdly, for the Platonist, possibilities testify directly to God, a morally concerned being; whereas for the Aristotelian they indirectly testify to a controlling God, since they are relevant to realizing Actualities apart from him and need him only in order to be able to be exterior to those Actualities. In partial agreement with the Platonists we are here maintaining that God without cessation offers relevant possibilities to Actualities, and sums up their partial realizations to a complete fulfillment by the end of a period. And in partial agreement with the Aristotelian we are also maintaining that those possibilities are kept exterior to the Actualities by God until they are completely fulfilled.

The argument that progress, evolution, dialectic offer evidence of the reality of governing possibilities under the control of a God specializes the view of a directional teleology. This begins with the consideration of any possibility whatsoever, and recognizes that any possibility which must be realized in time testifies to a temporally oriented God who keeps the realizable possibility exterior and relevant to realizing Actualities until fully realized.

4.20 A providential teleology begins with a cosmic possibility which indirectly testifies to a purposing God.
(See *2.18*, *3.07*)

THE FUTURE is a single possible which the various Actualities delimit, specialize, fragmentate. It is too wide for any Actuality and too temporal for God. Its proper correlate is cosmic Existence. Since a Future which will never be is not a future at all, it is essential that this cosmic possibility be realized. Nothing can guarantee its realization except a being capable of relating it to Existence, so as to exhaust it over the course of time either as a future possibility which Existence will attain, or as a normative possibility which measures the worth of Existence at every moment. The exhaustion of the Future in Existence is not essential to it.

Providence is primarily cosmic in import; it relates to the governance of the entire universe. It may have no delimited or anthropomorphic implications. To acknowledge it in its broadest sense is to point to a being cosmic in range and power, capable of making the Ideal function as a genuine Future for a perpetually vital Existence.

4.21 An architectural teleology begins with unified Existence as providing direct testimony to the reality of an effective God.
(See *3.01*, *3.03*, *3.102*)

EXISTENCE perpetually divides itself; it is forever placing part outside part, even opposing its own essence to the rest of itself. But without its essence it could not have a nature, be this rather than that, have a unity. Its essence is descriptive of it. But that essence, precisely because Existence is self-divisive, is not essential to it. For it to have the essence which is descriptive of it, it must look for aid outside itself. Actualities cannot provide this aid, for they are too limited in range and power. The Ideal cannot provide it either, for the Ideal is at the border of Existence, serving as its Future, and cannot therefore make the essence one with the all present Existence. Only God has the power to make the essence of Existence one with it, hold Existence together with its own essence so as to constitute a unified being with a nature. Since unity is essential and intrinsic to God, unified Existence provides direct testimony of the reality of God. Such testimony is wrongly specialized by those who take the regularity of some of the processes of Existence to provide direct testimony of the reality of God. Only a regularity cosmic in range, persistent in fact, and really unified with Existence could provide that testimony.

4.2 2   A mathematical teleology begins with phenomenalized Existence as offering indirect testimony to the reality of a cosmic God.
(See *1.09, 1.12, 1.22, 3.102, 4.17*)

THE BIBLE begins by speaking of God as hovering over uncharted Existence. It then goes on to indicate how he fragmentates it, localizes it, makes it ingredient in different types of being. The Existence he was supposed to confront initially is somewhat like Schopenhauer's unconscious or Bergson's *élan vital*, except that it lacks the forward thrust so characteristic of these modern views. The Cartesian vortices comes a little closer than the Bible does to these philosophic accounts; the theory of the ether comes a little closer than they do to the biblical. For modern physics Existence has a quite different nature. It is only a phenomenon, without being of its own, getting whatever characteristics it has, as a field, from the bodies said to be in the field. The older views were better, for they knew that Existence also had being. But in another sense, they were inferior, for they did not see that Existence is also a phenomenon with a nature determined by the bodies that make up the scientific world.

Actualities help determine the geometry of Existence. As they vary in grouping and activity that geometry varies. But they do not impose that geometry on it. The most that could be said, if one attended to Actualities alone, is that the geometry was an adventitious product of their conjoint presence. Since the geometry of Existence varies with the distribution of Actualities, it cannot be essential to Existence. Nor can it owe its presence to the Ideal, for this can only make Existence into an instance of itself. Only a cosmic God is able to make the independent and often oppositional Actualities have a single, persistent, harmonious effect on Existence in the form of a nonessential variable geometry. Such a geometry, constituting Existence as a phenomenon, offers indirect testimony to the reality of God. This view is partially stated by those who hold that God enables believers to constitute a "living" church.

4.23 A structuralized teleology begins with idealized Existence as providing indirect testimony to the reality of an ordering God.
(*See 2.99, 4.20*)

EXISTENCE is always in the present, though terminating in the Future. That Future is not essential to it, for it is outside it, at its limit. Still it is germane to Existence, enabling it to be *temporally present*, present in time. But to be present in time, it must be infected with Ideality, be characterizable as that which can be at a subsequent time, as that which has a Future.

No Actuality has the reach or the power to make the Future a factor in Existence. The Future can do this, but not without making Existence into just a locus, occasion for, or instance of itself. Only God has the power to bring them together in such a way that each retains its integrity. The result, since it is not a true unity, does not provide direct testimony of God. But it does offer indirect testimony of him, the being who alone has the power to allow the Future and Existence to be inseparable without compromising either.

When it is said that without God Existence would be chaotic, unordered, moving in no significant way, a faint and partial presentation of a structuralized teleological approach is being given. One then, instead of remarking on the nature of Existence as it is apart from the Future, stresses instead a possible consequence of the separation. Apart from the Future, Existence could be. It could even be intelligible, well ordered and one-directional. But it could not be in or constitute a present, for there is no present except in relation to a future.

III   COSMOLOGICAL   RELATIONS

4.24 There can be no teleological proofs of God.
(*See 1.81, 4.12*)

A TELEOLOGICAL approach provides testimony, direct or indirect. But it goes no further than to show the necessity for acknowledging an object, and then only as and so far as it is being testified to. It does not let us know what the object is as apart from what now testifies to it; it does not tell us what the object might be when not being testified to. Nor does it tell us whether or not the object is a final irreducible being. It gives us a premiss and thus implies a conclusion, but it does not relate us to that conclusion as that which could be affirmed in place of the premiss.

If a man has been strangled he provides testimony to a strangler, but to nothing more. We suppose there was such a strangler to explain the man's being choked while his hands were tied behind his back. But we do not know whether he was strangled by one who acted on his own or under compulsion. We do not know whether that strangler now exists or not. We suppose that he at least once had an independent existence, but only because we also assume that we can make valid inferences regarding the relation of hands to bodies, and bodies to Existence.

To prove the existence of God we must not only have a premiss but also a rule of inference, i.e., a warranted way of connecting that premiss with God as a conclusion; and we must then follow the route of that rule if we are to terminate in that conclusion. We must, in short, supplement the teleological approach to God with other approaches having other functions.

The classical three "proofs" of God, the teleological, the cosmological, and the ontological, are really three parts of one proof, and as such are mutually dependent. No one of them alone will yield a proof of God. Each needs the others if a proof is to be carried out. To speak of a genuine "teleological proof" then is but to speak of a proof involving the other types as well—and, of course, conversely.

Our use of the term "teleological" is not then altogether one with the more common use of it in the expression a "teleological proof" of God. The traditional "teleological proof" in fact is one which uses some specialized form of a teleological approach such as that the world has a beauty or excellence not essential to it, and then without further ado assumes a rule of inference and engages in an act of inferring to the object testified to. The fact of evil raises grave doubts regarding what this "proof" takes to be testimony. And even to one who accepts its testimony, it offers no warrant for the route its argument takes, or for the manner in which that route is in fact traversed.

All the modes of being can be proved by starting with and making use of the structure and activity of the others. If one of them could not be proved, it would be one which was altogether cut off from the rest; it would not be able to be together with them, and thus could not, with them, exhaust the whole of being. To be sure, we know beings and must know them apart from all proof. If we did not, our proofs could never be checked in an encounter, and our proving, for all we would then know, would be a misguided play with symbols signifying nothing. In fact, if by God we mean the *being* at whom our proof eventually arrives, we can have no testimony of his reality until we have finished our proof of him. A similar observation must be made with respect to the other modes of being as well. But if we also arrive at him and other beings through proofs, we will have learned how they are related to one another, how they support one another, and how truths and other values characterizing a knowledge of one can be validly transferred to the others.

In the foregoing examination of testimony we have ignored the case where two indirect testimonies are combined to give a single testimony. Although such combinations seem closer to what most people treat as testimony, and though the combination is no simple aggregation and makes a difference to the nature of what is testifying, the complication seems not worth special attention here. Putting these cases aside still leaves over many more proofs of God than seem to have been recognized in the literature.

4.25 There are three primary and six secondary cosmological approaches to God.
(See *1.81, 4.09*)

A PROOF moves from premiss to conclusion in accordance with a rule which justifies the substitution of the conclusion for the premiss. The rule required in a proof of God's existence must be capable of relating a teleological premiss, testifying to the reality of God, to God as a possible terminus of an inference, or of some other permitted process. Strictly speaking the rule should be independent in origin, justification, locus, use, and meaning from any particular testimony, though, of course, to be a rule governing a proof of God, it must always have God as the terminal term.

Each mode of being provides a *primary* rule in the form of some characteristic structure having God as a terminus. Since each mode of being is significantly qualified by two other modes of being, each mode of being also provides two *secondary* rules reflecting the pres-

ence and operation of the other modes. These secondary rules are no
less valid than the primary, differing from it only in that they express
the structure of a qualified rather than of a pure mode of being.

4.26 A formal cosmological approach to God relates some mode of being to him by means of the formal structure of possibility.
(*See 4.12, 4.25*)

FORMAL LOGIC is a subject, hidebound by tradition. It rarely recognizes more than one type of structure warranting a proof: a formal
structure reflecting the nature of possibility. And this abstract formal
structure, despite its universal applicability, is then denied a role except with respect to terms abstract and formal. If one were to accept
these conditions one could expect nothing from a proof but the derivation of an abstract formal result from abstract formal premisses
along an abstract formal route. The derivation of the premiss from
concrete material or experience, the acknowledgment of the conclusion as germane to something that occurs, and the very process of
deriving the conclusion would, on this account, lie entirely outside
the orbit of any proof. The structures logic recognizes are relations,
valid rules, governing proofs of all sorts, including that of the reality
of God, but they are not enough, by themselves, to yield a proof of
anything, even a tautology.

Possibility is the domain of logical relations of necessity. It is the
locus of entailments, of necessary connections between possible states
of affairs. The structure of the realm of possibility, whether this be
viewed as containing nothing but undivided Ideality or whether this
be viewed as already divided into limited possibilities pertinent to the
particular things in the world, is a fixed, universally applicable, prescriptive logic, whose structures provide legitimate routes for moving
from any item to any other, and thus from any item to God.

4.27 A devotional cosmological approach to God relates some mode of being to him by means of an individualized structure of possibility.
(*See 4.25, 4.26*)

FORMAL STRUCTURES of logic are specified and exemplified in Actualities. Man personalizes, delimits them, gives them another value

and function than that which they have in themselves. Any such individualized formal structure, when made to terminate in God, provides a secondary rule of inference to him. Such a rule is close to what is usually meant by the form of a proper religious attitude. Perhaps nothing expresses it so well as the structure of a prayer, for the structure of a prayer is a formal relation terminating in God as relevant to the nature of individual man. Just what are good, satisfactory prayers and what are not has never been adequately determined, in part because logicians have concentrated on more abstract and impersonal structures, and in part because religion is such a practical subject that major emphasis has always been placed on the activity of praying and the efficacy of the act, with a consequent ignoring of formal and theoretical issues. There are to be sure established prayers with quite definite structures, and those who are full members of churches are expected to make use of them, and at given times. But these prayers are usually thought to be important primarily for their content; whatever structures they may have are not justified by reference to any inherent rationale, but at best because of tradition, rhetoric, and supposed efficacy.

4.28   A naturalistic cosmological approach to God relates some mode of being to him by means of an existentialized structure of possibility.
(See *2.18, 3.03, 3.104, 4.25, 4.26*)

POSSIBILITY is infected by Existence, thereby attaining the status of a set of prescriptive laws which Existence is to exhibit. These laws have a structure, the very structure of possibility, but delimited, made germane to the ongoing scheme of things.

The prescriptive laws of nature are possibility tinged with Existence, possibility confined to the area of space-time. These laws have two sides. One side they show to Actualities, prescribing in advance what these can and will do. The other side they show to God, making it possible for him to act providentially. To make use of the laws of nature as a relation terminating in God is to have both sides at once in the guise of a secondary rule of inference to him.

4.29   An individualized cosmological approach to God
relates some mode of being to him by means of the
structure of Actuality.
(*See 4.12, 4.16, 4.25*)

ACTUALITIES have structures which can mediate between different
types of being. They, and particularly those that are men, can provide
primary rules which enable one to connect testimony, on behalf of
God, with God. The rule may be one exhibiting the structure of a
character or attitude. If the structure has God as one terminus, the
character or attitude of an Actuality is one of *reverence*. Such a structure has not had the attention it deserves; still it is known to all men
as one of the primary and perhaps the best way of relating testimony
to the God to which it testifies. Not the bad man or the indifferent
man but one who is reverential is able to mediate such simple testimony as that provided by the flowers in the field, and God. Without
that attitude of reverence the testimony provided by those flowers
will allow one to speculate or surmise, but will not relate one to God
in an individual way.

4.30   An institutionalized cosmological approach to God
relates some mode of being to him by means of the
structure of Actuality when qualified by Ideality.
(*See 2.16, 2.17, 4.25, 4.29*)

ACTUALITIES are infected with and inseparable from Ideality. They
are at once individuals and members of classes, kinds of beings. If
as individuals they have an attitude of reverence, they provide primary rules governing movements from some mode of being to God.
When those very individuals are members of some institution, a
church or group, they are qualified by common possibilities. These
possibilities, without abrogating the individuals' characters or attitudes, make the individuals into carriers of some more common feature or attitude. An Actuality, in the guise of a member of a church
or religious community has then, due to the qualifications provided
by possibility, a structure which enables him to relate some mode of
being to God. This structure can be used as a secondary rule in a
proof of him.

4.31   A worshipful cosmological approach to God relates some mode of being to him by means of the structure of Actuality when qualified by Existence.
(*See 3.38, 4.25, 4.30*)

EXISTENCE makes a difference to Actualities; it, by virtue of its continuity with the Existence in Actualities, imposes limitations, modifies activities, produces changes in those Actualities. A reverential worshipful Actuality, when qualified by Existence, provides a secondary rule serving to mediate a mode of being with God. This rule or structure has been acknowledged by the Stoics. They thought that a truly wise man was one who submitted to cosmic Existence, and who had a kind of attitude of worship towards an absolute fixed fire of truth in which that structure of wisdom terminated. This view is also expressed by Spinoza at the end of his *Ethics,* and indeed by all those who ask men to assume an attitude of natural piety towards all that lies beyond him and the Existence which affects and environs him.

4.32   A materialistic cosmological approach to God relates some mode of being to him by means of the structure of Existence.
(*See 3.02, 3.03–5, 3.15, 4.25, 4.30*)

MATTER for the philosophical materialist is quite immaterial; it is somewhat closer in nature to Plato's receptacle, the ether, or the space-time geometrized physics of modern relativity than it is to the hard atoms of Democritus or Lucretius. It is one in fact with what we have termed "Existence," a self-othering, perpetually expansive or productive domain. The structure of this expansive self-othering, treated as a kind of continuum without ultimate parts and with neither beginning nor ending, is isolated in a materialistic cosmological approach and used as a relation connecting some mode of being with God. Expressed in spatial terms this relation constitutes a theological space relating the other modes of being to God; expressed in temporal terms the relation constitutes the permanent structure of time in which every moment occurs; expressed in terms of energy the relation constitutes a cosmological constant to which specific things give limited and changing values.

4.33   An idealized cosmological approach to God relates some mode of being to him by means of the structure of Existence when qualified by Ideality.
(*See 3.104, 4.23, 4.28, 4.32*)

EXISTENCE, when qualified by the Ideal, is a tissue of the immanent laws of nature. These laws Peirce called habits in things—a perceptive observation, unduly restricted by him however to Actualities, and allowed to hide the fact that Existence has its own rhythm, apart from those "habits." The habits or immanent laws contrast with whatever prescriptive laws are imposed on Existence, either by some other mode of being or through an act of interpretation. To know the nature of the former kind of law is to know the rationale of the Existence that in fact environs us, and thus to be better able to adjust ourselves and our expectations to the course of nature.

The immanent laws of nature can function as secondary rules relating any mode of being to God. The Kantian view that the moral law mediates between the experiential world and a free spirit evidently offers a special case of such rules.

4.34   An historical cosmological approach to God relates some mode of being to him by means of the structure of Existence when qualified by Actualities.
(*See 4.22, 4.31, 4.32*)

EXISTENCE has an effect on Actualities, and they have an effect on it. By affecting it they conjointly qualify its structure and modify its course. The result is Existence as the perpetual matrix of historic phenomena. Existence in this guise is to be contrasted with Existence as a mere phenomenon. The former has its own integrity and effectiveness, with a rationale of its own, but one modified by Actualities; the latter has no other structure than that which has been exteriorly bestowed on it. The former, since the structure exhibits qualifications of Existence which Actualities themselves provide, offers testimony to the reality, not of God, but of Actualities. But the latter, since the structure characterizes Existence in ways beyond the power of Existence, Actuality, or Ideality to produce does provide testimony to the reality of God.

Existence when qualified by Actualities offers a secondary relation between a mode of being and God as well as indirect testimony to the reality of Actualities; phenomenal Existence offers indirect testimony to the reality of God, and also a secondary relation between some mode of being and Actualities. Both kinds of relation can serve as secondary rules in a proof, the one having a terminus in God, the other having a terminus in Actualities.

4.35 There can be no cosmological proofs of God.
(See *1.81, 4.12, 4.24*)

THE TERM "cosmological" used in connection with a proof of God has conventionally been understood to refer to a mode of argument which starts with any existence whatsoever and deduces that this must have had God as its cause. Such an argument looks as if it had avoided the usual teleological supposition that Existence is good or ordered or purposive. What the usual cosmological argument does is to treat Existence as though it were desirable but not intrinsically real, and therefore as though its presence offered testimony to the reality of a being concerned enough to make that desirable Existence be. But then it should first show that Existence has value, has no genuine reality, and that its presence could not be explained in terms of something other than God. The argument also holds itself rather narrowly to the use of only a formal relation between the existing beings and God, and then neglects to deal with the question as to how to make use of that formal relation in order to have God in the guise of an outcome or conclusion. If we understand by "a proof of God" a proof which takes its start with something that testifies to God, and ends with him as at the outcome of a movement along a validated route, a "cosmological proof" is no proof at all, but in fact at best only part of a proof. A cosmological approach to God can give only a relational structure which a proof must utilize; it does not enable us either to leave our testimony behind or to arrive at God; it must be supplemented by other approaches before a proof is possible. The resulting proof cannot properly be termed "cosmological" any more than it could properly be termed "teleological."

4.36 Teleological and cosmological approaches to God are supplementary.
(See *4.24, 4.35*)

A COSMOLOGICAL approach offers a relation which connects testimony with the object testified to. That relation should be defined in independence of the evidence, in order to assure us a terminus which can have a nature or being apart from the testifying feature. Conversely, testimony is needed if we are to make effective use of the relation. Without it there would be no opportunity, need, or desire to go through a proof. Only a world which bears the marks of God's power could lead us to him as a "cosmological" cause of it; only an independent, effective God could be the source of the features that offer direct testimony to him.

A teleological approach offers a premiss implying some conclusion; a cosmological approach offers a conclusion as implied by some premiss. Both are needed in order to have a premiss connected with a conclusion—using "premiss" and "conclusion" here to embrace not merely concepts, judgments, propositions, sentences, but beings as well.

4.37   A conjunction of teleological and cosmological approaches cannot provide a proof of God.
(*See 4.12, 4.36*)

GOD is not identical with what testifies to him; he is not merely an object of a testimony. Nor is he reducible to a term of some relation. Instead he stands out over against every other mode of being. A proof of him must in fact terminate in him, as one who is outside and over against what testifies to him and what relates that testimony to him. It must therefore go beyond what a conjunction of cosmological and teleological approaches could provide. To get to that mode of being which is God, we must move as well as begin and relate. This requires that he be detached from the structure of a proof through the agency of some mode of being distinct from him.

IV   ONTOLOGICAL DETACHMENTS

4.38   A proof of God requires an act of ontological detachment of him from the structure of a proof.
(*See 1.86, 1.87, 4.10–12, 4.37*)

IT WAS one of Kant's definitive insights that the so-called teleological and cosmological arguments could not reach the desired goal of proving the existence of God without the aid of the ontological argument. Kant, however, treated each of these arguments as though it were distinct and complete and then attempted to show that no one of them, and particularly the ontological argument, could arrive at the desired conclusion. He did not consider the possibility that what the arguments could not do separately they might be able to do together—a strange and perplexing oversight. As together the three traditional arguments no longer have their traditional form—nor make their traditional excessive claims. They are in fact parts of a more inclusive proof which has a strength not possible to its parts.

The teleological and cosmological approaches must supplement one another if there is to be a proof of God. The one provides the premiss while the other provides the rule relating that premiss to the desired conclusion. But if there be no detaching of the conclusion, which the cosmological approach relates to the teleological testifying premiss, there will be no proof in fact. Now, detachment is an activity, and like every activity follows a route. A good route, over which one can legitimately move to a conclusion, is offered by a formal structure expressible in logic. But there are other routes, much denser than the formal structures of logic, over which one can move with as much warrant as one can over those of logic. It is over these that artists move to the conclusion of their work and that religious men move to the conclusion of religious experience. Or, what comes to the same thing, there are media thicker than the medium of a logical mind, made use of by artists and religious men when engaged in their typical activities. Since the activities involve a passage from a beginning to an end in accordance with a rule which warrants the adoption of that end in place of the beginning, they can be viewed as varieties of inference. The outcome of the passage to a conclusion by logician, artist, and religious man results in the separating out of the conclusion from the relational structure of the rule, thereby converting a possible into an actual conclusion. The fact that the conclusions of the artist and religious man are not expressed in propositions, and that the natures of those conclusions may be accumulatively determined in the course of getting to them, does not affect the situation, but only kind of meaning and value that the conclusions might have for those who conclude to them.

4.39   There can be no ontological proofs of God.
(See 1.14, 4.12, 4.36, 4.38)

THE ONTOLOGICAL ARGUMENT attempts to prove that God exists, on the ground that since God is a perfect being and Existence is a perfection, a denial of the existence of God would involve a self-contradiction. One need not involve the argument in the controversy as to whether or not Existence is a predicate. That it is a predicate is I think clear (see 3.16). And whether it be a predicate or not, Existence is a perfection, an excellence, desirable, enhancing. This agreement with the main contention of the ontological argument, however, does not lead us to its conclusion. Quite the contrary. Since other beings than God exist, God cannot be absolutely perfect; he lacks the desirable existence that the others possess. What the traditional ontological argument proves is not the existence of God, but the existence of a cosmos in which a God can be at best but one item. To prove the existence of God the argument would have had to attend not to any kind of existence, yours or mine, a table's or an idea's, but only to God's kind. But then it would prove the existence of God only because it had assumed this to start with. If instead it started with God's nature and credited this with an appropriate existence, it would prove not the existence of God but the existence of that nature and thus only of a possibility, for this is what a mere nature is. A proof of God's existence, in opposition to the intent of the ontological argument, must start somewhere away from him and his existence, and move to him, not as a being already acknowledged to exist, nor to him in the guise of a mere nature or possibility, but to him as in fact existing. This requires one to make use of the teleological and cosmological approaches; the ontological can only supplement them in the guise of an act of detachment of the required conclusion.

4.40   There are three pure and six qualified modes of detaching God from a cosmological rule which begins with testimony to his existence.
(See 4.11, 4.38)

DETACHING is an activity, Existence operating on the conclusion of a rule. But there is not only Existence as such; there are also (existing) Actualities and an (existing) Possibility.

Work (see 4.47) is a means by which Existence serves to convert a possible conclusion regarding God's reality into an actual conclusion. It offers an agency by means of which God, as implied by some rule, is in fact detached from the rule, arrived at. *Faith* (see 4.44) offers a similar agency to be used by (existing) Actuality. Finally, an intellectual act of *assent* (see 4.41) offers a corresponding way by which (existing) Possibility serves to detach the conclusion, God. Each of these modes of detachment is creative in the sense that what was a merely relationally defined, possible conclusion is turned by it into one that is separate, determinate, put in place of the testifying beginning.

Each of the modes of detachment can be subject to qualifications imposed by other modes of being. There is thus not only something done by means of pure Existence (see 4.47) but also *good* works produced by Existence as qualified by Actuality (see 4.48) and *dedicated* work produced by Existence as qualified by Ideality (see 4.49). There is not only the detachment performed by Actualities in pure faith (see 4.44), but the readjustments achieved in *prayer* (see 4.45) and in *humility* (see 4.46). And there are not only inferences terminating in assents (see 4.41) but others which terminate in *acceptances* (see 4.42) and *acknowledgments* (see 4.43). These various activities are independent of one another, and independent as well of the kind of testimony that is available or the kind of rule that would warrant a beginning with that testimony and a terminating in God. Each deserves to be separately remarked.

What is normally termed a proof takes account only of the last group of inferences—those ending in assents, acceptances, or acknowledgments—since it attends only to that mode of detachment which uses the part of Existence that is operative in a rational mind. Such proofs get to a conclusion of a rather abstract sort. The others offer ways of moving to God in a more concrete and, if in a less intellectually then in a more religiously satisfying way. They prove in the way in which a man is proved in fire and pudding in the eating.

4.41   The existence of God can be logically inferred.
(*See 1.80–86, 4.40*)

INFERENCE is a creative, logical activity which attempts to transfer to some possible conclusion a desirable property possessed or guaranteed by the premiss. It does not give the conclusion its being; rather it enables it to be detached from a rule and thus to be faced as having a desirable property over against and outside the premiss and rule. This property should, when the inference begins with a true premiss and follows a legitimate route, coincide with that which the conclusion has apart from the act of inference. The proposition, "Socrates is mortal" does not become true by being deduced from "All men are mortal and Socrates is a man"; the deduction character- izes the proposition as "true," a property which we might not have been able, or might have found too difficult to know that it has. We infer truths about the other side of the moon and the movements of subatomic entities in similar ways, but in these cases we may never be able to know that the results to which we conclude are true except by going through the inferences. Just so, a properly grounded, valid logi- cal inference to some proposition regarding God may not be known to be true when held away from its proof.

There is always a risk in an act of inference, for even the *modus ponens* which says that if we assert "if p then q" and also assert "p," we can therefore justifiably assert "q," presupposes that the different "p's" and the different "q's" are in no important respect dissimilar. In opposition to idealists and existentialists, modern logicians simply assume that the transition from the internal relation of "if p then q" to the external relation "p therefore q" involves no significant change in the items related. That there is a difference of some sort between them, it would be absurd to deny, since it is the very intent of the rule of *modus ponens* to make us attend to it. It would be foolish to say that the difference is so great as to make the transition hopelessly and always illegitimate, for this would be tantamount to denying the legitimacy of every proof, and with it the legitimacy of any defense of this position. But it is proper to say that the difference in fact makes a significant difference in this case or that, or under such and such conditions. Every movement, logical or nonlogical, having an empiri- cal or other outcome, can be questioned. But if any one such transi- tion is in principle justifiable or questionable so is every other, unless there be a guarantee (see 4.56) that some process or other is without risk at all.

A logical inference to God need not begin with propositions or universals, or anything abstract; nor need it follow the route of a formal cosmological structure. But no matter where it begins or what route it follows it ends in an *assent* to, a remarking on some truth regarding God.

4.42 The existence of God can be accepted through an intellectual assent qualified by the self.
(*See 4.40, 4.41*)

A LOGICAL INFERENCE ends with an *assent* to the conclusion which has been warranted by some logical rule. If the conclusion is a presence or a nature or an action or a meaning, the assent is but an intellectual way of noting the presence, action, etc., apart from an encounter. But where the conclusion is a proposition the assent takes the form of an *affirmation*. These assents are sustained by a self. It is the self that uses the mind, that thinks, infers, assents, affirms.

The self always plays some role; it often ought to play a great role. This is particularly true in relation to some proofs of God. We seek not only to take an intellectual position with respect to God, but sometimes ought to determine a place for ourselves in relation to him. What is then needed is a qualification of an intellectualized proof by an awareness that the outcome should commit us in our innermost beings.

When we affirm a conclusion we characterize it as material to be used. It is that which has been established, and which thus may for the time being be put aside as not in question. When we *accept* a proposition we are ready to act on it; we place it within the frame of our tendencies to deal with other matters, we qualify the affirmation by subjugating it to our selves. And what is true of propositions is true of properties, acts, purposes. When we accept God as a purposive being, for example, we qualify our assent to his presence by an awareness that our selves are involved. The qualifications that the self imposes make a difference to the manner in which we and God then and thereafter stand with respect to one another. Acceptance is assent given subjective force, thrust forward into the context of human concerns, its object being thereby recognized to be portentous, big with meaning for us.

4.43   The existence of God can be acknowledged through an intellectual assent qualified by Existence.
(See 3.104, 4.40, 4.41)

ALL PROOFS are conducted by men, and thus are conducted inside the domain of Actuality. Still men, through their intellects, share in the realm of the Ideal, and, through their works, participate in an Existence outside themselves. It is legitimate therefore to speak of Existence qualifying an intellectual approach to the existence of God. Such qualification occurs in acts of sacrifice, where the individual loses or ignores himself to concentrate on some facet of Existence as providing a modifying note to his assent to God. The sacrifice need not involve the use of some particular object, nor need it involve some signal alteration in a thing. It can occur when there is an alteration in the quality of an assent by means of Existence.

Acknowledgement is a qualified assent, an assent in which the intellect is affected by Existence when this is represented by some sacrificed object, an object which is denied its normal function to become an agency for reaching God.

4.44   God can be reached through faith.
(See 4.40)

CONFRONTED with the terminus of a structure or rule of some sort, a man, instead of taking a pure or qualified intellectual approach to it, may alter his attitude, readjust himself to it. He may hold the terminus off from the rule in such a way that it stands over against him, not as something understood, but as his negative, as that which he is not. It is such a transition to God, the being who is not oneself, that characterizes a living faith.

Faith can follow a perfectly rational structure. It is not an anti-intellectual feat, a leap into the unknown, without warrant. Faith does go beyond reason, but only in the sense that the manner in which it arrives at, detaches, characterizes God is much bolder than that which the intellect tolerates. Indeed almost every act of faith is preceded by some kind of testimony and involves some recognition of the being testified to. He who was content with a faith which was grounded in no testimony or which followed no rule would be in the dark, knowing neither why nor how nor where to go.

Faith for the Protestant is usually thought of as a submission of oneself without reserve to God. For the Catholic it is an intellectual assent to what is revealed. These are specializations of the interpretation here given. A man of faith need not submit himself without reservation; nor need he suppose that there are any truths that have been revealed. But he does need testimony and he does need guidance, and that at which he ends does require of him more than conviction.

From the standpoint of an intellect unwilling to make use of any mode of detachment than that provided by *modus ponens,* faith goes much too far. But the converse is also true. From the standpoint of the detachment which faith provides, *modus ponens* is too bold, since it on the one hand subjugates God to private, finite affirmations, and on the other hand looks at his awesome majesty coldly, abstractly, and thus not at him as he really is. It would be foolish to choose between these ways of reaching God. Both are legitimate and satisfying, but for different purposes. Faith is the work of the self; assent of the intellect. The scope of the intellect is broader than that of the self in the sense that its rules are universally applicable and all its items are on a level. But the grasp of the self is more penetrating than that of the intellect; not only is the intellect its creature, but it can get to different things in different ways, changing its attitudes in accordance with their natures, and what these natures may mean to it.

4.45   God can be reached through prayer, a faith qualified by possibility.
(See 2.103, 4.27, 4.40, 4.44)

FAITH is essentially a private act; it occurs in the recesses of the self, involving a conversion or change of attitude towards that which is the terminus of some acceptable cosmological approach to God. Prayer, though often performed in public, is also radically personal. Unlike faith, however, it bears the mark of possibility, of what could be. It is a glorification, a petition, a supplication, a turning towards the being in whom one has faith, whom one can trust, but also from whom one can expect some appreciation of a possibility which one may fear or wish realized. That possibility qualifies the act of faith and thus makes a difference to the manner in which this terminates in God.

Prayer is faith restricted, confined, made to terminate in God, the

being whom one trusts to be operative with respect to whatever possibilities are relevant to oneself and others. Like faith, it can operate
in independence of any testimony and any rule. But it cannot be
counted on to reach God if it does not begin with relevant evidence
and does not relate this to God in some structural warrantable way.
A prayer which takes no account of what there might be to testify
to God, or which follows no acknowledged rule, whether this be
formally stated, credally given, or dogmatically affirmed, points nowhere and anywhere.

It is the neglect of the need to have proper starting points and adequate guides that permits so many prayers to be special pleas for help,
for the performance of miracles, or even at times for the sanctification
of wrong doing. To avoid these consequences many established religions prescribe the form of prayer that is acceptable. They build into
the prayer, as it were, the element of testimony and the factor of
structure. But then they run the opposite risk of reducing the prayer
to a pattern or structure to be followed mechanically. What is needed
is an independent testifying beginning, and an independent relation
connecting that beginning to God. Prayer can then serve its proper
function, be a dynamic, creative mode of reaching that terminus
through the thickness of an attitude of faith tinctured by what in fact
is possible.

Prayer is a kind of love, a basic relation connecting man with
God. All the other relations connecting man with God might, indeed, with little distortion be said to be so many different forms of
prayer. Now to love is first of all to expose oneself, to present oneself
naked before another, freed from irrelevance, facades, contingencies,
barriers, thereby risking injury and abuse. Prayer, an act of loving
God, is a means by which one exposes oneself, without qualification or
escape, to an infinite and awful majesty.

One's first encounter with God overwhelms, fills one with fear and
terror. God is felt to be one who could crush, and with right, anyone
who opened himself to him. The churches codify prayers partly because all church practices are primarily institutional experiments in
getting a proper relation to God, and like all experiments need to be
controlled, stabilized, and made common. They are codified partly
too because the churches know that prayer is an adventure in a daring,

dangerous effort to encounter God. But more important perhaps is the fact that they can then make more evident that the religious man's awesome God lifts up, preserves, and enhances while he correctly evaluates those who look to him, that he qualifies justice with mercy, forgives while he judges, and therefore need not be feared.

God in the guise of judge deals with the naked lover, the pitiable being who confronts him in prayer, firmly but with tenderness, saving all in him that can be saved. He puts aside all that is not of the very essence of the man, and thus puts aside most of that with which the nonpraying man identifies himself. Those who pray offer God nothing more or less than themselves, and with this he deals directly and gently. Those who pray therefore quickly pass from awe and fear, not to complacency and self-assurance, but to a confidence that he will not take advantage of one's weakness, that he will not altogether abandon one but will instead extract whatever good he can. Churches are not, however, indispensable. Good prayers can be privately or socially forged, provided that they are subjected to the limiting, structuring, and humanization of a memorable past, a present which is worth vivification, and a dedication to some worth-while pursuit.

4.46   God can be reached through humility, a faith qualified by Existence.

(*See 3.103, 4.31, 4.40, 4.44*)

WHEN one's attitude of faith is qualified by Existence, faith begins to express a cosmic power deeper and wider than oneself; one becomes aware of mysterious, subterranean forces. Faith then becomes not the simple trust of a Job or the prayer of an Abraham but the humility of a St. Francis, aware that God is a God not only for man but for everything in the universe.

Humility is no foolish rejection of oneself, a denial of one's worth, a cancelling out of all confidence, adventure, or even pride. Based on evidence of God's nature, conforming to some rule relating that evidence to him, it is superior to an act of self-rejection. It recognizes God's majesty. And it is sensitive to the fact that man is immersed in an Existence larger and grander than himself. It is the way we express most adequately the belief that if God created world and man he made them noble, and that if he did not create them, he is one who thinks that whatever good they embody ought to be appreciated and accepted, and are therefore to be encouraged, admired, enjoyed, not denigrated, denied, despised.

4.47   God can be reached through work.
(*See 4.40*)

EVERY ACT of detachment is due to the efficacy of Existence. And every detachment which occurs as a moment in a proof is performed by men. But the detachment which a man might perform may bear no mark of his nature or needs. To avoid this consequence it is desirable to engage in work.

All wholehearted immersion in work, since it leads to the subjugation of self to the processes and structures of nature, is a way of acting in accordance with the rhythms of Existence. He who acts in this way submits himself and his interests, his efforts and the value of his work, to Existence. He is thereby enabled to face God as a being in a dynamic relation to himself.

Any one of man's activities, engaged in for selfish reasons or not, can be treated as a representative of the whole of Existence. He who treats his own activities in this way makes an offering of those activities; he separates God off from a cosmological approach, not by exercising his role as an individual but by acting as a localized portion of Existence which he then represents. This approach is charmingly illustrated in the story of the juggler of Notre Dame, who offered his juggling as a way of expressing his adoration. He submitted himself to God through the agency of an activity, viewed as placing him in an existential relation to the divine. It is remarkable how everyone, young and old, educated and untutored, is ready to believe in the efficacy of the juggler's act. The point of course has been made in other ways; it is embodied in the Hassidic joyous dance before the lord and the Zen Buddhists' gestures and simple movements—in fact in the activities of all those who seek God selflessly apart from the constraints of some formal demand.

4.48   God can be reached through good works.
(*See 2.86, 2.99, 4.47*)

MUCH DISCUSSION of God is vitiated by the fact that men enter into it in a pragmatic spirit, to find out how to save their souls; there is a tendency on the part of many to neglect any issues or nuances which have no importance for this issue. But God is a being worth understanding on his own account, precisely because he is one of the basic realities of the cosmos. And one way of reaching him as a being—and not necessarily one who saves or forgives—is through the agency of works bearing the mark of our good intent.

Good works are the activities of Existence as qualified by a controlling, effective, actual ethical man. Such works have, in the popular mind, the capacity to make a man the object of God's favorable judgment. Of course no work of man could obligate God, guarantee salvation. This truth has led many theologians, particularly of the right, to deny any efficacy to good works; they unwarrantedly suppose that the only efficacy of importance is that which produces salvation. But there are other desirable functions, and some of these good work performs. Good work, e.g., will help one to learn to know God.

Works which reflect a bad intent or express a vice are, of course, just as existentially effective as good works. But they are not existentially effective in enabling one to reach God. For God of course both types of work, the good and the bad, are data for him to utilize, evaluate, and reorganize in his own way and according to his own standards; such activity on his part is independent of the activity of men seeking to reach him.

4.49 God can be reached through dedicated work.
(*See 2.102, 4.47*)

ORGANIZED RELIGIONS isolate special types of work as singularly effective in enabling a man to reach God. The work of the priests, of missions, of charity and love are not so much good works as dedicated works, works having an ideal intelligibility, works understood as sustaining and exhibiting what is possible and desirable, and capable of terminating in God. A priest might be a bad man, but his mass is as effective as is that of a priest with exemplary virtue. The mass is a kind of charity, a species of activity which is qualified by the presence of the Ideal, restricted perhaps to the good of a church or a religious community. Patriotism, work dedicated to the preservation of peace or the good of civilization, has an analogous import. It too can be used as an efficacious instrument enabling one to reach to God. And there are other less restricted types of dedicated work.

When a confidence in the attainability of God is combined with a lack of confidence in the efficacy of dedicated work, there is an appeal to magic. The magician claims to have special devices which not only reach to God but in fact compel him to behave in certain desired ways. But no basic mode of being can be compelled to do anything. Nor is any special device needed in order to detach God from a cosmological reference to him; any bit of work, recognized to exhibit something of the Ideal and used by a man for the purpose of enabling him to confront God, can be as effective as any other.

V   THE PRIMARY PROOFS OF GOD

4.50   Teleological and ontological approaches to God are supplementary.
(See 4.24, 4.38, 4.39)

A TELEOLOGICAL approach to God never terminates in him; it merely testifies to him. If there is to be a reaching to God through the intellect, in attitude or through works, it is necessary to make use of a power which will enable one to leave the testimony behind and turn to what is being testified. The teleological approach needs supplementation by the ontological. Conversely, the ontological approach needs supplementation by the teleological. One must begin with what points to God; otherwise one will not necessarily confront him. God must first be looked at in terms provided by experience, and then must be confronted in terms which transcend experience. The former condition is met by the teleological approach, the latter by the ontological.

4.51   Cosmological and ontological approaches to God are supplementary.
(See 4.35, 4.38, 4.39)

A COSMOLOGICAL approach to God relates two realms. As spanning both it neither leaves testimony behind nor gets to God as he is in himself; it has the two of them as correlative terms. A proof of God would require one to detach him from that relation, and such detaching is performed ontologically. Conversely, an ontological approach presupposes the cosmological. This relates the evidence with which one begins to the conclusion with which one would like to end; it translates the profane into the divine, the conditioned into the unconditioned, the finite into the infinite.

The act of detachment of course does not produce God; it can do nothing more than offer a context, a position, give specification to a possible intellectual assertion regarding him, an attitudinal submission to him, or an adventurous eliciting of him. Such outcomes are not alien to God's being, but they are also not identical with his being. No proof of God yields God himself; if it could a man could produce a real God out of an implied possible one. But a proof can bring one to his surface, to an abstract facet of him, exhibit something of his nature.

4.52   A proof of God begins teleologically, is validated cosmologically, and terminates ontologically.

(*See 4.12, 4.50, 4.51*)

GOD'S EXISTENCE does not follow from the fact or premiss that things exist, that the world has a certain nature, or that he is conceived to be perfect. It is shown to be relevant by teleological testimony, it is exhibited as possible by means of a cosmological structure, and is faced through the agency of an act of ontological detachment. We must make a teleological note of the presence of God in things, cosmologically relate him to those things, and ontologically face him apart from them. To be content with the first alone is to remain with one's data; to be content with the second alone is to have a structure having neither beginning nor end; to be content with the third alone is to be at a terminus without knowing how we got there or what its meaning is in relation to what we had initially accepted.

We are now in a position to present schemata of the main lines of proof of God, to be used by whoever does accept the testimony specified, does make use of the indicated rules, and does wish to go through the designated processes of detaching the desired conclusion.

4.53   There are nine basic ways of proving God's existence through faith.

(*See 4.15, 4.18, 4.21, 4.26, 4.29, 4.32, 4.44*)

A PROOF of God can begin with direct testimony of him, referring to him as the absolute Other, as evaluating, or as effective. These testimonies can be related to God by means of a structure provided by Possibility, Actuality, or Existence. The combination of these beginnings with these structures yields nine cases which can be subjected to the detaching activity of faith.

1 God the Other, when made the terminus of an implication,
   4.15   *4.26*
   can be confronted in faith.
      4.44
2 God the Evaluator, when made the terminus of an implication,
   4.18   *4.26*
   can be confronted in faith.
      4.44
3 God the Effective, when made the terminus of an implication,
   4.21   *4.26*
   can be confronted in faith.
      4.44

Each of these three proofs begins with one of three different types of testimony and arrives at God in one of three guises. All follow a logical structure relating the evidence on behalf of God to God in one of these guises. In all of them faith is the crucial factor by means of which God is detached from a structure terminating in him. These three proofs can be conveniently termed the *confessional* proofs of God the person, judge, and substance.

4 God the Other, when made the terminus of a reverential attitude,
   4.15   *4.29*
   can be confronted in faith.
      4.44
5 God the Evaluator, when made the terminus of a reverential at-
   4.18   *4.29*
   titude, can be confronted in faith.
      4.44
6 God the Effective, when made the terminus of a reverential at-
   4.21   *4.29*
   titude, can be confronted in faith.
      4.44

These three proofs differ from the foregoing only in that they follow a different type of route to go from the same beginnings to the same end. They offer us *religious* proofs of God in the guise of person, judge, or substance.

7 God the Other, when made the terminus of a continuum,
  4.15   *4.32*
  can be confronted in faith.
       4.44
8 God the Evaluator, when made the terminus of a continuum,
  4.18   *4.32*
  can be confronted in faith.
       4.44
9 God the Effective, when made the terminus of a continuum,
  4.21   *4.32*
  can be confronted in faith.
       4.44

These three proofs differ from the preceding six only in that they make use of the structure of Existence. They provide us with *theological* proofs of God in the guise of person, judge, and substance.

The nine proofs are on a footing; each begins with testimony as good as that provided by the others; each is related by one of three equally valid structures; and each reaches to God through an act of faith. But none of these proofs is usually pursued by the philosopher, since he seeks to prove God without taking account of any commitments or belief. The philosopher's interest is centered almost exclusively in the next set of nine proofs, and particularly in the first three proofs of that set.

4.54 There are nine basic ways of proving God's existence through a logical inference.
(See *4.15, 4.18, 4.21, 4.26, 4.29, 4.32, 4.41*)

THERE are three distinct types of direct testimony of God, referring to him as the absolute Other, as an evaluating being, and as effective. These testimonies can be related to God by means of a structure provided by Possibility, Actuality, or Existence. The combination of these beginnings with these structures yields nine cases which can be subjected to the detaching activity of an inference.

10 God the Other, when made the terminus of an implication,
   4.15   *4.26*
   can be reached through inference.
        4.41
11 God the Evaluator, when made the terminus of an implication,
   4.18   *4.26*
   can be reached through inference.
        4.41

12 God the Effective, when made the terminus of an implication,
      4.21   *4.26*
    can be reached through inference.
      4.41

   In these three cases the proof has the structure of a logical implication which an inference exemplifies in reaching the intellectual conclusion that God is Other, evaluator, or effective. These three are
the only proofs which are of interest to most philosophers, since they
wish to make use of only the thinnest of media and none but inferential modes of detachment. The three therefore constitute *rational*
proofs of God as person, judge, or substance. The other proofs are
just as sound and just as effective for other purposes and in terms of
other interests.

13 God the Other, when made the terminus of a reverential attitude,
      4.15   *4.29*
    can be reached through inference.
      4.41
14 God the Evaluator, when made the terminus of a reverential at-
      4.18   *4.29*
    titude, can be reached through inference.
      4.41
15 God the Effective, when made the terminus of a reverential at-
      4.21   *4.29*
    titude, can be reached through inference.
      4.41

   These three proofs differ from the foregoing in that the inference
detaches the conclusion from a more human thicker medium than
that provided by logical implication. They offer us *humanistic* proofs
of God in the guise of person, judge, or substance.

16 God the Other, when made the terminus of a continuum,
      4.15   *4.32*
    can be reached through inference.
      4.41
17 God the Evaluator, when made the terminus of a continuum,
      4.18   *4.32*
    can be reached through inference.
      4.41
18 God the Effective, when made the terminus of a continuum,
      4.21   *4.32*
    can be reached through inference.
      4.41

These three proofs differ from the preceding six in that they make use of the comparatively thick medium of Existence. They offer us *existential* proofs of God as person, judge, or substance.

These nine proofs should take the place of the traditional proofs of God; it is these alone which have the structure and mode of derivation which the history of thought has been inclined to accept as alone conceivably legitimate. Such proofs do not interest religious men as a rule, but they are no less valid and desirable (for other purposes) than are the preceding or succeeding nine proofs which do interest them.

4.55 There are nine basic ways of proving God's existence through work.
(See 4.15, 4.18, 4.21, 4.26, 4.29, 4.32, 4.47)

THERE are three distinct types of direct testimony of God, referring to him as the absolute Other, as an evaluating being, and as effective. These testimonies can be related to God by means of a structure provided by Possibility, Actuality, or Existence. The combination of these beginnings with these structures yields nine cases which can be subjected to the practical activity of detaching the conclusion from the structure warranting it.

19 God the Other, when made the terminus of an implication,
      4.15   *4.26*
   can be reached through work.
     4.47
20 God the Evaluator, when made the terminus of an implication,
      4.18   *4.26*
   can be reached through work.
     4.47
21 God the Effective, when made the terminus of an implication,
      4.21   *4.26*
   can be reached through work.
     4.47

In these three cases we have a logical structure, but instead of drawing an inference in terms of it, we act in accord with it. In this way we provide works which allow one to reach the logically implied divine Other, evaluator, or effective being. These are the proofs of interest to those who seek to first establish a rational ground for their acknowledgment of God and then attempt to arrive at the terminus

of such a rational justification, not through an intellectual but through
a practical act. They provide *practical* proofs of God.

22 God the Other, when made the terminus of a reverential attitude,
        4.15   *4.29*
    can be reached through work.
              4.47
23 God the Evaluator, when made the terminus of a reverential at-
        4.18   *4.29*
    titude, can be reached through work.
              4.47
24 God the Effective, when made the terminus of a reverential at-
        4.21   *4.29*
    titude, can be reached through work.
              4.47

These three proofs are of primary interest to the pious man who
combines reverence with the performance of meritorious works. They
provide *sacramental* proofs of God.

25 God the Other, when made the terminus of a continuum,
        4.15   *4.32*
    can be reached through work.
              4.47
26 God the Evaluator, when made the terminus of a continuum,
        4.18   *4.32*
    can be reached through work.
              4.47
27 God the Effective, when made the terminus of a continuum,
        4.21   *4.32*
    can be reached through work.
              4.47

These three proofs constitute the *daily* proofs of God which men
provide through their activities as sustained by an environing, law-
abiding, seamless Existence. The farmer, the worker, the mother, the
housewife, as they go about their daily tasks, unreflectively make use
of them.

4.56 All proofs of God are circular and question-begging.
(See *4.41, 4.52, 4.53–55*)

THERE can be no proof of God if one does not begin with adequate
testimony. Such testimony, however, depends upon features which
owe their presence to God. Were it otherwise, it would never direct

one to him. Nor is there a proof of God unless the evidence with which one begins is in fact related to him. Yet such relation, since it bridges the gap between the secular and the divine, can never be wholly confined inside the limits of any finite Actuality, an indeterminate Ideal or a self-divisive Existence; it must be a relation which bears the marks of a divine sustaining. Nor is there a proof of God unless there be a power sufficiently strong to permit of a detaching of him from a relation in such a way as to permit of the determination of him in the role of an effective being, a judge, or a substance. But nothing could bring about such detaching and determination unless it has the unlimited power of God behind it. Each one of the steps of a proof of God—premiss, rule, and concluding—presupposes God.

God is presupposed in the premiss, the rule, and the concluding of a proof of God. He is presupposed as well in *any* justifiable replacement of any premiss by a conclusion. The first of these contentions will be quite readily granted; the second as readily denied. Yet every act of concluding occurs outside and beyond both the premiss and validating rule, and there must be some assurance that, as so outside, it is legitimate. A legitimate concluding presupposes a power capable of identifying the possible and actual conclusion of a proof. Such is the power of God, a power which must be used or presupposed in every inference and other processes of proving, no matter where it begins or where it ends. We depend on him to guarantee that the difference between "if, then," and "therefore" is not significant. Without God one would have to hold that a juncture of logical rule and actual movement is proper or legitimate for quite arbitrary reasons. This Peirce and Royce faintly acknowledged in their theories that logic holds only for an unlimited community of inquirers, for the unity of such a community can be guaranteed by none but God.

The warrant of the use of both logical rules and inferences together is provided by God, not in his role of person, or even as active or concerned, but by him in the guise of an eternal unity presupposed by every other and functioning as the correlative of all Actuality and its primary representative, man. This is a consequence of the fact that logical rules and inferences are special cases of the Ideal and Existence, and that these can be said to be properly adjusted one to the other only so far as they are related in correlative, harmonized ways.

In strict truth one ought to affirm that every mode has a role to play in every proof. Every proof requires a singular, actual adoption of a premiss and thus presupposes Actuality; every proof requires the use of a general structure and thus presupposes Possibility; every proof makes use of an existential movement and thus presupposes Existence; every proof neutrally and legitimately identifies possible and actual conclusion and thus presupposes God. To prove any mode whatsoever one must not only use the other modes but presuppose the mode to be proved. The problem of a proof of God is not different in principle from the problem of proving any mode of being, and in the end, of proving anything whatsoever.

To prove the existence of some other mode of being than God, one must presuppose him as the guarantee that the process of concluding to the mode, despite its difference from, is in consonance with what formal rules require. God will also be used in connection with these other proofs in the form of a premiss, a validating rule, or an agency which permits the detaching of the terminus of a valid rule so as to obtain a genuine, distinct conclusion. Since what is finally concluded to will also be a being used in the proof, whatever virtues that being may have will be circularly presupposed in the very way in which the unity of a proof leading to God is presupposed in proving him.

Strictly speaking, no less than two other modes, functioning as harmonized correlatives, suffice to determine how a pair of modes ought to stand with respect to one another. Only together do they constitute a single *tertium quid* for the other two. This *tertium quid*, though constituted of two equally real modes, can be conveniently described primarily in terms of one of them. The only relations we men can provide are primarily to be described in terms of Actuality. On the other hand, because man is the constant factor in all our proofs, it is necessary to point up the truth that he operates together with some other mode.

We can say, for example, that a virtuous man, a man who has the proper relation to the Good, provides a test of the way in which God and Existence are to function in relation to one another. And we can say that a well-adjusted man, a man at home in Existence, defines just how God and the Ideal ought to take account of one another. With equal justice, we can say that a wise man, one who is alive to the reality of the eternal, provides a test of the way in which the realm of "if, then" is to stand with respect to the domain of "therefore."

But these cannot offer genuine tests except so far as virtue, adjustment, and wisdom operate together with the Good, Existence, and God.

4.57 A proof of God is satisfying only so far as God is encountered in other ways as well.

(*See 1.84, 1.87, 3.34, 3.54, 4.56*)

ALTHOUGH a conclusion may be justifiably detached and accredited with some feature which was originally possessed by or could be derived from the premiss, one is not satisfied with it until one can confront the conclusion in some other way as well. If we know it to have the feature only because this had been deduced, we do not know that it has the feature in fact. This we could not know unless we also knew that the world behaves in consonance with the demands of the deduction.

It is the presupposition of all reasoning—indeed of all legitimate transitions—that the facts will answer to what the reasoning concludes. But no one is entirely sure that this is the case, and even the most rigorous theoretical scientist therefore looks again and again to the facts for a certification of what he had formally proved. We reason to save time, money, energy or to get to truths experience cannot reach. Our inferences give us conclusions apart from experience. Those conclusions we seek to check wherever possible, even when we are confident of the validity of our reasoning and the rationale of the universe. And what is true of any proof is true of a proof of God. To reach him through inference, faith, or action is not yet to face him as a being who exists in independence of any proof of him. All proofs of God in the end are unsatisfying unless God in fact exhibits himself as having the nature, value, or function which one has concluded that he has. Until he so exhibits himself, a proof (even when this is achieved through the thick of Actuality or Existence), though it will enable a man to reach God, will not enable a man to know that he is being confronted by God.

All proofs are forms of *introduction;* they do not guarantee an *acquaintanceship.* This is true not only with respect to the proofs relating to God, but to those which relate to other modes of being, or to specifications of these. Since all of them present their conclusions freed from the limitations of a formal implication, all of them can be said to engage in a kind of artistic disengagement of a desirable component of a formal structure. But whereas the artist actually embeds his freed item in a more appropriate medium, the reasoner can at best only await for such a medium to present itself as that which can or does carry his freed conclusion. The proved being, when it confronts the reasoner, does for the conclusion proved something similar to what the artist must himself do for his freed component—give it an appropriate lodgement.

4.58   God's nature, as apart from proof, includes all that has been truly testified regarding him.
(See 4.15–23, 4.24, 4.57)

A PROOF enables one to know something reliable in advance of an encounter. If what is encountered does not have the features one has concluded it to have, the proof must have started with the wrong premiss, followed an unreliable route, detached the conclusion incorrectly, or exhibited a logic not sustained in fact. On the assumption that none of these alternatives holds, a proof must arrive at features which in fact prevail apart from that proof. God, on the basis of such an assumption, must therefore be characterized as the Absolute Other, judge and substance, who has the power to enable men to be both individual and human, who gives the past a needed Existence, who guarantees the realization of temporally relevant possibilities, who is providentially concerned with the world, who dictates that Existence have a single geometry, and who makes spatiotemporal Existence and the Future into inseparable correlatives.

In addition to these features, which are directly or indirectly testified to in ways that any man can note apart from all religious commitment or religious experience, there are features which have been accredited to God on the basis of revelation. Only a comparatively few men, however, claim to have had the benefit of such revelations. The rest can know nothing of the truth or falsehood of what this minority maintains, so far as the revelation tells them things in principle beyond the reach of any agency available to all men. And even if a revelation did nothing more than confirm what had been proved, the fact that such confirmation had occurred would not be known to everyone. There are men who are not religious; there are religious men who acknowledge no revelations; there are quite divergent religions affirming different revelations and different products of them; even inside a single religion there is considerable diversity in the understanding of what has been revealed.

For all men a proof of God can have some utility, telling something of what God is like apart from the act of proof, though not yet what it is like to be confronted by him. For those who believe themselves benefited by revelation, a proof can serve as a reminder, or as a way of articulating, communicating, or persuading. However, for them no proof is very important. If God has personally testified that he is, what he is, what he wants, and what he wills done, a proof can have only a limited value. It is more important for the rest of us. Understood in the broad sense of allowing for attitudinal and active, as well as intellectual modes of concluding, a proof is a primary way of getting to God, circular and question-begging though it be, and despite the fact that it falls dismally short of confronting us with him.

4.59 God's nature, as apart from proof, includes whatever is known of him through the agency of a systematic dialectic.

(See *1.14, 1.23, 1.92, 2.19, 3.99*)

A PROOF of God concludes to an existent being who possesses features and powers directly or indirectly testified to. The very fact that there is testimony, a method for using it, and a process of going from it to its original source, points up the truth that God is less than all being, that he is, indeed, but one of four basic modes of being. Since each mode of being is known to have features, needs, and functions supplementing those possessed by the rest, other truths about God can be obtained without recourse to testimony. Such a contention presupposes that one has already proved that God exists—or what is the same thing, in addition to conclusions derivable from testimony offered by a given mode of being, there are conclusions derivable from the dialectical truth that other modes of being are dependent on the presence of the given mode. A mode of being is, only so far as it is not the whole of being.

Each mode of being is a being only because there are others. Pure being altogether is not; the only beings there can be are beings together. Whatever beings there are must assume one of a set of inseparable but independent roles. God has one of these roles, and is therefore possessed of features and functions which are knowable in the light of what the other modes must obtain from him and he from them in order for all of them to be at all.

4.60 Our most adequate idea of God is self-engendered.
(*See 1.52, 1.74, 4.15, 4.57, 4.58, 4.59*)

DESPITE the fact that multiple gods have been acknowledged at some time by various religions in the past, and apparently even by the Hindus in the present, and despite the fact that there are those who speak of God as infinite and others who refer to him as necessarily finite, we can say something about God that is universally applicable. For all, he is the most perfect of beings, the supreme being, either because he has more perfection than any other can have or because he alone has perfection.

God must also be said to be a substantial unity. This unity is no object of an idle idea. It is the terminus of all possible longing and need, the counterpart of ourselves who are finite, defective, and unsatisfied, entraining the emotions of joy and fear, satisfaction and wonder. To grasp something of its enormity we must retreat far within ourselves into our lonely privacies, for it is only thus that we come to recognize ourselves as essentially others, inevitably pointing to him who is our permanent counterpart. We all have a dim awareness of him, for all of us, no matter how superficially we think or live, are thrown back again and again into the recesses of our being and thereby become aware that something eternal must be if we are to be what we are.

Our awareness is not a full awareness of God if it is not an awareness of one who is distinct not only from ourselves but from all else— all other Actualities, the Ideal they seek to realize, and the Existence in which they are. The most adequate idea of God is one which puts him over against all else as a unity large enough to encompass not only Actual individuals but the Ideal and Existence as well. For us to have an adequate idea of him we must solidify what we grasp of ourselves in our privacies with what we discern of other beings. The idea of God is an idea engendered by uniting what we discern in ourselves with what we discern of the Ideal and Existence, while vitally recognizing that outcome to have a single counterpoise.

Distinct from Actualities, Ideality, and Existence, God lacks the essential features of these. Singular, he is, despite his individuality, no contingent, striving Actuality. Determinate and inward, he is, despite his perfection, no mere Ideal. Not spatiotemporal, he is, despite his Existence, simple.

Undivided, the counterpart of our idea of him, God's being is distinct from his actual individuality, his ideal essence and his vital existence. His being is all of these together, one and undistinguished. Absolute in comprehensiveness, he is limited in excellence, since he is without the reality which the other modes possess. Finite, since there are others, he is yet internally infinite, able to encompass all.

VI   GOD AND THE OTHER MODES

4.61   Theoanalysis is the art of dealing with other realities in theological terms.

(*See 1.13, 1.73, 2.14, 2.19, 2.97*)

EACH MODE of being not only provides testimony regarding the others but offers a basis in terms of which one can analyze them. All of the modes together explicate the meaning of the entire cosmos; each offers an explanation, clarification, a way of approaching and dealing with the others.

In the terms provided by Actualities, other modes of being are essentially beings standing over against all else, limited and limiting, possessed of needs and substantiality. In the terms provided by the Ideal, other modes are essentially subjugating and subjugated powers. In the terms provided by Existence, other modes are essentially dynamic, active, productive, and produced. In the terms provided by God, other modes are unitary, inclusive, or controlling realities.

Since each mode of being is approached from three distinct perspectives, it could well be argued that each is in fact not a single being but a plurality, having at least three members. And, if account be taken of the fact that there are many Actualities, each of which is occupied with the other modes of being, one could go on to maintain that there are at least as many instances of these other modes of being as there are Actualities. There is point in doing this. Although we have persistently spoken of Ideality, Existence, and God as though they were single, it is also, as a matter of fact, true that each encompasses a distinct type of plurality at least equal in magnitude to that which is characteristic of Actualities. The Ideal contains a plurality of stresses relevant to Actualities and the other modes of being. Existence perpetually divides, but also terminates at the various Actualities and the other modes. And finally God, in knowing himself, distinguishes within himself the Actualities and the other modes as well. Because of what we ourselves are, we are primarily aware of the plurality of Actualities and only secondarily of Actuality as such, but in the case of other modes we first know some one item in the plurality, and learn about the others only when we come to know of the mode as a singular being. Beneath the outward calm which the modes in ther singularity present to us we can faintly discern worlds of activity, as rich, as complex, and as interesting as the world of Actualities.

It is to be noted, however, that Actuality has being only as sustained by particular Actualities. The plurality of Actualities is substantial; Actuality as such is comparatively abstract. When then it is said that Actuality interplays with other modes this is only shorthand for saying either that some Actualities represent all Actualities, or that all Actualities interact with all else. Men perform the first function; Actualities, when constituting a natural world, the second.

God, in contrast with Actuality, is substantial in his singularity; the plurality in him is carried by him, and is comparatively abstract. The Ideal is somewhat like God in that its unitary nature has priority. But that unitary nature unlike God's is not over against the plurality; its plurality is not different in type or power from it as singular. Existence, in contrast, is somewhat like Actuality in that its plurality has a kind of priority. But that plurality unlike Actuality's, is not over against the unity; it is the very being of it, not different in type or power from it. The only plurality that is absolutely necessary is the plurality of the modes of being. Two of those modes—Actuality and Existence—encompass a plurality of realities; the other two— Ideality and God—encompass a plurality of distinctions.

Each member of the plurality in Actuality is an instance of it and a constituent of it; each member of the plurality in God reproduces him and has a counterpart outside him; each member of the plurality in the Ideal specializes it and can be given a role outside it; and each member of the plurality in Existence is a limit for it, and helps constitute it.

It is also the case that all complex Actualities have a kind of plurality within them. This, like the pluralities in the Ideal, Existence, and God, is a sustained plurality, but unlike the others is made up of items which can have some being apart from what sustains it. Within Actuality then there are many real Actualities, themselves encompassing subordinate Actualities. Within other modes there are many parts, some of which are quite complex, but no one of which encompasses genuine subordinate items, capable of fully standing apart from those parts. Subdivisions of Actuality can have genuine parts; subdivisions of the other modes cannot.

Theoanalysis looks at the modes of Actuality, Ideality, and Existence in terms which have primary and exemplary application to God, the being who is radically one. Most religions, once they have attended to God's nature, engage in theoanalysis to some extent; they make some attempt to restate the nature of things as "images" of God. But this attempt to deal with other modes of being in theological terms is perhaps the special province of the Franciscan school. It deserves exploitation and development.

4.62   In theoanalytic terms, Actualities are God's self-identity endlessly multiplied and combined.
(See *1.47, 1.96, 4.61*)

EACH BEING is self-identical. It is what it is. But the self-identity of God is different from the self-identity of other beings. Each mode of being in fact has its own way of being self-identical. This is evidently so with respect to Actualities in contrast with God. "Aristotle is Aristotle" says that the law of identity holds of Aristotle. That law holds also of Kant. "Kant is Kant" is just as true as "Aristotle is Aristotle." The same law holds in both cases, the two differing only in the kind of filling they provide for it. That filling is distinct from, over against the law, enabling the law to be illustrated in these two distinct cases. Neither the substantial Aristotle nor the substantial Kant is identifiable with the law. But the case of God is different. "God is God" is an assertion different in kind from "Aristotle is Aristotle." In his case the law of identity is not rooted in an alien substance; it is his substance. Only God's being is adequate to the meaning of the law of identity.

Because God offers the law of identity a locus where it has a being completely appropriate to its meaning, God is rightly designatable as *the* self-identical. He and the law of identity are one. "Aristotle is Aristotle" on the other hand expresses a tautology after the fact, an analytic result of the synthesis of the distinct being of Aristotle with the law of identity. When we affirm that "Aristotle is Aristotle" we are forced to go outside Aristotle to the law of identity, and outside the law of identity to Aristotle, whereas when we affirm that "God is God" we remain within God and the law, accepting both fully and at once.

In God the filling of the law of identity is one with the law itself. All other beings stand over against the law of identity; they are not therefore as intelligible as the law itself. They subject the law of identity to conditions, root it in something else. Yet this something else must itself be self-identical, already exhibit that law. When we separate off the law of identity from Actuality we are left with a residue in which we can find the law once again, and so on without end. From God's perspective each Actuality, instead of being describable as the law of identity with an alien filling is properly describable as that law endlessly repeated, and thus as God himself endlessly multiplied. Repeating God's own self-identity, the Actualities nonetheless differ from God, since the identities that constitute them are alongside one another, whereas God is one simple self-identity.

"Aristotle is Aristotle" is recognized by all to be trivial because it fails to reveal anything about Aristotle as a being in nature. We get not much further when we say that Aristotle is distinct from Kant, but we then at least deal with him as a distinct, substantial Actuality, with his own individual unique unity. But from a theoanalytic standpoint, an adequate analysis of both shows them to be different sets of repetitions of God.

There is a host of identities associated with the identity "Aristotle is Aristotle." These constitute its filling. The nature of that filling and the way the identity is united with it is distinctive. One Actuality in fact is to be distinguished from all others by the way in which it combines repetitions of the law of identity. Theoanalytically viewed, each Actuality offers a distinctive exterior conjunction of repetitions of the divine.

4.63   In theoanalytic terms, the Ideal is all-encompassing.
(See 2.100, 4.61)

PLATO quite clearly distinguished God and the Good in his *Timaeus*. His insight was blurred by later theologians, perhaps be-cause they thought that theoanalysis required the denial of the in-dependent reality of the Good or Ideal, rather than a characteriza-tion of it in theological terms. Be that as it may, God's essence is an all-inclusive essence. Even those who speak of him as finite tend to hold that he is at the apex of the universe, doing excellently what the rest do deficiently, completely knowing or remembering and perhaps even struggling or suffering with all things whatsoever. Since God is only one of four basic realities, he is evidently a limited being. Like the others he needs the rest in order to be himself. Un-like them though he can also meaningfully contain all the others as part of his very essence. For him the Ideal is an avenue for express-ing his essence. In theoanalytic terms, the Ideal is a singular meaning which contains every other as a limited case, and through which there-fore God can know and guide whatever there be.

4.64   In theoanalytic terms, Existence is creativity.
(See 3.11, 4.61)

GOD is rich beyond expression. Were he sunk wholly within himself he would be purely potential. To be himself to the full his being must be made explicit, exteriorized. This is exactly the work that Existence does for him.

Viewed theoanalytically, Existence is no blind, sheer exteriorizing; it is God himself making himself manifest everywhere, exhibiting his power in all possible directions. It is God expressing himself, fulgurating perpetually, making himself evident in the guise of space, time, energy, with their plurality of actual terminal points and Future. Each of these manifestations vanishes as soon as it becomes; viewed theoanalytically Existence has no persistence except the persistence of being perpetually remade. This Descartes clearly saw, and incisively focused on in his observation that conservation and creation are one and the same. But he failed to recognize that this is only a theoanalytic result, and does not do full justice to the nature of Existence as it stands outside God and other modes. Apart from God Existence persists and acts. Like the other modes of being Existence is more than what it can be theoanalytically shown to be.

4.65   God's nature, mind, and expression are one with the being, knowledge, and creation of all there is.
(*See 4.62–64*)

Aristotle acutely remarked that God knows only himself, for nothing else is worthy of his attention. Aristotle, however, failed to see that this applies only to his direct knowledge, and that in knowing himself God thereby knows the nature of all else, and in knowing all else knows himself.

Plotinus recognized that all that happens is the expression of God. However, he seemed to think that God's remaining forever in himself precludes there being anything real outside him. But God's self-expression repeats the pattern of what is in fact not God.

Spinoza urged that God is a being of which everything else is but a delimited, negative particle. He seemed to think that this admission precluded the affirmation that anything else was real. As a consequence he did not know what to say regarding the reality of particular things, without which there would be no world of experience, common sense or science. He treated all things theoanalytically, forgetting that these first had to be, before they could be so treated.

Theoanalytically an Actuality is God's nature repeated endlessly, the Ideal is his essence exteriorized and occupied with all else, and Existence is his self-expressive production of himself in a plurality of guises. In being himself he is these others, in knowing himself he knows them, and in expressing himself he makes them, they all the while remaining apart from and independent of him. When God is, knows, or acts he but—to speak theoanalytically—multiplies himself.

4.66   God internally reproduces other modes of being.
(See *4.62, 4.65*)

ACTUALITIES are not merely sets of identities. They are individual substances. If God is to know them he must deal with them in theo-analytic terms. To grasp them as the substances that they are he must add to the identities, into which they are analyzable, a power of combining those identities in different limited ways. Only thus will he, while remaining in himself, be able to do justice to the substantial reality of Actualities. Similarly, the Ideal is not only inclusive but has a definite nature of its own, imposing limitations on what could be included in, or how things are to be subordinated to it. If God is to grasp the nature of the Ideal, he must confine its role to that of a principle of evaluation. He will then be able to know it to be more germane to the differences among things than a mere encompassing essence could be. Finally, God's activity of self-expression is endless in reach and spontaneity. It is too variegated and fertile to be able to do justice to Existence except so far as he adds to his self-expression the qualifications of the particular order that in fact governs the course of the existent universe. The results of theoanalysis, in short, must be subjected to limitations, restrictions, qualifications if it is to be made appropriate to the full being of Actualities, Ideality, and Existence.

4.67   God has a direct awareness of exterior Actualities.
(See *4.15, 4.66*)

TO HAVE an adequate grasp of Actualities God must, in addition to apprehending the set of identities into which they can be analyzed, and which are nothing but himself multiplied, take account of the manner in which those identities are unified to make single actual beings. But he cannot know what type of unification to impose on sets of identities unless he has some grasp of what Actualities in fact are. Actualities, moreover, are constantly coming into being and passing away; they change and move, act and react. He has no knowledge of them unless he allows himself to be guided in his act of combining identities by what he knows of the Actualities apart from such combination. His knowledge of those Actualities is no knowledge of identities somehow exteriorily combined. It is a grasp of the Actualities as substantial individuals, because it is guided by the Actualities themselves.

God analyzes and reconstitutes Actualities in consonance with what they in fact are apart from him. As he sweeps over himself, he re-divides himself into multiple identities, which he then and there unites in different combinations, in consonance with what he discerns out-side him. His awareness that the Actualities are exterior to him, with their own centers, is one with his awareness that they are his others. Since they, as limited, transitory, multiple, can be only limited, relative, fluctuating others, and since otherness is a symmetrical rela-tion, they make him possess the nonessential status of a limited relative other.

Both Actualities and God are thus at once *relative* and *absolute* others, others which vary in terms of one another, and others which are constants for one another. In the former guise they are occupied with, involved with one another, in the latter they are all inward, but over against one another. God's direct awareness of exterior Actualities is an awareness of them as relative others. To be aware of them as absolute others he must reflect on what must be in order that he should be their Absolute Other. This means that Actualities must be potential abstractive subdivisions in him which contrast with his singular concrete unity, and that he can separate out these Actu-alities in an act of self-awareness. He can always find testimony in himself to the reality of Actualities outside by noting the subdivisions he makes in himself.

4.68   God has an indirect awareness of Actualities in relation to the Ideal.

(*See 1.118, 2.21, 4.16, 4.63*)

GOD is aware that Actualities are occupied with the Ideal which they need to and ought to realize in the guise of the Good. As a consequence he not only reconstructs them in himself as individuals, but as beings who seek and need the Ideal in the guise of the Good.

God's reconstruction is completive; he adds to the Actualities that part of the Ideal they failed to embody. This completive activity occurs both outside where the Actualities now are, and also in-side himself. The first of these is the completion of making Actuali-ties members of classes, kinds of things when and while they are individuals, with the consequence that they indirectly testify to him. The second of these is his private completion of the Actualities, his satisfying them by bestowing on them the Good they failed in fact to realize. To engage in the first of these completive activities without the second is to give Actualities only the degree of completion they, as the concrete beings which they are, can at the moment tolerate. To engage in the second of these activities without the first is to satisfy Actualities not as individual, spatiotemporal substances in a world apart from him, but only as reconstituted or eternalized beings.

4.69   God has an indirect awareness of Actualities in relation to Existence.

(*See 3.41, 4.17, 4.67–68*)

ACTUALITIES become de-existentialized at every moment. The resultant facts would perish utterly were they then not preserved. Such preservation occurs both where they are and inside God. As occurring where they are, it is a preservation which has to do not with the present, but with the past. God endows past facts with an existence so as to enable those facts to have a permanence, forever outside of and over against whatever Actualities exist in the changing present. Apart from him the facts are related to the present by a dense series of facts terminating in the present; he enables them to exclude and be excluded by the present. Since Existence has in fact moved away from the facts constituting the past, never to be brought back into them even by an infinitely powerful being, the only way in which God could make the past have being is by isolating a nondynamic facet of Existence, and bestowing this on the past facts. The past facts thus divinely existentialized offer indirect testimony of God, the being who alone has power enough to make even a phase of real Existence integral to the facts from which that Existence has forever departed.

Actualities are preserved by God in the guise of others, as beings possessing universal features, and as past facts. Because he is an irreducible unitary being, the Actualities can stand apart from him as his others. Because he is occupied with them as needing the Good, they can continue to be apart from him, striving to make the Good and its subordinate universals one with themselves. And because he is occupied with Actualities permanently, because he seeks to have them be always, despite the fact that they have only finite spans, they can be past forever.

Actualities in turn offer God data for his reconstituting activities. When and as he preserves them apart from himself he reconstructs them within himself. As apart from him, they have their own integrity, and he can preserve them there only as past facts; as in him, they are data which he preserves while enriching, completing them. God completes Actualities in himself by uniting them with Ideality and Existence in a way not possible to them when apart from him. When apart from him they are unpurged, unreconstituted, not yet harmonized in themselves or with one another; in him they are made part of more perfect wholes.

4.70 God has a direct awareness of a normative Ideal.
(See 2.09, 2.14, 2.100, 4.18)

THE IDEAL is at once exterior and relevant to God. It is exterior because it is an irreducible mode of being; it is relevant because he needs it in order to be at all. Were it merely exterior, it would not have any particular bearing on what he is or does; were it merely relevant, it would not necessarily measure him, determine his worth. God in knowing himself to be perfect knows that the Ideal is different from himself, for he then knows himself to be measured in terms not provided by himself. When and as he takes account of the Ideal as exterior and relevant to himself, and when and as he reproduces it within himself in order to grasp it in theoanalytic terms, he is also aware that it is a principle of value capable of measuring Actualities and Existence as well.

Actualities and Existence do not exhaust the Ideal. This means either that the Ideal holds itself apart from them or that God holds it there. Now the Ideal does not hold itself apart. In fact it tries to subjugate them, make them into instances of itself. To function as a principle of value measuring their worth it must remain outside them, and yet characterize them as more or less defective. This requires it to have the help of God.

God can make an adequate application of the Ideal to himself. He can enable it to function as a valuational structure or meaning for his own intent. It is then that he finds it not only to have a nature of its own, resisting him, but a nature which can serve to measure the worth of whatever else there be. It is its capacity to measure the worth of Actuality and Existence which enables the Ideal to provide direct testimony for the existence of God, since the applicability of the Ideal to them is due to him, an evaluating being, himself measured by that Ideal.

Each mode of being, of course, offers a kind of norm for all the others. But each also needs the help of the others in order to function as a norm. Even God himself can provide a norm of unity for, say, Actuality and Ideality, only so far as Existence makes him pertinent to them. And the application of the Ideal to him must depend on the ability of Actuality and Existence to make a domain of intelligible structure pertinent to him, a being otherwise neither intelligible nor excellent.

4.71 God has an indirect awareness of the Ideal in relation to Actualities.
(*See 2.13, 3.92, 4.19, 4.70*)

THE IDEAL has a normative role with respect to Actualities. Actualities may not live up to it, and their work must, if the Ideal is to be a genuine possibility, be supplemented by other beings. The Ideal also has a nonnormative role with respect to Actualities in the form of a set of prospects which are to be realized in the course of time through the activity of those Actualities. God's awareness of the Ideal as relevant to the particular Actualities that in fact exist in the course of time is an awareness of the Ideal, mediated by an awareness of Actualities. Such an indirect awareness of the Ideal, the grasp of it as that which is to be exhausted in the course of history, is one with the production of the indirect testimony to the existence of God, since it involves a divine delimitation of the Ideal in the light of the nature, needs, and capacities of Actualities.

4.72 God has an indirect awareness of the Ideal in relation to Existence.
(*See 2.13, 4.20, 4.28, 4.70*)

THE IDEAL has a cosmic, temporal role as the Future facing Existence. Were there to be an end to Existence's restless surging, that role would then and there vanish. This is a limitation on the Ideal, not within the capacity of Existence (which it beckons), of Actuality (whose individual needs it transcends), or of the Ideal itself (which has inexhaustible power and range, evaluative of but never merely a prospect for Existence). It is a limitation which requires the action of a cosmic power. God, when he approaches the Ideal in terms of Existence is aware of it as a Future to be exhausted in time, and makes it provide indirect testimony of himself.

4.73   God has a direct awareness of an extensive Existence.
(See 4.21, 4.65, 4.66)

GOD sweeps over the infinite range of his being in new ways at every moment and thereby conforms to the Actualities that happen to be, and of which he is aware. He also analyzes himself into multiple loci of self-identities, thereby reproducing the Actualities that are apart from him. He is also aware of the Ideal as a measure of himself and all else, reproducing it in himself in the form of an all-encompassing absolute value. At the same time he is aware of Existence as actively separating Actualities from one another and from the Ideal, and both of these from himself, when and as he reproduces that Existence in his act of complete self-expression. He is aware that Existence is perpetually separating itself and all else from him, and he maintains a hold on it only by imposing on it the unity which it needs.

4.74   God has an indirect awareness of Existence in relation to Actualities.
(See 3.100, 4.22, 4.73)

BY APPROACHING Existence through the mediation of Actualities, God is aware of it as having a variable geometry, as affected in its nature by the stresses of the Actualities which are related across it. This awareness is an awareness of the outcome of his own activity, for it is he who so imposes the Actualities on Existence as to provide it with a single variable pattern, and incidentally indirect testimony of his own existence.

4.75   God has an indirect awareness of Existence in relation to the Ideal.
(See 4.23, 4.73, 4.74)

THE IDEAL in the guise of the Future enables Existence to have the status of something present in time. God's awareness of Existence through the mediation of the Ideal is thus an awareness of it as temporal. This indirect awareness occurs together with his indirect awareness of Existence as spatial, and his direct awareness of it as energizing. Existence thereby becomes for him his counterpoise, a mode of being which is primarily divisive, requiring his own internal endless self-division in order to be reproduced, and his imposition of his own unity on it in order that it be able to have a nature of its own, offering indirect testimony to his existence.

4.76 God is omnipotently omniscient, providential, and self-expressive.
(See 4.66, 4.67, 4.70, 4.73)

GOD cannot know what cannot be known. He cannot know round squares. Nor can he know the future in its concreteness, for there is no such future to know.

God cannot know what would be destroyed by his knowing. He does not know Actualities from within themselves, for this requires him to be them in fact, and thereby cheat them of their independence. Nor does he know the Ideal in its ultimacy, for this measures him and his knowledge and must therefore remain exterior to him. Nor does he know Existence in its vital oppositionality, for this Existence forever retreats before him. He does know all of them, but only by reproducing them within himself, guided by his awareness of them as they are by themselves and in relation to one another. Since the full reproduction of anything requires nothing less than infinite power, God's omniscience is one with his omnipotence.

God is concerned with the Ideal as capable of measuring the worth of all else. He makes an effort to have that Ideal realized as a norm. But he cannot dictate its satisfaction in others while they stand apart from him, without thereby denying to them independence of being and power. To satisfy it he must enhance the self-divisions of himself so as to make the result be a fulfillment of the Ideal. By so satisfying the Ideal within himself God providentially fulfills Actualities and Existence, completing the work that they themselves do in connection with that Ideal. Since providential fulfillment of whatever there be requires nothing less than infinite power, God's providence is one with his omnipotence.

God expresses himself in an endless number of ways, thereby

doing justice not only to the plurality of Actualities that there are in fact and to the Ideal as the measure of them all, but to Existence as divisible without limit. This self-expression of God is one with his reproduction in himself of whatever else there be. Since such an activity requires nothing less than infinite power, God's self-expression is one with his omnipotence.

4.77 Actualities relate God's reproductions to the objects of his awareness.

(See 1.67, 4.29, 4.66, 4.67–75, 4.76)

GOD is directly and indirectly aware of Ideality, Existence, and Actuality. This awareness is a kind of adumbrative accompaniment of his providential, self-expressive, omnipotent, reproductive act of knowing. The awareness guides these internal activities, thereby producing testimony in God of the objects of which he is aware. He does not encounter them in being aware of them. To have such an encounter he must move from the testimony to the Actualities, the Ideal, and Existence themselves. This movement can be guided by the structures of Actualities. These provide primary and secondary relations between his internal being and activities, and what is outside him.

It is the claim of prophets that they provide God with a vehicle for the relating of his intent, purpose, truth to other men. But this conception of the prophetic role is too narrow, on the one side, and too bold on the other. It neglects the fact that God needs a vehicle to connect him not only with men but with all Actualities, as well as with the Ideal and Existence. And it supposes that God has an intent which he seeks to communicate. It forgets that, like us, he has a need to prove and thus to know the existence of other modes of being, to which he testifies and which he might encounter.

4.78 The Ideal relates God's reproductions to the objects of his awareness.

(See 4.26, 4.67–75, 4.76)

GOD knows and thinks in himself and by himself, but not in complete indifference to or in defiance of the requirements of logic. He can think without slip or error; his range of interests and his choice of formal routes are enormously wider, and his flexibility and subtlety are unquestionably greater than that possible to any man. But for all that his arguments are to be tested for validity in the same way as are the arguments of men. For God to come to correct outcomes it is necessary that he submit to the conditions embodied in the Ideal which stands over against him and other modes of being. By doing this he will be able to reach the other modes in rationally certifiable ways. No one of course knows how God thinks, and just what formal structure his arguments have. But as one who is aware of other modes of being, in their role of guides for his own omnipotent omniscience, providence, and self-expression, he is one who must seek to prove their existence. If he did not, he would not have an opportunity to determine the accuracy of his reproductions, and would not know even as much about the totality of being as is possible to a philosopher.

4.79 Existence relates God's reproductions to the objects of his awareness.

(*See 3.37, 4.32, 4.67–75, 4.76*)

HE WHO supposes that God creates all else out of nothing is faced with a dilemma. Either God makes the others be, or he does not. If he does not, he does not in fact create them; but if he does make them be, they are, and so far have no need of him. A theory of the creation of real beings can go no further than to affirm that the origin of those beings, the fact that they have come to be and not the fact that they are, requires a reference to a creating God. But there is no coming to be of Ideality, Existence, or Actuality; there is only the coming to be of new applications of Ideality, of new presents sustained by Existence, and of new individual cases of Actuality.

God's reproductiveness is one with his self-expression. Viewed as terminating in modes of being outside him, it must follow the route provided by the domain where activity can occur. This is Existence. Existence has a being to which all activity must conform. Both in its unqualified and its two subordinate qualified forms it provides God with a stabilized will, a structure which connects what he has reproduced with what he adumbratively discerns to be outside him. His will, unlike his self-expression, but like the will of man, has a relational nature, and can operate only so far as it conforms to the conditions of Existence.

4.80   God arrives at the other three modes of being through the agency of love.
(See 4.10, 4.44)

BY FAITH a man can move, along the route of some relational, validating structure, to the being of God. The reciprocal of that movement, performed by God, is love. That love, the West has too often assumed, is pointed at men alone, in the face of its accepted biblical observations that God finds all his creation good, and watches over every part. Nor has it usually been understood to encompass the Ideal or Existence, with the consequence that the Ideal inevitably assumes the guise of a brute, predestined end, and Existence is taken to be an impenetrable irrationality. The insight expressed in the account of Christ functioning as an actual vehicle for God's love for men needs to be extended therefore so as to make it worthy of a being whose loving concern extends to all that is.

God's love has a primary and two subordinate forms; in all three cases it goes through the resisting medium of Actuality, and reaches to the other modes. Christianity has trouble with the problem of evil partly because it supposes that this love is not carried by any medium and is therefore irresistible. To account for atheists and heretics its theologians have had to suppose that God is niggardly, cautious, calculating, that he does not bestow his love until what he loves has put itself into a proper mood or posture, or comes at the right time. But there is no need to limit the occasions or range of God's love; he can love all and always. Beginning with his guided reproductive knowledge, he moves through the medium of an Actuality to end with what he would like to encounter. The point is partly seen by those who affirm that God's love is manifest in the love a man shows to other men.

4.81   God arrives at the other three modes of being through the agency of divine understanding.
(See 4.10, 4.41)

THERE can be valid inferences terminating in God. These inferences enable one to qualify a possible conclusion in advance of experience. Their reciprocal is divine understanding, the assent to beings as purified and ennobled. Like the inferences, the divine understanding, while keeping within some given and warranting structure, goes beyond what such a structure provides. Unlike the inferences, instead of characterizing the outcome with some such qualification as "truth," "goodness," "probability," it refines them, sifts out irrelevancies and distortions to arrive at them as they are in their purity. It goes too far when it is precipitate, altering too quickly and radically the nature of the beings in which it terminates; it does not go far enough when it is cautious or conservative, and fails to free the beings from all that is irrelevant. It is appropriate only when it takes account of the way in which the Ideal is modified by Actuality and Existence.

4.82 God arrives at the other three modes of being through the agency of grace.
(*See 4.10, 4.47*)

WORK offers a good means by which men in fact can arrive at God, providing they begin with what testifies to him, and follow the route of some validating structure relating that testimony to him. The reciprocal of such work is grace, the expression of God's power in such a way as to make the other modes of being into loci of testimony regarding him. God's grace detaches beings from the relation which connects them to his guided reproductive knowledge of them. Like work, it has an unqualified and two qualified forms; like work it requires activity which is beyond the power of a mere mind. It is primarily an act serving not to make things be— since they are already—but to make them better, completed through the possession of divinely bestowed, nonessential traits. Since the other modes of being always possess these nonessential traits, God's grace must be understood to be irresistible, a grace forever operative and unavoidable. Such grace of course is not incompatible with the need for man to act, and even to prepare himself for the receipt of some divine benefaction.

4.83 Beginning with God, there are nine primary ways of proving the existence of each mode of being.
(*See 4.08, 4.53–56, 4.67, 4.70, 4.73, 4.77–82*)

GOD's direct awareness of the other three modes can be related to those modes in one of three primary ways; those modes can then be detached from those relations in three primary ways. Since any one of the three acts of detachment can be used on each relation, there are evidently nine ways, beginning with God, for proving the reality of some other mode of being. God, for example, is directly aware of Actualities. His guided reproductive knowledge of them can be related to those Actualities through the agency of one of three structures, and can then be detached from the structure through an act of love, understanding, or grace. In addition to these nine primary ways of arriving at Actualities from the standpoint of God, there are twice as many secondary ways, having to do with structures and inferences which express something of the effect of one mode on another.

Taking account only of the primary modes of proof, there are, beginning with God, nine ways of proving the reality of some one mode. Beginning with God there is evidently then a total of twenty-seven proofs of the other three modes. These twenty-seven, together with the twenty-seven proofs of God previously sketched, make a total of fifty-four primary proofs which either begin or end with God. There remain fifty-four further primary proofs that begin and end with some mode of being other than God. Ending with Actuality, Ideality, or Existence, they start from one of the other two, make use of the structure of the other two or of God, and detach the terminus of the structure by means of one of the other two or God. Most compendiously; there are four possible endings, each of which can be related in one of three ways with three beginnings and can be detached from the relation in one of three ways. This totality of 108 primary proofs of the modes of being requires that the mode with which we end be not explicitly used in the course of the proofs. It, however, does allow for the use of the same mode as a beginning, to connect the beginning with the end, and to provide for an act of detaching of the desired outcome. It thus allows one not only to start with Actuality, for example, but to use this to provide the structure of a proof and the agency for detaching a conclusion. Modi-fication of these conditions will of course yield a smaller or larger number of primary proofs.

All of the proofs are necessarily incomplete since they do not explicitly make use of what is concluded to. Those which end with Actualities make no adequate provision for the uniqueness of the outcome; those which terminate in Ideality make no adequate provision for the formal validation of the argument; those which terminate in Existence make no adequate provision for the derivation; those which terminate in God make no adequate provision for the unity of the argument. These failures are due to the fact that each mode of being has a definite role to perform in a valid proof, but which it cannot perform if acknowledged only as the outcome of a proof. On the other hand, all the modes are presupposed in every proof. As a consequence a proof of any is necessarily circular. All of the proofs too are only anticipatory of what one might directly encounter apart from all proof. Still, they are useful. They do permit one to know truths about the various modes before those modes are definitely experienced.

4.84 God needs and makes use of Actualities.
(See *1.14, 2.86, 4.15, 4.60*)

THE TRADITIONAL VIEW is that God needs nothing. He is thought to be absolutely perfect, containing within himself all excellencies and realities. Such a view makes it impossible to acknowledge the independent reality and excellence of anything else. In good part it is a view which rests on the confusion between the idea of God as a supreme being and the idea of him as an all-inclusive being. God is supreme in that there is no other superior to him, but such supremacy is consistent with his having needs of his own, to be satisfied through the aid of other beings.

Acting to realize the Good, infected by and infecting Existence, Actualities provide God with so many different avenues through which he can make his nature, intent, and demands known. Without those Actualities he would be able to act, but not in many different individualized ways at the same time. Without them he would be able to occupy himself with the Ideal, but not as the terminus of a plurality of distinct efforts and concerns. Without them he would be able to diversify his activities over Existence but not in a focused way, through a plurality of independent individual beings.

The more perfect an Actuality is, the more receptive it is of God's excellence, the more able it is to accept the work of God as its own. Since the most perfect of Actualities is a virtuous man, God looks to the virtuous as best enabling him to be effective in this world of

ours. And only such men can accept the work of God as their own.
The others must radically reinterpret the meaning of that work before
they can make it one with themselves.

4.85 God needs and makes use of the Ideal.
(See *2.100, 2.103, 3.106, 4.18, 4.60*)

THE INJUNCTION that men are to be as perfect as God himself
is evidently to be understood in some metaphorical sense, since it
requires that men not only try to live up to a standard which is completely beyond their finite reach, but one which is not necessarily
pertinent to their natures. God is not an Actuality, even the most flaw-
less of Actualities, but quite a distinct kind of being. And even if he
were just the most excellent of Actualities, he would not provide
a proper measure of what it is they ought to do, but only a measure
of the degree to which they fall short of *his* perfection. If God is to
dictate what Actualities are to do in this spatiotemporal world, he
must deal with them in terms which are relevant to them, and not
merely appropriate to himself. He must approach them through the
avenue of a providentially determined Good, and for this purpose
he needs the Ideal. He needs the Ideal also in order to enable him
to guide the cosmic whole of Existence as it moves through time. But
in addition he needs the Ideal by itself as that which enables him
to have and realize a divine intent. Without the Ideal he would be
sunk within himself, realizing nothing. He needs the Ideal in the
guise of a Principle of Perfection, to enable him to be evaluated as
excellent and purposive.

4.86 God needs and makes use of Existence.
(See *3.08, 3.102, 3.105, 4.21, 4.60*)

ONLY SO far as a being exists can it act. Since God engages in
acts of self-expression and reorders himself in an effort to realize the
Principle of Perfection, he must have Existence within him. But
Existence is also outside him, a domain of space, time, and energy,
endlessly dividing itself and expanding. God has need of it. Without
Existence God could express himself through Actualities and through
the Ideal, but he would not be omnipresent, active at every point of
space and time, since neither the Actual nor the Ideal is everywhere.
Also, though Existence is turbulent and perpetually changing, it is

irreducible, inextinguishable. Only it is persistent enough, vital enough, extensive enough, divided enough to be capable of satisfying God's need to be everywhere. It alone provides him with endless and perpetual opportunities to express himself, to have a spatiotemporal role.

4.87 God preserves Actualities.
(*See 4.17, 4.62, 4.66, 4.84*)

ACTUALITIES are so many individual items which stand over against God as other than he, striving to realize the Good in the course of time, and passing away in the guise of facts. They are needed by God and satisfy him to some extent. He reproduces them in himself, is aware of them, and proves their existence. He endows them with nonessential features. He also encounters and preserves them. God is the being with maximum retentiveness, who seeks to give every Actuality a place somewhere in his economy. He is the apex of the universe, facing the entire realm of present Actualities as a datum of an awareness, the entire realm of past factuality as a datum for a purged, divinized reconstitution of them, and the entire realm of possible Actuality as a datum in a private evaluation of the worth of the world. Absolute in comprehensiveness, limited in reality, supreme but not alone in the universe, he must preserve Actualities to remain a being who forever knows what has been, to enable him to see the Ideal in its role as the Good, and to enable him to grasp Existence as a transitory, vitalizing field.

4.88 God preserves whatever excellencies can be obtained from Actualities.
(*See 4.69, 4.87*)

EVIL is frustrating. Debilitation, conflict, destruction are the very antithesis of the excellence which is God. Since every Actuality is a mixture of good and evil, with excellencies and defects, the divine preservation of any would require a dividing off of a good accommodatable and a bad rejected part, or it would require a transformation of the Actualities until they were purged of the evil they contain. Since God is the source of unity and not of division, he cannot simply reject the evil in beings and acknowledge only what is good in them. He must reconstitute them to make them better than they were. He must preserve them not as they in fact are but as they in principle are. This he does by overcoming their internal self-defeating oppositions, by purging and transforming them. The better the beings the less transformation they will need in order to be accommodated by God. The better the things therefore the more they are in God in the very guise they have apart from him.

God can know evil, even though he knows and reproduces in himself only the goodness in things, which is to say, things so far as they are in harmony in themselves and with one another. He knows evil by recognizing that his knowledge of Actualities is more abstract than it need be. He knows the evil in them by knowing the kind of knowledge he has of them, by knowing that the good in them is not concrete enough to be entirely good. He senses their resistance when he deals with them as data. His conservation of the values of Actualities is not accomplished by tearing those values or the Actualities out of space-time, but by privately reconstituting the Actualities, thereby transforming them until they can find a place within a reconstructed harmony of all Actualities. Only when they are in that state do they deserve to be preserved, as part of the very being of God.

Divine judgment is one with divine punishment and divine rehabilitation. So far as a being is evil it needs to be radically transformed before it can be part of God's economy. Evil is given lodgement in him only as transformed into good. Such transformation involves a rejection, a nonpreservation, a letting go, and in this sense a forgetting of what the thing is. Divine punishment for evil is divine forgetfulness. God punishes by not letting the thing have a being for him except as purged, reassessed, transformed, made part of an eternal harmony. When he preserves the past, to be sure, he preserves it entire, making no distinction between good and bad. It is only when he reconstitutes it that he transcends the evil in it.

4.89   God establishes the Ideal as a perpetual standard of value.

(See 2.19, 2.21, 2.100, 3.92, 4.70, 4.85)

THE IDEAL is a prospect for Actualities and Existence, necessarily realized over the course of time. It also has a normative role with respect to them, measuring their worth. In the latter guise, it must not only be held apart from Actualities and Existence, but must pertain to them.

At every moment God reinstates the Ideal as an absolute measure of all the modes, and thus one having an application even to himself. Without such a measure, not only would God not be characterizable as excellent, but he could not be evaluated as better than the others. By retreating within himself while continuing to hold on to the Ideal, he faces it as a measure for himself and every other mode of being.

4.90 God provides the Ideal with satisfying Actualities and Existence.

(See *1.118, 2.14, 2.21, 2.22, 2.99, 2.104, 3.104, 4.85, 4.89*)

ACTUALITIES and Existence are not all they ought to be. They may never by themselves attain the status of being as excellent as it is possible for them to be. Such failure will be the result of the way in which they in fact function, due either to some internal lack or some external circumstance. Whichever it be, it involves a failure to satisfy the Ideal. But if the Ideal cannot in fact be fully realized in them, it is just so far, as a matter of fact, unrealizable. Since their failure to fully realize the Ideal that ought to be realized marks them as a defective, and since such failure is inevitable in this universe, we are faced with the paradox that Actuality and Existence are criticizable for failing to do what they could not possibly do. Or, perhaps more sharply, the Ideal in the guise of the Good is beyond the power of man, that finite, frustrated, ignorant, maladjusted being, to realize fully. But if this is in every way beyond his power, it is paradoxical and also wrong to charge him with ethical failure.

One can be obligated to do only what could possibly be done. But what will never be done anywhere is that which in fact cannot be done. Consequently, what men fail to do in this world must either be done by some other being to whom they can attach themselves, or must be done by themselves in some other realm. It is because there are possibilities which may not be realized in any Actualities that it makes sense to say of the entire course of the universe that, in whole and in part, it is defective, that it does not measure up to the require-ments of an absolute standard. This is what the Platonist so clearly sees and says. It is one of the cornerstones of his view that the Good need not be embodied in this world, that it has its own intrinsic dignity and worth. The task of things is to measure up to it, and so far as they fail they are defective.

Kant in a Platonic spirit insisted that virtue did not entail happiness, but he also knew that his account would be incomplete if he did not show that in the end perfect virtue was joined with perfect happiness. To make good the deficiency of his system he had to postulate the immortality of the soul and the existence of an interested God. Hegel pointed up Kant's makeshift solution with the observation that the Ideal was not so miserable and feeble a being as to be itself incapable of achieving an adequate realization in this world. For him the Ideal was not only realizable but realized; a Kantian virtue inevitably entrained a happiness. Hegel's solution, however, precluded him from affirming that the universe might never be all it could have been. And this is essentially the outcome to which Marx, Peirce, Dewey, Nelson Goodman, and others, who have no room for real, unrealized possibilities, must eventually come. None of them can possibly forge a place for an ethics with genuine obligations towards good objectives which men might forever fail to bring to pass.

The Good ought to be realized; it can be realized; it must be realized. Since it may not be realized here it must be realized elsewhere. Such realization is required by the nature of the Good. Not by postulation, but in the very nature of things, a happiness which completes virtue must follow on it. Not by postulation, but in the very nature of things, there must be a God who guarantees realization of the Good.

Ethically the Good need not be fully realized in this world; ontologically it must be realized somewhere, somehow. The very fact that the Good is part of the cosmos requires that there be at least another being which makes its inevitable realization possible. Kant is right; this world of ours may never see the full realization of the Good. But Hegel is also right; the Good is necessarily realized. Kant is right also in remarking that God helps realize the Good; Hegel on his side is surely also right in remarking that the realization of the Good is required by it. Kant failed to see that a God who fulfills an unavoidable task must be real. Hegel failed to see that the realization of the Good may occur somewhere other than here in history.

These alternatives are in fact not exclusive. God reconstitutes all Actualities, and Existence as well, making them as good and unified as it is possible for them to be. Such reconstituting is an act of integrating them with the Ideal they had not but ought to have embodied. The transformations do not go the whole way of making Actuality and Existence do full justice to the Ideal, for Actuality and Existence are resistant, recalcitrant, insistent on themselves over against the Ideal. Consequently, God must add to the transformed improved realities something of his own excellence; only then can he give satisfaction to the unsatisfied residuum of the Ideal. The total result a man can make his own by submitting himself to God, the considerate being who supplements, completes, who sees to it that all deficiencies are made good.

4.91 God unifies Existence.
(*See 3.01, 3.08, 4.73, 4.86*)

God is perpetually aware of Existence as separating itself from itself and from him. To be in himself over against all other modes, including the whole of Existence, and in order to be able to act on all other modes, including Existence, he must maintain his grip on it. And it needs him to provide it with a persistent essence. As he sweeps over the whole of his being, redividing himself into identities, he reproduces the whole of Existence in the shape of an infinite set of simple loci. This reproduction is governed by his own unity and the need to express this in the guise of identities. He thereby makes Existence have an integral essence, an essence which enables it to be a unified Existence. As standing apart from him Existence has only an *opposed* essence, an essence from which it is perpetually escaping; but as reconstituted by God, Existence has a fixed and *permanent* essence, an essence from which there is no escape.

4.92 God eternalizes Existence as his private extensionality.
(*See 3.03–5, 4.66, 4.91*)

BY ANALYZING himself into an infinite number of distinct points, God reproduces Existence with a fixed and permanent essence. Such reproduction would be inadequate unless at the same time God preserved the very extensionality of Existence. Unlike the evil in things this extensionality is desirable, worth God's preservation, for it makes possible a multiplication of distinct activities and effects.

The idea of an extended God is today still perhaps as repugnant as it was when Spinoza revived and transformed the Hebraic and Arabic view that a divinized extension is the common matter which underlies the Aristotelian four elements. But, as Spinoza remarked, the extension which is in God is not a divisible extension in the sense that one part of it could be separated off from another, divided in any way; it is an extension which is not to be separated from God's single unifying essence.

4.93   God supplements the work performed by any pair of modes on behalf of a third.
(See *2.14, 2.21, 2.104, 3.12–14, 3.106, 4.84–92*)

THE PRIMARY NEED of Actualities is preservation. This is partially given by God in the guise of an absolutizing Other, by the Ideal which provides them with a locus for their generic, indispensable features, and by Existence which dates them and keeps them oriented to a present. The primary need of Ideality is to be all-encompassing, and this result it partly obtains from Actuality in the guise of a realized Good, from Existence as a realized Future, and from God as a realized Principle of Perfection. The primary need of Existence is organization, and this it partly obtains from Actualities which function as its termini, from the Ideal through subordination, and from God through the bounded repetition of his unity. Each mode of being needs the contribution made by the other three; what any two of them fail to do must be done by the third, which means that the third must, in addition to its own work with respect to the first, take on the burden of doing what the others neglected to do. Thus, Existence and the Ideal both contribute to the completion and satisfaction of Actuality. Their resistance to Actuality would result in an inescapable demand which could not be satisfied were it not that God assumes the burden of satisfying Actuality when he reconstitutes it together with the Ideal and Existence.

God must give Actualities not only a purged reconstituted permanent being in him but must do this in such a way that they get the value and concordance which the Ideal and Existence should have provided but did not in fact provide. He must also give the Ideal the status of a Principle of Perfection, but one which is infected by the Good that the Actualities failed to exhibit and by the Future which Existence did not embody. And finally he must give Existence an essence, but one which also bestows on the Existence the intelligibility and control which the Ideal and Actualities should have given but did not in fact give to it.

4.94 Each mode completes work God should do on behalf of other modes.

(*See 3.14, 3.106, 4.05, 4.93*)

GOD'S primary task with respect to Actualities is to preserve them; his primary task with respect to Ideality is to enable it to be a realized principle of value; his primary task with respect to Existence is to give it an essence. Each of these modes resists him; to none of them does he give himself entirely. What he as a consequence fails to do with respect to any one mode devolves on the other two. When the Ideal transforms Actualities into instances of itself, and when Existence subjects Actualities to a cosmic co-ordination, they enable Actualities to acquire an intelligible and space-timed permanence which God did not give them. Similarly, when Actualities and Existence realize the Ideal, they also give it an application and fulfillment which it ought to have had but does not get from God, since he retreats from it to be within himself. And finally, when Actualities terminate Existence, and Ideality subordinates it, they make integral to it the essence which God does not entirely succeed in imposing on it. Severally, the modes are not sufficient one for the other; but none demands the impossible, and what any particular mode fails to do on behalf of another is necessarily performed by others.

VII   RELIGION

4.95 All the modes of being merge with the being which is God.

(*See 4.01, 4.60*)

NO ACTUALITY ever achieves the state of being altogether over against God. All are to some degree merged with him. And what is true of Actualities is true of Existence and Ideality. They merge with

God, and also with one another and Actuality. He who begins with any one of them has some acquaintance then with every other. Each of course has a being and a nature at which we can only point and cannot fully and directly grasp. Dialectical speculation and proofs of various sorts will reach to these other modes, but do not confront us with them. These other modes in turn, in their different ways, reach to us but cannot make us confront them.

From the very beginning of his conscious life a man is dimly aware of a standard of value, a vital ongoing, and a unity which are other than himself and with which he inchoately merges. Possessed of a unique value he is also comparably better or worse than others; existing on his own, he is caught within a larger dynamic world; living in history he is at the same time outside history. As he matures he more or less separates himself out over against these factors with which he merged, at the same time that he focuses on one of them as the primary correlate of himself and all else. Focusing on the standard he sees himself and all else facing a cosmic destiny; focusing on the process, he sees himself and all else to be subject to a relentless cosmic force; focusing on the unity, he sees himself and all else to be over against a supreme being. His achievement of self-consciousness is one with his awareness that the Ideal is effective, that Existence is dynamic, and that God is his Other.

4.96 A religious man seeks God as apart from him, convinced that the search will be successful.

(See 1.28, 2.86, 4.15, 4.40, 4.53, 4.55, 4.95)

THE ESSENCE of all personalized concern for God, no matter what its being, form, process, or stated end is: Seek and you shall find. A religious man seeks God with all his being; he is blessed if he finds him. To every request, criticism, objection, and doubt he has one constant rejoinder: Seek again, again, and again; you will be answered. For him everything else is exegesis, the function of which is to show that the search is inescapable and universal, and that the finding is unavoidable.

The various ways of searching for God are so many different forms of proof of him. A religious man is one who prefers those proofs which involve faith and works rather than logical inference. He adds to these a confidence that there will be an end to his quest,

that he will somewhere and somehow find God in the sense that he
will in fact be confronted by him.

4.97 The search for God is provoked by evil, tragedy, sorrow, pain.
(See 4.88, 4.96)

IT IS POSSIBLE for men to set out to seek God when they are
joyous. Usually though they begin when they are sad; tragedy, pain,
evil, sorrow provide the normal initial stimulus for a search for him.
It is when men see what they cherish pass away that they turn to
God for an assurance that it still remains. They turn to him as the great
preserver, the being who will redress every wrong, who will make
good every claim, who will perfect beings to the degree that their
natures, achievements, and capacities permit.

The *occasion* for the search for God is a concern for whatever is
in fact good in this world. The *reason* one looks to him is that one is
confident that he preserves the values which nature would otherwise
allow to perish. Men turn to God in the light of a genuine concern
for the good in everything there may be. But because no one can
ever fully grasp every value, no one can fully grasp God as the locus
of them all, preserved forever. Religious confidence outruns dialectical justification.

4.98 God can be sought and found anywhere.
(See 4.14, 4.95, 4.96)

EVERY MODE of being bears the marks of God; each offers direct
and indirect testimony that he exists. God can therefore be sought
in every being. He will not be found there in *propria persona*, to be
sure, but a beginning will there be provided for a movement to him
in fact. And since every being merges with him, he can be reached
without the need of a leap into or across an infinite abyss. It is only
when we seek to reach God as he is in and by himself that we are
forced to move an infinite distance.

Under the pressure of tragedy, the religious man, as a rule, first retreats within himself, and then recognizes himself to be an other who
cannot remain in this guise except so far as he is the reciprocal of an
Absolute Other, for whom he longs and in whom all excellence is
preserved and enhanced. He wants to confront and be confronted by

God, and he seeks him wherever this longing points. If wise and fortunate, he constrains his longing according to the structure and procedure of a reliable proof. Those who do not seek to confront God but rather to lose themselves in him or to become one with him are engaged, not so much in a religious quest, as in an effort to have a mystical experience. The latter should be preceded by the former, if one is to know where and how to move wisely and well.

Of course, if one takes the beginning of a longing for God to be the beginning of a search for him, it is not the case that the search for him can begin anywhere. But one retreats before one longs. Since a man is constantly involved with other Actualities and other modes of being, he can be said to begin a search for God whenever he begins to free himself from an involvement with these Actualities and modes. And if a man takes the finding of God to be the outcome of a proof which directly gets to him as apart from the other modes of being, then it is also not the case that the search for him will end anywhere. But since one proves God through the agency of Actualities, Ideality, and Existence, and since God, when proved through these means, is not necessarily distant from them, a finding of God can take place anywhere. Such finding, too, since it is not necessarily without a reciprocal giving by God of himself, may involve an encounter with him. This of course will take place wherever God presents himself—and this can be anywhere.

4.99   The search for God can never come to an absolute end.

(See *4.53–55, 4.58, 4.59, 4.95, 4.97*)

THERE is no one unique way to get to God. He can be sought through logic and works, through prayer and reverie, in fear and trembling, or in jubilation. And since we do merge with him always, he can be found immediately, at every moment. But the most effective way of being aware of him and what he means for man is to long for him with a sorrow sustained by confidence. The more one is alert to tragedy, if only in the shape of the passage of value, and the more confident one is that it is redeemed, that there is a "divine comedy" following on the daily tragedy, the more certainly does one point to and arrive at what subtends, reconstitutes, and eternalizes the other modes, satisfying each by integrating it, in a perfected form, with the others.

God is the unity present in all things; to know oneself or anything else as a unity is therefore to have some grasp of God. This is not a knowledge of him in his concreteness, but of his nature as exhibited outside himself. In himself he cannot be reached; like every other being his center is inviolable, not capable of being penetrated from without. The search for God can never therefore come to an absolute end; his inwardness can never be fully plumbed. One can never reach him as he exists in himself, an eternal being, permeated with value, conserving all that is excellent. But neither can he wholly probe our depths and reach us as we exist in and by ourselves.

4.100   God reaches to and finds every other being.
(*See 4.67–75, 4.80–83, 4.95*)

ARISTOTLE thought that the relation of the world and God went in only one direction; the world depended on him, pointed towards him, but he made no reference, had no relation to it. Christianity, particularly in its Augustinian phase, makes the one way relationship go in the opposite direction. Man, for it, cannot really get to God except so far as God reaches down to him and lifts him up. God is related to man but man is not related to God, it thinks, not because God is dependent on man, but rather because man is impotent, incapable of being related to God, and perhaps even incapable of existing, except so far as God sustains him. The views should supplement one another. This Meister Eckhart recognized when he remarked, "God needs me as much as I need him." The relation holding between God and man—and more generally, the relation holding between any modes—does not run in one direction only.

God is aware of the other modes of being; he can reconstitute them in himself; he can prove them; he can provide them with testimony of himself; he can be aware of them. He is ingredient in them, and they are ingredient in him. And he knows that he is other than they, a true, eternal unity without internal conflict. He also knows that there are constantly new Actualities, new realizations of the Ideal, new transformations of Existence, and that these are receptive of him in various degrees. The resistance which God feels they exhibit to his reconstructive activity dictates the direction in which his acts of knowledge and production are to follow. He thus knows where to make contact with other beings outside himself. And since he can encounter them as surely as they can encounter him, and since they no less than

he are both receptive to and resistant, he knows when, and something
of the degree to which he has made contact with them.

4.101   God and men are related in a common field.
(See 4.15, 4.67, 4.95, 4.99–100)

GOD makes all Actualities have the status of absolute permanent
others; they reciprocate and give him the status of a relative Other,
an Other occupied with them in their changing transitory forms. He
and they thus are double others, absolute and steady, and relative
and variable. He is initially an Absolute Other and endows them with
this status; they are initially relative others who, because they require
him to alter the way in which he knows and deals with them, make him
into a relative other. The relation of absolute otherness constitutes a
field between them. When this field is quickened by their desire for
one another, the field becomes the field of their relative vital interplay.

4.102   The mystic traverses the field he constitutes with God.
(See 4.98, 4.101)

THE MYSTIC submits himself to God so as to obtain the joy of being
completely one with what he takes to be alone of value. He tries to
empty his being into his longing for God so as to lose himself in that
unity in which every other has a place. He can reach his goal of
course only so far as God is receptive to him. And so far as God can
receive him, God can receive the field which they together constitute.
When the mystic returns from his experience, he should return as a
being who has been purged by God. He should have a new sense of
value and mission. Consequently he should be able to change the
nature of the field that they before had together constituted, since he
can now infect it with his experience of God's goodness. A mystic is to
be known by his mastery of the field which he and God constitute and
through which they act.

4.103   God completes the work of man.
(See 1.118, 2.13, 2.14, 3.92, 3.94, 4.93)

THE POSSIBILITY of being a feudal man had to be fulfilled during
medieval time with its particular economy, religion, etc. The man
and the time come to be and pass away together. Before the medieval

period is over the possibility of being a feudal man is not altogether fulfilled. What guarantees the fulfillment of the possibility by the close of the period? Nothing could guarantee such fulfillment except a power which either restructures the possibility constantly so that it is exhaustively expressed over a period, or completes it at the very close of the period. God makes the different realizations of a possibility over the course of time add up to the full realization of that possibility. He does not arrange that the possibility be satisfied only at the end of a period; possibilities are usually steadily realized over a stretch of time. God sees to it that the structures projected at the beginning of subdivisions of history are exhausted by the end of them. It is he who makes the work of individuals, peoples, epochs, and civilizations, into the work of one mankind over one history.

There are also normative possibilities which never may be realized at any time. In terms of these, every part, and the whole of history can be judged. The Greeks cannot be rightly criticized for not doing the things Romans did and could; but they and the Romans can both be rightly criticized for not having adequately realized the normative possibility of being good men. God is needed to make possible the single judgment that all the different peoples in the course of time have been more or less defective. And since what ought to be must be realized, or define a task which is in fact impossible, he must assure the satisfaction of the norms which men fail to satisfy.

God's *justice* is expressed in his acceptance of the good which things possess; his *mercy* is expressed in his preservation of that good; his *forgiveness* is expressed in his cancellation of the debt that evil owes. He is to be worshipped because he completes the work of men.

4.104 Trust is the belief that what man takes to be good is good in God's sight.
(*See 4.90, 4.97, 4.103*)

GOD makes good man's (and Existence's) failures on behalf of the Good. But no one knows whether the additions which he provides are solely supplementary or transformative of what men do, and of the Good that is relevant to them. Nor does any one know whether or not what men take to be a fulfillment of the Good is a fulfillment in God's sight. No one knows whether or not what men find to be good he finds to be evil; no one knows whether or not he dismisses what they think they ought to adopt, and adopts what they think they ought to dismiss. The story of Cain and Abel underscores this fact, pointing up the truth that God has his own ways of determining what is good and bad, not evident to men. The story of Job teaches a similar lesson; in the end God gives no reasons for his acts and evaluations.

The religious man trusts that God's justice, mercy, and forgiveness are like man's, but carried to an absolute limit. A member of a religion trusts that God's salvation, justice, mercy, and forgiveness accrue most readily or exclusively to those who believe and practice in accordance with that religion's demands. The two trusts are independent but not incompatible. A religious member of a religion trusts that what man takes to be good God does, and that this good comprises what the religion sanctions. But he does not, in this life, know whether this is true or not.

4.105 Ethics and peremptory religion make independent demands.
(See 1.118, 4.104)

THAT God does satisfy the Good not satisfied by Actualities, even when helped out by Existence, we know. But we do not know whether what we, as ethical men, take to be the Good is identical with what he takes to be the Good. We may have misconstrued just what ought-to-be, or he may satisfy it only within a context, only as supplemented and modified by him in such a way as to make it have quite a different import from what it had before.

In the end men must look to God to complete their work, but this God and his work is not to be defined in ethical terms. There is no need to refer to God in ethics then except at the point where all human and natural powers fail, and then one cannot be sure that what he does will sustain what ethics demands. And in any case what he does on behalf of the Good becomes a man's, only so far as man accepts that work as his own, translates it into ethical terms.

Understanding by a peremptory religion a devotional discipline which requires of man only what God demands, and by ethics a rational discipline which requires man to realize the Good everywhere, it is evident that they are independent enterprises. Each in fact offers standards in terms of which the other can be criticized. Over the course of history each has served to force modifications in the defense, elaboration, and practice of the other. Our ethical temper is no longer that of the Greeks, and our religious spirit is not as parochial or petulant as it was in previous decades. But in the end we are forced to say that from the standpoint of ethics, religious demands are often arbitrary and sometimes even corrupt and unethical, and that from the standpoint of religion, ethics is derivative, and perhaps even effete, incomplete and too humanistic. Ethics and religion are not to be reconciled by supposing that that alone is ethically right that is commanded by God, or that God commands only what is ethically right. The first of these alternatives denies rationality to ethics, denies that there are things we men ought to do just because we are free, worldly men, facing an unsatisfied Good, and for no other reason. The second of these alternatives supposes that God's commands are all ethically right, thereby making a reference to God quite unnecessary for an ethics. And both alternatives suppose somewhat arbitrarily that God is a being who commands.

Religious trust offers one form of a reconciliation of religion and ethics, but only on the supposition that God endorses what the religion does, even when he adds to or transforms what it takes to be the Good. The acceptance by an ethical man of the work of God as man's own, can be offered as a second form of reconciliation of the two disciplines, but only on the supposition that God satisfies the very Good that ethical men actually face, even when he transforms them and places their Good within a larger context. Both answers are evidently biased and inadequate to one or the other of the reconciled elements. Neither can therefore finally satisfy.

4.106 Scientific and religious claims are independent.
(See *1.90, 4.97, 4.105*)

THE RELATION of science and religion is analogous to that of ethics and religion, except that ethics attends to the Ideal whereas science attends to Existence, and that the problem of their reconciliation relates primarily to truth and not to values.

From the standpoint of science, religion makes unverifiable and imprecise claims; from the standpoint of religion, science ignores the richness of experience. They cannot be reconciled by supposing that what is scientifically true is only what is endorsed by a religion, or by supposing that what is religiously true is only what a science certifies. The first of these alternatives denies autonomy, rationality, and free inquiry to science; the second makes these same denials with respect to religion. A reconciliation though may be found in the recognition that truth is one. This one truth might be taken to be the truth of religion which the truths of science are to complete and conform to. Or it might be thought to be the truth of science which the truths of religion are to complete and conform to. These however are evidently biased answers, pointing to a truth beyond both.

4.107   Psychology and religion are grounded in independent attitudes.
(*See 1.50, 4.99, 4.105*)

THE RELATION of psychology and religion is analogous to that of ethics or science to religion, except that psychology—or as it is now called, psychiatry—concerns itself with an Actual self rather than with the Ideal or Existence, and that the reconciliation involves an adjustment of attitudes rather than of values or truth.

From the standpoint of psychology or psychiatry, religion imposes too heavy a burden on the self, and offers an answer which cannot be checked or controlled. From the standpoint of religion, psychology or psychiatry takes too narrow a view of the self, and gives it a momentary rather than a lasting peace. They cannot be reconciled by supposing that religion alone determines what makes for human happiness, or that a true religion is to be defined as one which promotes happiness. The first of these alternatives denies the this-worldly nature of human concerns and what satisfies them; the second denies the other-wordly import of religion and the fact that its demands may involve unrelinquishable but difficult and perhaps unending tasks. But a reconciliation may be found in an attitude which points beyond both.

4.108   A proper adjudication requires neutrality.
(*See 4.105–7*)

OPPOSITION is a symmetrical relation. It requires that there be two sides, each denying, rejecting, negating the other. Let us term two sides A and B, and let us term the languages which do justice to the structure, divisions, meaning of A and B, languages *a* and *b*. As complete and independent, *a* and *b* are logically distinct, co-ordinate languages; each makes distinctions the other does not acknowledge. From the standpoint of language *a*, language *b* is to be said to speak *meaninglessly* so far as it makes distinctions which *a* does not permit, and is to be said to speak *confusedly* so far as it fails to make the distinctions that *a* makes or requires. From the standpoint of *b* similar observations are to be made regarding language *a*. In summary this is essentially the structure of all polemics. We find it today in philosophy exploited by positivists and analysts, particularly with respect to metaphysics and theology. The criticism is just from the standpoint of the language these critics adopt. Metaphysics is nonsense and confused in terms of the criteria offered by symbolic logic and elementary philosophy of science as to just what constitutes a well-formed sentence and a proper term, usage, or meaning. What these critics fail to see is that from the standpoint of the language of metaphysics or theology their own language can be criticized with the same degree of justice. From such a standpoint it is evident that positivists and analysts sometimes fail to make needed distinctions (e.g., between Actuality and Existence, between Ideality and God, or between logic and mathematics) and sometimes make unnecessary distinctions (e.g., between sheer absurdity and perfect clarity, or between scientific knowledge and truth) and are therefore rightly chargeable with discoursing in a manner both confused and nonsensical. An occasional theologian and metaphysician has seen the point and has in this vein criticized his opponents as severely as they criticized him. But neither side enjoys a preferential status. They are on a par. Each is subject to criticism by the other as surely as it is qualified to criticize that other. And since there are more than two domains or two languages, each side is guilty of failing to distinguish what even from its own side ought to be quite different types of "nonsense" and "confusion."

An adjudication of an opposition which does not unwarrantedly favor one side over another must assume a position neutral to both. Unlike biased reconciliations which attempt to do justice to both sides by adopting one side and then having the other complete and conform to it, a genuine reconciliation requires one to stand outside them both, making them measure up to a neutral standard.

4.109   A genuinely neutral treatment of what is the case
is at once prescriptive and descriptive of all the modes.
(See 4.56, 4.108)

A CONFLICT can be adequately adjudicated only if there is a standard which is neutral to the contending parties, does not compromise
their independence or their distinctive natures, and can be satisfied by both sides. That standard ought to be exhibited by
both of them, always. If they never did exhibit it, the standard would
be effete, impotent, idle. And if there were a time when they did not
exhibit it, in some way and to some degree, that time could be followed by another and another and another, and so on without end,
so that the standard might never be exhibited in fact. The adjudicating
standard is prescriptive, brooking no failure. How is this possible? At
least five answers have some plausibility.

1. The opposing items might, as a matter of pure contingency,
happen to be together in such a way as to exhibit the adjudicating
principle, and this state of affairs might just happen to continue
forever. 2. History and inquiry might be self-corrective, so that a
deviation from the standard in one direction was compensated for by
others through the use of the self-corrective process of history or a
self-corrective method of induction. 3. There might be a predestined
end where all oppositions were eventually overcome; until then there
would be no really determinate items which were opposed, but only
opposition or struggle, which precluded a distinctive nature to what
was involved in it. 4. There could be a power outside all oppositions
which imposed the standard on them and evaluated the degree to
which they measured up to it, the evaluation serving to overcome
whatever discrepancies in fact existed. 5. Every moment and case
could be an illustration, a way of exhibiting the standard to some degree.

These five answers come closer and closer to a satisfactory solution.
None, however, does full justice to the fact that a genuine reconciliation of a conflict requires that the adjudicative principle be always
exemplified, but in such a way that a distinction can be made between
a better and a worse adjudication. What is needed is something like
a combination of the fourth and fifth answers. The standard must be
at once prescriptive and descriptive. The condition is met in the

recognition that all oppositions, no matter what their degree and nature, must somehow be together, and must therefore exhibit the meaning of togetherness. The togetherness, as that which must be exhibited, is fixed, inescapable, prescriptive; but as that which is exhibited, it is descriptive, changing in character from case to case. The
two sides are inseparable. Both are constituted of the very items which
are together, the one having them externally together in a steady way,
thereby allowing them to exercise the role of a sheer plurality, while
the other merges them in a fluctuatable way, from a minimum where
they are independent items to a maximum where they are interwoven
and hardly distinguishable.

Religion offers but one of many legitimate ways of expressing in
demand, in claim, or through attitude, something of the nature, presence, intent, or being of God. It and the other legitimate ways of
knowing and acting can be reconciled only in a neutral domain. A
religion should consequently reject the temptation to take itself as
ultimate—a self-denial which should also be practiced by other disciplines. To do less than this is to usurp the role of what enables them
to be over against and yet with one another.

The neutral domain is a *tertium quid* constituted by two modes of
being or representatives of them. Ethics and religion are reconciled in
a *tertium quid* constituted of a unity of Actuality and Existence, or
in its representative, the *well-adjusted* man. Science and religion are
similarly reconciled in a juncture of Actuality and Ideality, i.e., in a
representative *virtuous* man, whereas psychology and religion need
the mediation of a unified Existence and Ideality, or its representative, the *historically tempered* man. The reconciling requires that the
disciplines keep apace with one another, altering their rhythms and
modifying their punctuation while keeping their distance, until they
express in opposite correlative ways nothing more or less than the
being which reconciles them. At one moment this discipline must give
way, and at another moment the other. Convenience, experience,
sometimes experiment, and occasionally genius determine just what
is to be changed, and when. But sooner or later both of the opposed
disciplines will be forced to change their ways in accordance with
the dictates of practical judgment, or of an ethical or civilized life.

In 4.56 it was seen that Ideality and Existence (e.g., in the form of
an opposed set of logical prescriptions and actual inference) can be

reconciled by a *wise* man. The reconciliation of cases of the Actual and the Ideal (e.g., psychology and logic) and the Actual and Existence (e.g., psychology and physics) are the province of the *scientific* and the *religious* man respectively.

The types of men evidently pair off with one another—the historically oriented with the wise, the virtuous with the scientific, the well-adjusted with the religious. From the perspective of one the other is a limit which can never be achieved. But all of them can exist together. This is possible only so far as the modes of being can be together. To refer to that togetherness is to refer to what is in one sense less and in another more than all the modes, since it is just all the modes together. It makes little difference whether we call it a reality, the rationale of the universe, a cosmic *élan*, or the living immanent God. What is important is that it is a position neutral to the modes and to the men who exemplify them. This position lacks the reality of a genuine mode of being; it is abstract to the very degree that it is one and multiple to the very degree that it is concrete.

A single undivided neutral position for the four modes of being could have concreteness only so far as the modes were without unity. The neutral position for all of them has four exhaustive polarities, answering to the demands of each of them. Each of these polarities offers a different way in which the four modes can be neutrally together. But there is no power which forces those polarities to make a single unity. Fortunately no such unity is needed. The modes of being need no reconciliation since they, together in a fourfold way, exhaust whatever there is or could be.

PART II

The Negative Route

CHAPTER 5

The Adequacy

OF A PHILOSOPHY

I   PHILOSOPHY AND OTHER APPROACHES

THE ACTS of an actual man exhibit him as more than a mind, even when he does nothing more than think. His knowing inevitably bears the marks of his bias; his knowledge of things cannot therefore be entirely neutral. There is nothing like sheer knowing; but the higher up in the hierarchy of abstractions we go, the more clearly we can approach the stage where we can cognize things perfectly and neutrally, but abstractly. It is this limit which a philosophic system seeks to reach, subject to the qualification that no significant differences in things be transcended or blurred. An organic unity of general principles and categoreal observations, philosophy deals with things not in their concreteness and individuality but as kinds, natures, meanings, structures, as instances or illustrations of basic modes of being. It recognizes that knowledge is a strategy which enables a man to get, though only in the abstract, what otherwise could not be reached, mastered, retained, manipulated, and related, and that it is desirable to engage in this strategy more persistently and over a larger territory than nonphilosophic enterprises will or can. Philosophy is the agency employed by some Actualities to master whatever there be.

Each mode of being has its characteristic bias, affecting the way in which it deals with all else. For Actualities, other modes of being are essentially others; for the Ideal they are instances of itself; for Existence they are so many different termini; and for God they are himself reproduced. If we take our stand with Actuality we tend to negate the other modes of being; if we take up the position of Ideality we tend to subordinate them; if we are in Existence we tend to maintain extensive relations with them; and if we take the position of God we tend to synthesize them. From the perspective of the Actual all the other modes are distinct from it; from that of Ideality they are included in it: from that of Existence they are apart from one another within it; and from that of God they are conjoined in him. The logic of Actuality is "this not that"; of Ideality, "if this, then that"; of Existence, "this, therefore that"; and of God, "this and that."

What knowledge is for Actuality, appreciation is for God, evaluation is for Ideality and co-ordination is for Existence. These are strategies enabling the respective modes to encompass the others neutrally, through a sacrifice of their own characteristic concrete stresses; equally, they are ways of releasing the mode from involvement in others, of freeing it from its role as a part of a many and allowing it to stand over against those others, to become a one for a many. Genuine alternatives to cognition, they are the proper and inevitable expressions of efforts at neutrality, from other positions than that of a cognizing Actuality. From the perspective of those other positions, knowledge is a more limited and distortive way of apprehending the rest than appreciation, evaluation, or co-ordination would be.

In the endeavor to make the others part of itself so that it can be complete, self-contained, the master of what conditions it, each being deals concretely with the others from its own particular perspective. But this prevents it from getting to the others as they are in themselves. To grasp what they are in themselves it is necessary for it to transcend the bias which it has by virtue of its particular nature, functions, need, position, and substantiality. The price to be paid for neutrality is abstractness.

A study which starts from the standpoint of some other mode of being than Actuality must then avoid confounding its legitimate claim to universality (which must be framed inside a noncognitive characteristic way of dealing with others) with the illegitimate claim that it can satisfactorily cognize those others. Only he who starts from the standpoint of Actuality can know the others adequately. He, however, makes a mistake similar to the others if he supposes that he could fully appreciate, evaluate, or co-ordinate those other modes of being. Precisely because his knowledge contains appreciation, evaluation, and co-ordination as subordinate and qualified cases of itself, he ought to know that he cannot, in his knowledge, do full justice to the other viewpoints in their concreteness. His philosophy, and the domain of Actuality which sustains it, must be recognized to be instances of such other disciplines as religion, mathematics, and art—disciplines to be exploited by men who take the position of God, the Ideal, or Existence respectively. Like philosophy, no one of these is free from bias, no one of these gets to the other modes in their concreteness. The best religious expression is inadequate to the concrete being of Actualities, Ideality, and Existence, both because it is abstract and because it abstracts only appreciatively. The best philosophy, similarly, is inadequate to the concrete being of Ideality, Existence, and God, both because it is abstract and because it abstracts only cognitively. Each discipline fails to do justice even to the particular mode of being which it abstractly expresses, though it does more justice to this than it does to the others.

Only he who begins from the perspective of Actualities will be able to pursue the ideal of pure knowledge without limit. But he ought to recognize that his knowledge involves an abstraction from the full concreteness of Actuality itself, that it cannot get to the modes of being in their full concreteness, and that it offers but one way of apprehending whatever there be. A pure cognizing philosophy, one having no noncognitive elements, is a fiction, for no Actuality is entirely cut off from all the other modes. Still one can approximate to the pure state beyond any preassignable degree.

There are four proper approaches to the totality of being. Only one, knowledge, is appropriate to Actuality and to the philosophy which expresses it. A philosophy, however, should recognize the value of appreciation, evaluation, and co-ordination; it should acknowledge that these express powers and virtues other than but not inferior to knowledge. Just as a philosophy will, when held over against them, wrongly claim to know other modes of being as they are in themselves, and to be able to dispense with the kind of approaches which they ground, so they, as over against it, will claim to grasp Actuality and the rest by other means, and to be able to dispense with or to make satisfactory use of cognition. We cannot, however, sunder cognition from these other approaches.

If we are willing to speak of "knowledge" when cognition not only subjugates other ways of dealing with being, but is also subjugated by them, we can legitimately say that an approach which begins from some position other than Actuality can provide a genuine philosophy alternative to and as comprehensive as one which begins with Actuality. Each of these other philosophies will subjugate cognition to some other mode of apprehension. By assuming the position of the other modes of being in Chapters 2, 3, and 4, these alternative philosophies can be given a place alongside one which assumes the position of Actuality and stresses cognition.

Once it be recognized that each mode of being grounds its own characteristic way of apprehending, and that this is not entirely separable from other modes of apprehending, there is perhaps little danger in an attempt which, while sensitive to the different natures, stresses, and activities of the various modes, deals with all the modes with a primary stress on one type of apprehension. This is what philosophers traditionally do, and this is what has, for the most part, been done in the previous chapters: all the modes have been dealt with as primarily objects of cognition. But it is one thing to persist in a single type of apprehension and quite another to take account of only one mode of being.

A study which remains with only one mode of being, no matter which, is no better or worse off than one which remains with some other. A philosophy which takes account only of Ideality is not better off than one which instead starts and remains with, say, Actuality. A nominalism, for example, by limiting itself to Actualities, denies knowledge the range it achieves through its abstractness. The nominalism will therefore not do more justice to the facts than is possible in an idealism, a materialism, or a monism, which, starting from the perspective of some other mode of being, tries to take cognition as the most appropriate way of dealing with all else.

A nominalist acknowledges only Actualities to be real, denying any status to the Ideal or to Existence; if with Occam or Luther he acknowledges a God, that God is thought to be a being like himself, though of course of a higher order and of a greater degree of excellence. The absolute idealist, particularly a post-Hegelian, has a philosophy which recognizes the reality only of the Ideal; the Actual is viewed by him as a congeries of universals, Existence is denied to have any being apart from the Actual, and God is either dismissed as unreal, or identified with the Ideal itself. The materialist, in contrast, has a philosophy which acknowledges only Existence. Actuality is for him a limited version of this, the Ideal is a kind of shadow thrown off by it, and God is but a word marking a confusion. For the vedantistic monist, God alone is real, and Actuality, Ideality, and Existence are illusions, errors, delimited partial ways of philosophically referring to God. The nominalist, idealist, materialist, and monist would do more justice to their chosen positions if they recognized that these did not permit of the best cognition; but even if they took up more appropriate attitudes, their denial of the reality of other modes would still leave them with incomplete accounts.

Interesting versions of these four types are obtainable with the recognition of the presence of one mode of being in another. Thus, when Actuality is recognized to contain something of the Ideal, it becomes *"oughtified,"* a being within which the Ideal is to be found in the shape of an individual conscience or moral consciousness. Or it may be recognized to be *existentialized,* infected by Existence and thereby made to manifest a kind of cosmic unconscious. Or it may be recognized to be *eternalized,* seen to possess something of the divine within it, to be the image of God.

Similarly, when the Ideal is seen to be infected in part by the Actual, it can be acknowledged to be a kind of Platonic form, an ought *"is-ified"* and individuated. Or it can be treated as *existential-ized,* so permeated by Existence as to become a kind of Platonic world-soul. Or it can be acknowledged to be *eternalized,* to have within it something of God, in which case it assumes the guise of a Providence.

Existence also can be *"oughtified,"* treated as already having within it something of the Ideal. This is the way it is thought of by those who speak of the living law, or of a collective moral consciousness, or of the best of all possible worlds. Or Existence can be viewed as *infected* by Actuality, in which case it is given definiteness and in-dividuality. This is the line taken by those who subscribe to a rela-tivity physics with its world lines and cosmic constants of energy. And finally Existence can be treated as *eternalized,* as qualified by divinity. This is what is done when one takes prime or dialectical matter, as outside time and space, to be the basic reality.

God can be said to be *actualized,* made to take the shape of an Actuality, as in an incarnation. Or he can be taken to be *"oughtified,"* made the locus of the Ideal, in which case he is viewed as judge—or where he is thought of as turned inward, as essentially mind. And finally, God can be taken to be *existentialized*, one whose essence is the act of existing, as the Thomists say.

In these new versions, each one of the modes is recognized to contain something of the others, so that he who begins with one of them has, in some sense, all the others. But the same difficulty that confronted the views that held there was only one mode of being, confronts these new versions. These too in fact adopt the position of only one mode and presuppose the reality of the others.

Combinations of these new versions provide views which, unlike those just listed, have considerable plausibility and explanatory power. Many types of combination are possible. A promising type treats one mode as the cause of the other, or as its test or measure. This can have any one of twenty-four cases, derived from the six pairs: Actuality and Ideality, Actuality and Existence, Actuality and God, Ideality and Existence, Ideality and God, Existence and God. The first pair can serve us as a model for the rest. In personalism idealized Actualities are treated as *causes* of actualized Ideals; neoplatonism reverses the stress and treats actualized Ideals as causes of idealized Actualities. In Jamesean pragmatism, idealized Actualities serve to *measure* actualized Ideals; Bradleyan idealism reverses this and treats actualized Ideals as the measure of idealized Actualities. None of these recognizes all four modes to be on a footing, at once exterior to and interior to the others. Yet such recognition is necessary if we are to do justice to the facts. Nothing less is needed than a study which not only deals with each mode by itself but takes account of the fact that each mode is involved with every other. This is what the foregoing chapters were designed to provide.

II THE PHILOSOPHIC WHOLE
AND ITS PARTS

A philosophic system approaches the world primarily through cognition. It then evidently has over against it those disciplines which approach the cosmos in other ways. It also has over against it other philosophies which, though they do engage in cognition, say only part of what it does. It also has over against it the philosophies which disagree with it, and also whatever particular denials there be of its own particular assertions. A philosophic system which recognizes less than four modes of being is incomplete, but one which, while taking care of them, does not deal with its opponents or with the denials of its truths, is inadequate.

Every philosophic system implicitly claims to be all-inclusive. It therefore must find a place for the views which oppose it. Every philosophic assertion, affrmative or negative, must find its justification in it. The system must then have a place not only for every philosophic truth but must account in principle at least for every philosophic error, denial, negation as well. It must be able to say that there are philosophic errors which others commit, and that there are partial or different accounts of the very facts with which it deals. If it could not at least in principle account for, find a place for, explain such views, it would fail to allow for all the facts. The principles of an adequate philosophy must accommodate all others as instances of itself; if it is illustrated by whatever there be, it must be illustrated even by what opposes it.

It is a mistake for a philosopher to claim to have a true, inclusive, adequate system and yet try to think of himself, say, as a naturalist for whom idealism is false or nonsensical (or conversely), unless he can provide a naturalistic (or idealistic) account of how the falsehood or nonsense arises, and can endow that falsehood or nonsense with some kind of naturalistic (or idealistic) status. The positivist meets half of this challenge when he defines Heideggerian metaphysics as nonsense, for he explains how it arises from what he thinks is a mistaken use of such terms as "nothing," "being," "is." But not until there is room in the positivistic system for the reality of confusion and nonsense, not until he can show how the Heideggerians are positivists in a poor sort of way, can he claim that the whole truth is contained in principle within the positivistic philosophy. If instead he does not wish to make the claim that he has the whole philosophic truth, he must acknowledge that he and his opponents may divide it between them, and that the two of them may be encompassable within a more inclusive scheme, which may judge either or both of them to have little truth or value.

It is not enough, however, for an adequate philosophy to treat opposing views as subordinate parts of itself. It must recognize that they, as philosophies, also claim to be true and even to be all-inclusive. No philosophy is adequate unless it explains how and why the others make such claims. It must enter sympathetically into the spirit of those other views, and come to understand how they also must claim to be adequate, and why they must therefore contend that they accommodate it. It is arbitrary to dismiss other philosophies as foolish or mistaken; one must show how these foolish or mistaken views not only illustrate one's own principles but, as so illustrating them, inevitably urge themselves as views superior to one's own. To take our tiresome example again, no positivist answer to metaphysics is plausible unless it can show not only that its supposed nonsense is a case of positivist truth (regarding the outcome of a misuse of language or logic), but that it is the kind of nonsense which necessarily claims to include the truth of positivism as a subordinate part. This latter condition the positivist cannot meet. By insisting that his opponent talks utter nonsense, he prevents himself from allowing that his opponent makes any claim at all. But then he should realize that his opponent does not and cannot oppose him, and need not therefore be answered. The positivist would do more justice to his own position if he were to give more credit to his opponent's. Instead of charging his opponent with talking nonsense he should show that the opponent does nothing more than positivistic work, but so badly that he thinks he does all of it, and this primarily because he uses terms ambiguously. But this is a tactic which the opponent can employ as well. He can claim that positivists too are metaphysicians, but poor ones, and this primarily because they are superficial. Neither has a right to settle the matter between them, for there is no hope for justice where plaintiff and judge are one. To adjudicate their quarrel one must go outside the area of both and recognize tests and truths neither acknowledges.

The polemics which dot the history of philosophy are bitter but ineffective. No one is persuaded by the arguments of other philosophers in good part because no one finds his views properly presented by those other philosophers. He finds himself refuted inside another system which has no way of allowing him to be over against that system. And yet this is where he is, and even where that other system claims him to be. If a philosopher, on behalf of his system's claim to truth and adequacy, maintains that his opponents are no other than himself in some form, possessing part of the very truth that he himself supposedly has in a more adequate way, he must still recognize that that partial truth opposes and is opposed by the whole. What has only part of the truth has it in such a way as to claim, falsely, that it has the whole, and that it therefore includes the very system which claims to include it. As having part of the truth which it puts in opposition to the whole it defines that whole to lack something, to be a whole only in an abstract sense, and thus from another point of view to be itself only a part, having less than all the truth.

The existence of warring philosophic systems is proof enough that no one of them says all that needs be said. Rejection of the rest by each is what one might expect from partial systems falsely claiming to be all-inclusive. The claim that there are no items outside one of these systems is an error made inside it, but reflecting the presence and power of what is outside. Only that system can justly claim to be adequate which includes all the rest as partial illustrations of itself, and shows why they, in turn, claim it to be a special case of themselves. Nothing, the system in effect must show, is wholly wrong, wholly outside it, wholly nonsense. It must show that its opponents' errors are in a way inevitable, as a consequence of an overinsistence on the need to grasp the system part by part, and thus in opposition to itself as a unity. The contentions which go counter to a system must illustrate it. They are the expressions of the system's elements treated as standing away from it, and as such, because ignoring the claims of all else, necessarily maintaining that they offer the whole truth, and consequently that they ought, and do, cancel and replace the given system.

The point can perhaps be best focused on if we attend to the following distinctions:

1. The separate *parts* of the system. In the present case the parts are the various theses presented in Chapters 1 through 4, viewed as separate, distinct items. A part will be symbolized by an "x" or a "y".

2. The *assemblage* of the parts of the system. In the present case the assemblage consists of the 441 numbered theses of Chapters 1 through 4, viewed as a single mass, with the items no longer separate from one another. The assemblage will be as symbolized as "x.y".

3. The *structure* of the system. In the present case the structure consists of the four main divisions, marked out as chapters, of the six to ten subdivisions in those divisions, marked out with subheadings, and of the interconnection of the various theses as made partly evident by the cross references. The whole structure will be symbolized by ",".

4. The *unity* of the system. In the present case the unity is exhibited in the way in which the assemblage and the structure are together. The unity will be symbolized by a "V".

5. The *whole* system. In the present case the whole system is an interlocked, unified totality of the assemblage, the structure and the unity. The assemblage, structure, and unity are all the *elements* of the whole, comparable to the parts x and y which make up an assemblage. This will be symbolized as "x,y V x.y" or alternatively as "pq" where "p" and "q" are symbols of real elements in the cosmos, referred to in a philosophic system.

6. The *negations* of the system. These are formal, philosophic denials of the parts, the assemblage, the structure, the unity or the whole. They will be symbolized as "–x" and "–y".

7. The *rejections* of the system. These are the negations carried by something which is not a cognition—the thinker, the world, experience. They will be symbolized as "–X" and "–Y".

8. The *experience* over against the system. This experience is correlative with the system. Where we have a whole system, experience must be understood as possible experience, experience as extendable without limit to encompass the counterpart of every stress and distinction in the system. This will be symbolized by "X,Y".

9. The *understood cosmos,* which is the whole made up of the whole system and experience. The system and the experience connect the items in the cosmos in correlative ways. This will be symbolized by "pq ⟷ X,Y," where ⟷ represents the correlativity.

There are no genuine separate parts in the system. Each part demands that there be others. It is organically related to the others in a structure; thus "x" is a part of the structured unity "x,y", and also a part of the assemblage "x.y". "x,y" and "x.y" in turn are both abstractions from the whole, "x,y V x.y", where they are related by the unity, V, of the system. That unity has no separate being; its being consists in the relating of these items to one another. If we try to isolate the

"V" we get an indeterminate relation, an unrealized possibility; this becomes determinate and realized only when the "x,y" and "x.y" specify it in correlative ways.

It is possible to hold "x" and "x,y" and "x.y" and "V" apart from the whole system, "x,y V x.y", only by standing outside the system, i.e., taking a stand in experience. This is exactly where all rejections, "–X" and "–Y", of the system must be located. These rejections achieve the form of negations, of denials of what is asserted, become "–x" and "–y", only by being brought into the system, for the system is the locus of all assertions, in principle and sometimes in fact. But to bring the rejections into the system they must be identified with one of the parts of it, thereby being made into positive elements constituting the whole. They have the status of negations only when dealt with as parts which, while inside the system, stand over against it. This they can do because they are specifications of the unity of the system, "V", when this has been isolated from the system and made to stand over against it. The excluded negations of the system's theses, then, are so many incompatible specifications of the unity of that system. "–x" and "–y" can offer negations opposed to what the system affirms, only because they are incompatible specifications of the system's isolated "V". x and y are compatible specifications of this V. When the x and y are united in "x,y" and "x.y", they exhaustively determine that "V", and thereby yield the whole system "x,y V x.y".

"–x" offers a negation of "–y" as well as of "x", "y", "x,y", and "x.y". It is a negative of "–y" because it claims to be the exhaustive specification of "V". It is the explicit negative of "x", related to it by the relation of otherness. Since that "x" cannot be separated from "y", "–x" denies not only "x" but "x,y" and "x.y"; and since "y" is inseparable from "x", it denies "y" as well. But "–x" cannot *negate* "x,y V x.y", the whole system. It can, though, stand outside the whole system, "x,y V x.y", but only if made into a *rejection*, "–X". It then becomes one with the whole of experience, the correlate of the system.

A negation of the system presupposes the system; the negation is a specification of one of the components of that system, the "V". But the negation makes the mistake of treating this "V" as though it could be torn away from its role in "x,y V x.y". The negation exists only in the guise of a specific relation between the positive structure and assemblage, "x,y" and "x.y", but instead of functioning between them, sets itself over against them. The negation of the system is the unity of the system, "V", claiming to embrace all there is. That negation, "–x", is incompatible with any other specification of the "V", with "–y", for example. If one wished to assert both "–x" and "–y" one would have to abstract from their specificity and thus reduce them to the "V". The "V" is both "–x" and "–y" but as undistinguished; they, from diverse positions, generalize into it. Consequently, if any one of the theses in the Chapters 1 to 4 is held outside the system, it would be more accurate to formulate it as its own negative; that negative offers one of a number of incompatible specifications of the unity of the system, "V", when that unity is isolated and given a status apart from the system.

From the standpoint of the unity, "V", every item is a specification of it. By being separated off from the system, through the help of experience, "x" becomes identical with "–X" and thus can have the role of a rejection of itself. By turning away from experience, "–X" loses its power to reject, to become one with "x" in "x,y" and "x.y". "–x" opposes the system only because some element in the system, to wit "V", has already been made to stand apart from the system, an act which is possible only because there is an experience outside the system where one can stand and oppose it. In the end then a denial of a system's assertions, like the separated items of a system, but reflect the fact that a system does not exhaust the universe.

All denials of a philosophic system in effect say that there is an experience outside the philosophic system. Thus far they are not in error. They become erroneous when they are made to contradict what the system says, for then they become part of the system and lose whatever power they had to make it possible for them to stand outside, and there oppose the system.

To say that some assertion is in error is to say that it is not yet an integral part of the system. When it stands outside the system, each part is in fact the negative of itself as in that system. To say on the other hand that the unity "V" or the fragments "x,y" or "x.y" are unsatisfactory is but to say that these are not the whole system. Made to stand over against the system and over against the "x" and "y", these items are abstractions which have no other truth except that of enabling the "x" and "y" to be so interrelated that they constitute a system. The entire system involves a utilization of the parts in such a way that they involve one another, thereby precluding their standing outside the whole. The system has a unitary truth, exhausted in the systematic interrelationship of its parts.

The theses of Chapters 1, 2, 3, and 4 are to be understood as co-ordinate and supplementary, related both by "," and by "." (as well as by two others ">" and ".·." not relevant to this discussion). If we hold the theses apart from one another as self-sufficient, they turn out not only to be negations of one another and of "x.y", "V", "x,y" but also to reject the entire system "x,y V x.y". Taken severally they deny all that we have contended for; taken together they qualify one another. Taken as supplementary they constitute the system, "x,y V x.y". If we deny every one of the assertions made in the system we tear the system apart, but thereby learn something of the nature of the experience outside the system. When seen to interrelate the items in the system, each negation, which is the "V" made absolutely concrete and specific, is seen to be a way of helping us present the system "x,y V x.y". The negations of the theses in short, are part of the system; they function as negations, however, only when made too specific, given too much independence, treated as terms instead of as relations.

Hegel rightly insisted that the truth of the whole system was not to be found by just cancelling out its parts, but only by interrelating them with one another, thereby altering the contentions of each. However, he thought that the unity of the whole, "V", was somehow more concrete than its parts; he ignored other elements such as "x,y" and "x.y", and seemed to identify the system with the world. But his primary error was to hold that the act of rejection was inside rather than over against his system.

The numbered assertions in the previous chapters must be understood to express ways in which the modes of being implicate one another. They are incapable, in the end, of being dealt with in isolation. But they can in fact be made to stand apart from the system, if rooted in an experience, "X,Y", outside the system. They then will assume the role of correlates of the very system which they claim to reject.

The system includes all assertions, even denials of itself, but only by making them mutually muted parts of itself, on the one side, and by putting its being over against them on the other. If one then denies what has been said in Chapters 1–4, one will in effect be calling attention to the reality of what, in effect, is the larger cosmos, "X,Y ⟵⟶ pq", which includes that experience "X.Y" and the philosophic system, "pq". It would be a mistake to suppose that the system is thereby in any way challenged. The system "pq", does not claim to be "X,Y", or "X,Y ⟵⟶ pq".

The truths of the system are interrelated in claim though distinct in meaning. They can and do receive their own justifications and clarifications. Together they represent a single organic whole, portraying the nature of the reality outside the system; at the same time they articulate the whole system and thereby categorize that outside reality. The system is an explication of what lies outside it, in the sense that it reflects this; it also offers an explanation of what lies outside, for it presents this with a comprehensive, relevant, abstract account in which co-ordinate parts are distinguished while interrelated.

To make evident that there is warrant for the rejection of the system by the correlative experience (and conversely), it is desirable to restate the pivotal assertions of the previous chapters, give a summary reason why each ought to be accepted, and some indication of how the negation of it might be defended. Each one of the negations, "–x", "–y", reflects the fact that experience, "X,Y", is not in the system, "pq". This experience (where alone the isolated unity "V" can have being) rejects the philosophic system "x,y V x.y" in which that "V" is a functional, integral part, only so far as the "V", when isolated, rejects itself in its role of integral part of that system. It is, in short, only when experience gives being to the isolated unity of the system that there can be rejections of the system. The denials that follow but express the nature of those rejections when brought back into the system, and dealt with severally, and thus atomically. Dealt with as interrelated parts of a single whole, they reappear as the numbered assertions of the previous chapters.

CHAPTER 6

A NEGATIVE APPROACH TO

Actuality

1.01   An Actuality is a being in space. *Otherwise it could not be encountered.*

AGAINST: An Actuality has an inside. That inside is not in space. The self, the mind, the will, the center of a being are not spatial, and yet they are it most truly. It is only because we define an Actuality in terms of its outside and locate its inside as at the place where the outside lets it be, that we can speak of the Actuality as spatial.

1.02   Some Actualities are active. *Otherwise nothing would be produced.*

AGAINST: In itself no Actuality is active; it is just what it is, and that is the end of the matter. Activity is the Actuality already beside itself—indeed already about to be transformed into an effect.

1.03   "Some Actualities are active" is necessarily true. *Otherwise it could be denied without absurdity.*

AGAINST: This proposition has no necessity in itself but only as involving the action of a thinker; it is true only so far as he and that of which he speaks are viewed in relation to what is beyond them.

1.04.   Some Actualities cannot act. *Otherwise there would be no aggregates or wholes which were beings in space.*

AGAINST: This can be denied in two ways. If we recognize only primary Actualities all can act; if we stay inside each, none can act. It is only because we acknowledge Actualities without a genuine interiority that it is possible to maintain that some Actualities cannot act.

1.05   There are two types of primary or active Actuality: simple and complex. *Otherwise there would be no quanta and no organisms.*

AGAINST: In itself every Actuality is simple, a unity, divided in no way. As occupying space, every Actuality is complex, with part exterior to part. There are then not two types but only one type of primary Actuality. And if account is taken of the reality of God, neither of these types is really primary. From the standpoint of God, all Actualities are derivatives from his being.

1.06   Actualities are temporal beings. *Otherwise they would not be capable of action or have careers.*

AGAINST: So far as a being is in one moment it is not in another; it is, therefore, only so far as it is not in time. There is a time for it only so far as it is contained within a frame larger than itself; in itself it might contain time, but is not temporal.

1.07   Actualities have characteristic natures which enable them to be known and distinguished. *Otherwise they would not be capable of action or have careers.*

AGAINST: To distinguish a nature is to divide a being which is in fact undivided. And we know and distinguish things not by their natures but by signal marks and usages and locations. A reference to natures is a reference to what is common, universal, and is precisely that which misses the Actuality as it is, in the concrete, where it is distinguished by virtue of its own effort at distinctiveness, and not by virtue of some abstractable feature.

1.08   Primary Actualities are distinctive, persistent, resistant, insistent beings in space and time. *Otherwise there would be nothing which could interact.*

AGAINST: These are characterizations of the Actualities from without; in themselves Actualities are root and final, in no way comparable. To speak of them as persistent, resistant, and insistent is to look at them inside a more inclusive domain, and is thus not to treat them as Actualities.

1.09 There are primary beings which are not Actualities. *Otherwise there would not be irreducible possibilities, a field, or eternity.*

AGAINST : We, as Actualities, are final; we are the beginning of all inquiry and the end. What is other than ourselves is derivative, secondary, for there cannot be more than one primary type of being. The contention supposes that one can start with Actualities and yet go outside them in such a way as to find what is just as real. The supposition of the equal reality of other modes of being is possible only from a neutral standpoint which takes no one of them to be final. But each is final in itself, while derivative in terms of others. Each is on a footing with the others from a perspective which is so abstract as to be the perspective of nothing, thereby allowing for a purality of beings only because it has nothing to say for any one of them.

1.10 There are derivative modes of being. *Otherwise there would be no space, time, qualities, or compounds.*

AGAINST : A derivative mode of being is in effect no being at all; to be derivative is to have one's being in something else. The supposition that there are derivative modes of being looks at a facet of a being from the outside and detaches it as though it could stand by itself.

1.11 There must be possibilities. *Otherwise an Actuality would not be able to continue or pass away.*

AGAINST : What is possible is not yet; to treat a possibility as though it were a being is to treat that, which is only in relation to the world of Actualities, as though it could stand apart from that world.

1.12 There must be a field. *Otherwise Actualities could not be co-present.*

AGAINST : A field is a domain of relations; but relations are, only by virtue of the Actualities they connect; they are abstractions, *entia rationis*. To speak of a domain of them is to confound the distinguished with the distinct. It is to look at relations from some position outside Actualities themselves, despite the fact that we are Actualities and can do no more than look at things from the perspective of Actualities.

1.13 There must be an eternal being. *Otherwise the objective worth of Actualities could not be measured.*

AGAINST: From the standpoint of time and time-embedded beings, the eternal is but an abstraction, a fixating of what is momentarily held in the mind. It is the product of a mistaken attempt to see the world from some other perspective than that of Actuality.

1.14 No Actuality can be absolutely perfect. *Otherwise an Actuality would not lack the reality possessed by other beings.*

AGAINST: Every Actuality is perfect in itself; it is what it is. It needs no more than it has, to be what it is. To speak of its imperfection is to speak of it in alien terms.

1.15 Beings condition one another. *Otherwise a being would not define the others as lacking the reality it possesses.*

AGAINST: A being is final, substantial, irreducible, self-contained; it neither affects nor is affected; for a being to be subject to others is for it to lose its finality, its status as a real being.

1.16 Each Actuality is unified. *Otherwise it would be a many, without a single nature.*

AGAINST: Characterizations of an Actuality are modes of dealing with it from without; the Actuality is no more a unity than it is a plurality.

1.17 Actualities engage in acts of self-adjustment. *Otherwise they would not remain unities.*

AGAINST: No self-adjustment is necessary; and if it were, it would have nothing to operate on. Self-adjustment is a characterization which testifies to the fact that an Actuality is not being taken seriously in itself; it wrongly supposes that there can be a real entrance into the recesses of a being.

1.18   Actualities affect other beings. *Otherwise they would not be able to retain the natures they have.*

AGAINST: To be able to affect others an Actuality must go outside itself. This is absurd, since wherever it acts it is and must remain in itself. No affecting of others is possible in a world where one takes Actualities seriously.

1.19   To be at its best an Actuality must adjust itself to others. *Otherwise it would not deal with them as capable of satisfying it, competing with it, needing it, and standing over against it.*

AGAINST: There is no better or worse state for an Actuality to be. In itself an Actuality is what it is; no measure of it in other terms has any compulsive value.

1.20   Each Actuality attempts to subordinate and accommodate others. *Otherwise it would not adjust itself to them.*

AGAINST: Not only need an Actuality not adjust itself to others, but so far as those others are final they cannot be subjugated or accommodated by it. Each is what it is and over against all else, neither yielding to nor dominating anything outside, nor endeavoring to be concordant with it. For it to be at all is for it to be what it is, and with whatever else there be.

1.21   An Actuality seeks to adjust itself to possibilities. *Otherwise possibilities would not be generic meanings which set the conditions for future actualization.*

AGAINST: Possibilities are indeterminate and exert no compulsion. No Actuality need accommodate them. If it had to, it would not be able, since possibilities are in another domain outside the reach of the actions of anything else.

1.22   An Actuality seeks to make the field integral to itself and to submit to it. *Otherwise it would not be part of one universe with others.*

AGAINST: A field, since it is only a tissue of relations, can exert no compulsion. Nor is there any way in which an Actuality can make integral to itself what is by nature outside it.

1.23   An Actuality strives to act on and adjust itself to eternity. *Otherwise it would lack genuine unity.*

AGAINST: An eternity, since it is outside of time, can exert no compulsion. Nor can any act, since it is in time, reach to it. There can be no adjusting to eternity by what is intrinsically temporal.

1.24   An Actuality engages in all efforts at adjustment together. *Otherwise it would not be that which endeavors to overcome its fourfold condition.*

AGAINST: The consideration of each type of demand excludes a consideration of the others. The demands are incomparable precisely because they are oriented in different types of being, and no Actuality can adjust itself with respect to all of them in any way.

1.25   All four efforts qualify one another. *Otherwise the various modes of being would not need one another.*

AGAINST: Each effort occurs without reference to the others; it is in no way qualified by those others. If it could be so qualified it would not be able to act independently of them, be the effort of an Actuality over against others.

1.26   An Actuality's attempt to deal with other Actualities is qualified by its attempt to deal with possibility. *Otherwise other Actualities would not be dealt with as governed by a relevant possibility.*

AGAINST: Actualities interact in a direct, brute way; possibilities are, for them, effete at best. Nothing can control an Actuality but what is Actual.

1.27   The attempt of an Actuality to deal with other Actualities is qualified by its attempt to deal with the field. *Otherwise other Actualities would not be dealt with as contemporaries.*

AGAINST: Other Actualities are dealt with without regard for their status as contemporaries. Moreover if action takes time, that which is acted on is precisely what is not contemporary. And if an Actuality had to deal with another as a contemporary there would be no need for it to deal with the field but merely to work through it. It is wrong to deny the sufficiency of a world of distinct Actualities. Actualities are merely over against one another, the unmediated termini of one another's actions.

1.28   The attempt of an Actuality to deal with other Actualities is qualified by its attempt to deal with eternity. *Otherwise other Actualities would not be encompassed within a common unity.*

AGAINST: Eternity cannot be reached through any act in time. Nor need there be a common unity other than that which is constituted by the acts of Actualities with respect to one another. Only the refusal to deal with Actualities, as constituting an interacting set of beings, forces a recognition of something outside them.

1.29   Each Actuality attempts to turn all other Actualities into concordant beings under the common aegis of a possibility, a field, and an eternity. *Otherwise these modes of being would not be pertinent to Actualities.*

AGAINST: None of these is pertinent to Actualities. If any one was, it would not require the Actualities to deal with it, but would instead itself affect the Actualities. Whatever other modes of being there are, are only qualifications of and in Actualities.

1.30   Each Actuality uses other Actualities. *Otherwise it would not be able to qualify the import of possibility, field, and eternity.*

AGAINST: An Actuality is what it is; it does not use nor can it use any other. Each is final, irreducible, never really subject to another Actuality. And if it were, this would not require one Actuality, which makes use of some other, to affect a different mode of being. Subjugation is direct, and makes no reference to anything other than mastering and mastered Actualities.

1.31   Some Actualities can change without losing identity. *Otherwise they would not be substances.*

AGAINST: To maintain an identity is to be selfsame, but to be selfsame is not to change. If there is any identity in changing Actualities it must lie outside the area of change, and thus be outside time. The Actualities would by that fact be divided into two parts, having nothing to do with one another. At any moment an Actuality is what it is. It cannot change, but just is.

1.32   It is not of the essence of an Actuality to occupy a particular region of space. *Otherwise it would not be capable of motion.*

AGAINST: To move is to change, to be subject to new characterizations, or it is to be involved in relations having nothing to do with the essence of an Actuality. In the former case it is of the essence of an Actuality to be at the place where it is; in the latter case, the Actuality will cease to be an essentially spatial being. In itself an Actuality is where and what it is, nothing more and nothing less.

1.33   Not everything is eternal. *Otherwise there would be no causality.*

AGAINST: What is not eternal is not fixed, and what is not fixed is not intelligible. Whatever be the case it is true that it is so, and that truth does not alter with time. But even if one were to affirm that everything was eternal, it still would not follow that there would be no causality. Causality would then express the relation of logical necessitation which held forever. Only where it is denied that the future is already full-bodied does it make sense to suppose that causality requires time.

1.34   There is causality. *Otherwise we could not explain why some things come to be; nor could we explain how we got the idea of causality.*

AGAINST: Each being is self-explanatory, in the sense that whatever reasons there be for it are in it. To try to explain it by looking outside it is to remain outside it, and is thus not to do justice to it. Also, if an explanation were found outside, this would not be one with finding its cause. Whatever happens may be the adventitious fulguration of some more basic reality. Or it may just happen, and can be 'explained' only by imposing adventitious frames upon it, enabling us to handle it and to be shrewd with respect to what might happen in the future.

1.35 The category of causality is an inexpugnable, unrejectable way of ordering what occurs and what we encounter. *Otherwise it would not be definitive of occurrences and consequently of experience.*
A G A I N S T : Since the idea of causality has often been rejected, it cannot be unrejectable. Since items can be ordered in many ways, as mathematicians have made evident, causality is not the only agency for ordering them. And since things occur by themselves, as distinct from anything that went before or may come after, causality cannot be definitive of them, nor of the experience they constitute. Only the false supposition that Actualities are produced from antecedent Actualities in the course of time forces an acknowledgment of causality.

1.36 When a cause is actual, its effect is only possible. *Otherwise the effect would not occur later than the cause.*
A G A I N S T : Effects are not later than their causes; the head indents the pillow by lying on it. And if effects were later than their causes they would define those causes not to be real causes, for when those causes are in existence they have no actual effects. But a cause without an effect is not a real cause.

1.37 To know a possible effect we must infer to it from its cause. *Otherwise it would not have a cause.*
A G A I N S T : A possible effect has its nature, and that nature can be known without referring to what might have caused it. Moreover, it might not have been caused at all; it might always have been. Only the false supposition that a possible effect is the effect of an actual cause requires one to treat it in terms of a cause.

1.38 At least some effects are deducible from their causes. *Otherwise there would be no predictive sciences.*
A G A I N S T : There are no predictive sciences, but only sciences

which have been more successful than others in guessing the routes
the world will take. And so far as the sciences predict they do not
deduce effects, but derive them inductively and only with probability.

1.39   An actual effect occurs subsequent to its cause.
Otherwise causation would not take time.

A G A I N S T : Were an effect to take place subsequent to its cause,
the necessity for it would be lost. And in any case, effects must occur
with their causes, or those causes would just so far be ineffective. Detach the effect from the cause and the cause is without its effect, and is
thus a cause no longer.

1.40   A possible effect is distinct from itself as actualized.
*Otherwise there would be no difference between a
predicted and an occurring effect.*

A G A I N S T : To know what effect will ensue on a cause is to
know a possible effect. If that effect is not identical with the effect that
ensues we, though knowing the possible effect, will then not know
the effect that is the effect in fact. The possible effect is identical with
the effect in fact, and this is already implicit in the cause.

1.41   What explains a possible effect does not suffice to
explain an actual effect. *Otherwise there would not be a
difference between the two.*

A G A I N S T : If the possible effect did not explain the actual effect,
that effect would require something else to explain it, or it would be
inexplicable. But if something else is required to explain it, this would
be part of the cause, which will then ground both the possible and
the actual effects. Were the actual effect, on the other hand, to be
inexplicably different from the possible effect, that difference could
not be known, or if known could not be understood, and thus could
not be said to be part of the explained effect.

1.42   Production is intelligible but not deducible.
Otherwise it would be irrational or unnecessary.

A G A I N S T : Since a production takes time and has its being in its
unfolding, it is in fact unintelligible. To treat it as intelligible is to
convert an existence into an essence, the temporal into the spatial, an
inward duration into an external structure. He who holds that pro-

duction is intelligible but not deducible falsely denies that essences are linked one with the other, permitting of the derivation of one from the other. He also unwarrantedly supposes that what is deduced lies outside the reach of an understanding of a premiss.

1.43   An actual effect is produced by that which transcends, is outside the cause. *Otherwise it could be derived from the cause alone.*

A G A I N S T :   A cause is no fixed point, but a moving agent, terminating in an effect. The reference to something other than the cause depends on a mistaken prior detachment of cause from effect, a wrong denial of the simultaneity of cause and effect, the false supposition of an intelligible production, and the error of separating the idea of productivity from that of cause.

1.44   An actual effect is necessitated. *Otherwise the cause which makes it possible and the production which makes that possibility actual would not suffice to make it be what it is.*

A G A I N S T :   A necessitated effect would be deducible and would be present when what necessitates it is present. But then no production would be needed. 'Effects' just come to be; they are all contingent. No one of them need have been.

1.45   An Actuality makes an effort to change in the face of insuperable obstacles. *Otherwise it would not tend to be reduced in nature nor try to maintain itself in existence.*

A G A I N S T :   An Actuality is what it is. There is no need and no way for it to change except by giving way to something else. A change is not something it seeks to produce, and certainly not in order to avoid reduction in nature or maintenance in existence. Taken in itself the Actuality remains what it is until externally overcome.

1.46   Man is the product of evolution. *Otherwise he has always been, or he has come to be inexplicably.*

A G A I N S T :   It is of the essence of man to have a mind transcending local needs; not reducible to the body, that mind cannot be accounted for by any bodily changes. Since he is one being, man cannot be accounted for except by going outside the world and its

evolutionary course. His nature is a delimited form of possibility, forever in being; when an individual instances that nature a man is all
at once. Until then it is not a man at all, not even potentially, since
there is nothing in it or in the world pointing to a result that can, or
will, or ought to be.

1.47 A man has self-identity. *Otherwise the changes in
his judgment, mind, and will would be changes of nothing,
a mere sequence of happenings.*
AGAINST: So far as a man changes he is not what he was. If he
remains selfsame, whatever changes occur are adventitious, exterior,
not affecting him, and are therefore not his changes. Men have self-
identity but only because they are private beings, untouched by
change or time.

1.48 A man can discipline himself. *Otherwise he would
not be able to curb tendencies in his body and his mind.*
AGAINST: To discipline oneself is to be over against oneself;
to be over against oneself is to be two beings and not one, and therefore not to be able to discipline oneself.

1.49 A man can evaluate himself in terms not exemplified
by him. *Otherwise he would not be able to judge himself
to be defective, bad, guilty.*
AGAINST: To judge oneself in terms one has not exemplified is
to judge oneself in alien terms. From an alien perspective anything is
deficient; being what it is, it cannot satisfy criteria which have to do
with what it is not.

1.50 A man has a self. *Otherwise he would not be able
to persist over time, to defy his body and his mind, and to
employ a standard of judgment.*
AGAINST: A man is a being with a body; a self is other than
this, and, so far as it is other, either a man is divided into two or that
self is not his. Moreover, the self can become self-conscious, can express itself in time, and where once innocent can become guilty. But
then it is a being which changes, leaving nothing over to persist.

1.51   A self is expressed as a life of a body. *Otherwise when the self ceases to express itself in this way, the body would not die.*

A G A I N S T : Animals are alive and so are plants, and these presumably have no selves. Life is integral to an organic body, and is not something put into it from without.

1.52   The self is immortal. *Otherwise it would not have its own essence and existence.*

A G A I N S T : A self without a body is not the self of a man. An immortal self is not a human self. Also a self without a body has no size and thus can be nowhere; it has no agents for action and thus cannot be effective in time. A detached self is nothing.

1.53   Sometimes the self expresses itself as a mind. *Otherwise we would not have knowledge, and thus would have no knowledge of the self.*

A G A I N S T : A mind operates as part of an organism; it is affected by bodily changes and determines bodily changes. It is no agent of a self over against the body, but of the body as a whole. This can know whatever self there be without becoming a mind; it can know through a feeling, i.e., through an immediate grasp of its own self-centeredness.

1.54   The mind is not a body. *Otherwise it would have size, shape, color, a capacity to move about, and be able to compel some body to change or to move.*

A G A I N S T : A mind is where and what its objects are; if it knows a body it is a body. It has no shape or color only because it can have or be *any* shape or color.

1.55   The mind is not a function of the body. *Otherwise it would not be able to imagine and infer what is beyond the reach of any body.*

A G A I N S T : Imagination and inference can go beyond the reach of the body by adding steps from the point where the body has reached. But this does not mean that they are not functions of the body. Also, error is not beyond the province of a mere body, yet it points the body to what is not and therefore to what is not within the reach of the body. Illusions, distortions, miscalculations, are evidently bodily determined. 'Mind' is in fact but a phase of the body distinguished for various purposes.

1.56 The mind can encounter sensuous content. *Otherwise it would not make use of the senses.*

A G A I N S T : The senses are part of the body and cannot be employed by what is supposedly nonbodily in nature or function. And so far as the mind is a way the body functions through various organs, it serves to produce rather than to encounter sensuous content. The sensuous is not separable from a sensing and thus from a body, and is therefore not something that can be encountered.

1.57 Perception yields content, which is in part sensuous, is judged and accepted, and may be believed. *Otherwise perception would not be an activity of the self making use of the mind.*

A G A I N S T : The sensuous and the judged, the accepted and believed, are quite distinct in nature, and cannot be made to form a single whole. And perception, since it is an act and does implicate the perceiver in a changing world, cannot be performed by a supposedly constant self. Each content is what it is; each act is distinct from every other. Perception is a single, undivided act of a body in relation to a distant body, tracing the incipient action which the perceiver tends to perform with respect to that distant body. Instead of reporting an objective fact, it just projects a subjective tendency.

1.58 Through perception, an external world can be truly known. *Otherwise we would never know we had made a perceptual error.*

A G A I N S T : If we could know we had made a perceptual error we could avoid it. Also, a perceptual world reflects the nature of the perceiver, the kind of organs he has, and the conditions under which he perceives. What it tells us is something about the perceiver rather than about a world beyond.

1.59   Perception involves the use of nonsensuous content. *Otherwise it would not provide knowledge of an external world.*

A G A I N S T : Since perception involves the use of the senses, it cannot make use of nonsensuous content without being divided into two distinct, quite independent acts with independent contents. The external world is not a world freed from sensed content; in fact what is nonsensuous is precisely that which is either not known through perception, or what cannot tell us about an encountered or encounterable external world.

1.60   A perceived Actuality has a location, to be pointed to, indicated, not sensuously undergone. *Otherwise it would not be known while over against the perceiver.*

A G A I N S T : Things are located in relation to ourselves, and can be known to be so located only so far as they are sensed to be there. To be over against the perceiver is to be over against him as that which is experienceable by him, and thus as that which is mediated through his senses.

1.61   Perception involves the contemplation of a universal, distinct from but not alien to the sensuous. *Otherwise it would not yield something intelligible.*

A G A I N S T : There are no universals in fact, but only concrete particular or individual beings. If perception involved the contemplation of universals it would involve the contemplation of what was not the case. And since the sensuous is that which exists only when and as sensed, it is other than, alien to what is merely contemplated in the form of a universal, for this is detached from experience, unaffected by organs or time.

1.62   Indicateds and contemplateds are had as independent, but also as mutually pertinent. *Otherwise their union would not be both desirable and reasonable.*

A G A I N S T : It is not desirable to unite what is disparate; it is not reasonable to unite items from quite distinct realms. Indicateds and contemplateds are not pertinent to one another, for the one re-

lates to what is singular and the other to what is universal, and these
have no bearing on one another. And we do make errors, showing
that the indicated and contemplated are distinct but not mutually
pertinent. We can unite them only by dealing with them from without, subjecting them to an irrelevant tie.

1.63   The indicated and contemplated are aspects of the
object veridically perceived. *Otherwise we could not,
through their agency, know what was the case.*

AGAINST: The object perceived is one seamless unit; it contains no indicated and no contemplated. To know by means of an indicated and a contemplated is to know by means of an isolated location and an isolated universal, which are outside the object and which
therefore could conceivably be credited to other objects.

1.64   Perception provides knowledge through a union of
indicated and contemplated. *Otherwise it would not
represent the objective unity of that indicated and
contemplated.*

AGAINST: A union of indicated and contemplated, since it
is a union of quite disparate contents obtained in independent ways, is
a union which is surely arbitrary and perhaps impossible. Also, an
object is not a unity of indicated and contemplated; it has being before
and apart from these. To know by means of an indicated and contemplated is to know by means of that which is less than, outside the
object; no union of these can express what the object is apart from
them.

1.65   A perception is not identical with its object.
Otherwise there would be no perception of Actualities.

AGAINST: What a thing is, is what it is perceived to be.
Otherwise we would have to be able to know objects in nonperceptual ways. But such objects could not be experienced, encountered. We could not know that they existed and thus were
Actualities in fact. An object unperceived is in no way known to be.
All knowledge is oriented in a perceiver and is mediated through the
senses; it terminates in the object, which is only when and as perceived.

1.66   While perceiving we know that the perceived is not the real object. *Otherwise we would not know there was more to the object than we perceive of it.*

AGAINST: If the object is not what is perceived to be, there can be no veridical perception. If we know there is more to the object than we perceive of it we must engage in some act additional to perception. But this nonperceptual additional act need not alight on anything related to the perceptual. If it did, the fact could not be known either by perception or by the additional act. Perception terminates in the perceived, leaving no residuum, except for one who is self-contradictorily at once in and out of the act of perceiving.

1.67   An Actuality is adumbrated when and as an indicated and contemplated are united in a judgment. *Otherwise it would not be known to be external to the judgment.*

AGAINST: An Actuality is known only when and as known. While judged it cannot be had as not judged. Either then the adumbrated is part of the judgment or it is outside the judgment and thus cannot be known in the judgment. To know there is something external to the judgment one would, self-contradictorily, have to be at once inside and outside the judgment.

1.68   The adumbrated conveys knowledge. *Otherwise we would not know that we were ignorant, that the perception is not the object, or be able to test the judgment for truth or falsehood.*

AGAINST: To know that one is ignorant is to be confronted with an emptiness which is known to be filled apart from us, or it is to be acquainted with an object which we do not know. But if we are confronted with an emptiness we then do not know that it is filled; and if we are acquainted with an object, we know it. Ignorance expresses merely a disposition on our part to know more. Also, so far as we judge, we cannot test our judgment. And so far as we do test it, we either face a need to test the test and so on endlessly, or somehow can have certainty immediately, and therefore need no test. The object perceived is exhausted in the sensuous encounter; if there be anything else we cannot know it.

1.69 Perceptual content grounds generalizations, specifications, and other inferences. *Otherwise other judgments and contemplateds would not be derivable from perceptual judgments and contemplateds.*

AGAINST: Perceptual content has no endurance, substantiality, or independence. If it grounded generalizations, etc., these would be deprived of that ground at once. Moreover, generalizations, etc. are acts requiring powers quite distinct from perception, with a legitimacy quite independent of perception's.

1.70 An idea has an empirical meaning if there is a perceptual contemplated from which the idea can be derived. *Otherwise there would be no relation between empirical and perceptual meanings.*

AGAINST: Each perception has its own unity. It has only contingent relations to others, and these are insufficient to ground a meaning of any sort.

1.71 The meaning of an idea is any other, perceptual or not, as qualified by that conceivable transformation which would convert it into the former. *Otherwise there would be no relating of all meanings.*

AGAINST: All meanings are not related; we have no systematic knowledge of everything. Nor would a transformation of one idea give the meaning of another. An idea needs no transformation in order to have a meaning; if it did, there would be no initial idea to ground the transformation. Each idea has its own meaning.

1.72 An idea of something nonempirical can be transformed into an idea of something empirical by subjecting it to the conditions of experience. *Otherwise there would be some other condition differentiating them.*

AGAINST: To transform the nonempirical into the empirical is to alter it radically. What differentiates the two is nothing which can be overcome. The nonempirical is distinct, self-enclosed, untransformable into the empirical. If it could be so transformed we could make realities out of fictions.

1.73 An idea of the empirical is transformable into an idea of the nonempirical by freeing it from the conditions of experience. *Otherwise there would be some other condition differentiating them.*

AGAINST: No condition differentiates the two kinds of ideas. If there were such a condition, it would not enable us to transform one into the other. If it could, we would be able to derive the idea of God from the idea of a piece of chalk or from the idea of a bit of dirt, from the ugly, the evil, the erroneous, and the sinful.

1.74 What is independent of experience can be understood in terms of the empirical, and conversely. *Otherwise they would not have related meanings.*

AGAINST: Since the empirical and the nonempirical are opposed in origin, content, and meaning, neither can be understood in terms of the other. To view one in terms of the other is to deal with it in irrelevant ways.

1.75 Different types of transformation provide supplementary ways of defining the meaning of a given idea. *Otherwise there would be some ideas isolated from all others.*

AGAINST: Every idea has its own integrity; it has its own nature, existence, career, and is therefore, as just that idea, isolated from all others. None can help another. None can be defined in terms of any other.

1.76 Memory reverses transformations produced by the passage of time. *Otherwise there would be no appreciation of the present as that which has an explanation in what we once encountered.*

AGAINST: The passage of time can never be recovered, and surely cannot be re-traversed in reverse except in a subsequent time. But then it is no longer. A memory does not terminate in what is past; it is a present content unwarrantedly claiming to report a past unreachable fact.

1.77 Expectation is a waiting for determinations for some idea. *Otherwise there would be no warranted position to take with respect to the future.*

AGAINST: Strictly speaking, waiting cannot be with respect to the future, outside a present; one waits only in the present for something present. And if one could wait for something in the future, that still would provide no warrant for a present expectation. Awaiting is resting, not getting somewhere ahead of time in order to locate what might produce determinations in an idea we have. Also, we can and do provide our own determinations for our ideas. Expectation is a present content felt as incomplete, and nothing more.

1.78 Ideas can be imagined. *Otherwise there would be no new ideas produced.*

AGAINST: The imagination produces nothing. It reorganizes what is perceptually encountered. All its material is perceptually given; what it produces and entertains is at least implicitly perceived.

1.79 Thinking is the act of transforming an idea or judgment into another. *Otherwise it would not link premiss and conclusion.*

AGAINST: To think is just to pass from one idea to some other idea. Not all thinking is logical. And logical thinking is not a transforming but a replacing. To transform an idea is to change it.

1.80 A sound inference is a thinking which terminates in the warranted qualification of an idea. *Otherwise it would not be an instrument for discovery and validation.*

AGAINST: Inferences are unreliable; they need testing by logic. In themselves they are psychological processes, warranting nothing.

1.81 Inference is governed by rules, conformity to which determines the warrant of a transferred or transformed qualification. *Otherwise logic would not be necessary or desirable.*

AGAINST: If the rules do not warrant the conclusion, they are unnecessary; if they do, the inference is unnecessary. Logic merely formulates what is already known to be a satisfactory inference.

1.82   All thinking exemplifies rules, and terminates in necessitated conclusions. *Otherwise it would not be at once formal and productive.*

A G A I N S T : There is random thinking, disorganized thinking, fresh thinking, for which no rules exist. And conclusions can be avoided; any one can be denied. Premiss, thought, conclusion has each its own reality. Neither separately nor together do they yield necessities.

1.83   A particular conclusion has content, meaning, implications beyond that expressed in a general rule. *Otherwise it could not be concluded to.*

A G A I N S T : One concludes only to general outcomes. And if one did validly conclude to a particular conclusion, one must have followed a valid rule.

1.84   A process of moving to a conclusion ends with what is not wholly predictable. *Otherwise it would not terminate in a conclusion.*

A G A I N S T : To terminate in what is not wholly predictable is to terminate in the irrational. An adequate knowledge of the premiss does provide a knowledge of what can be rightly concluded to.

1.85   Premiss and rule together define only a possible conclusion. *Otherwise it would not be necessary to produce an actual conclusion by going through a process in time.*

A G A I N S T : A logical conclusion follows from premiss and rule together. That conclusion is necessitated; it is an actual not a possible conclusion.

1.86   All inference is logically necessitated and creatively free. *Otherwise it would not be governed by a logical rule and come to conclusions not established by that rule alone.*

A G A I N S T : What is necessitated is not free, and what is free is not necessitated. Logical conclusions are necessitated; they are or-

ganically united with their premiss. Psychologically arrived conclusions are necessitated by the nature of the psychology of the
thinker, but this necessity is not logical. Only some inferences then
are logically necessitated, and none of them is creatively free.

1.87 All making is rational as well as creative.
*Otherwise it would not attain an outcome through
a free process exemplifying a rule.*
AGAINST: What is made is freely made; rules governing
making are but guides, props, not justifications of what is done. The
justification of the made is the excellence of it, not the process by
which it was obtained.

1.88 To produce well is to engage in an art; to
produce for an enjoyment which awakens an awareness
of an adumbrated is to engage in a fine art. *Otherwise
art would not be desirable, and fine art would not be
pleasurable and informative.*
AGAINST: Art is the last opacity for the human spirit. It is
misconstrued when viewed in terms of how it serves desire or knowledge, or when it is treated in terms of production rather than achievement.

1.89 Inquiry is a chain of inferences designed to
reach a source of desired judgments or their elements.
*Otherwise it would not be rational, creative, persistent,
and informative.*
AGAINST: Inquiry begins and ends in knowledge, and cannot
therefore be properly defined in terms of a source, in terms of what
is outside judgment or knowledge. And, since whatever source one
might reach in inquiry is something known and judged, inquiry can
find nothing except items of knowledge or judgment.

1.90 A science is an inquiry well conducted. *Otherwise
it would not be an art which is persistent, informative,
creative, and rational.*
AGAINST: Art and science are quite distinct, with different
origins, requirements, media, objectives, tests, and modes of expression. And a mere well-conducted inquiry might be directed at any-

thing. But science relates to what is open to verifiable prediction and can be precisely stated.

1.91   Philosophy is at once a science and an art. *Otherwise it would not creatively inquire into the essential features of valid knowledge and genuine being.*

A G A I N S T : Philosophy lacks the precision of science; it also lacks the imagination and freedom of art. In fact, the nature of things is most adequately learned from the sciences and the arts, leaving for philosophy no genuine work of its own.

1.92   Philosophy's method is speculative; i.e., it infers to presuppositions. Its argument is primarily dialectic; i.e., it infers to what would complete the already known. And its attitude is at once sympathetic and critical. *Otherwise it would not be primary, systematic, and self-reflective.*

A G A I N S T : A presupposition of the empirical is empirical, and is to be found by empirically oriented methods. Dialectic infers to what need not be the case; sympathy is the proper concern of aesthetics. Philosophy can have no other method than analysis; this enables it to clarify what is already known. It cannot even criticize, since it knows no facts.

1.93   Philosophy is a circular enterprise. *Otherwise its account of essential features would not presuppose a correct grasp of the nature of real beings and the real world which these beings are engaged in knowing, and conversely.*

A G A I N S T : A systematic philosophy is circular, which is to say it has neither entrance nor exit, and can be about nothing but itself. A nonsystematic philosophy is about the world or knowledge. But since it stands away from what it knows, it fails to do justice to the world or to knowledge.

1.94   The essentials of any cognition are expressed in a category or principle embodied in whatever is apprehended. *Otherwise there would no unity to knowledge.*

AGAINST: Knowledge is so complex and multiform that any category appropriate to all items would be radically indeterminate. Universal relevance requires absolute amorphousness, and this cannot give the essentials of what is necessarily determinate.

1.95 The primary category is inescapable. *Otherwise there could be some item which might not be encompassed by it.*

AGAINST: If it is possible that a category be not used, or possible for it to be rejected, it is not inescapable. But we do not use a category when we sleep, and we can reject it as soon as we focus on it.

1.96 The category embodies the law of contradiction. *Otherwise the law would not be a truth exemplified by everything.*

AGAINST: We contradict ourselves. All becoming involves the juncture of one thing and its negative. The law of contradiction cannot therefore be exemplified by everything. A category, moreover, must be more significant and discriminatory than a mere logical law could be. It has a nature of its own, not to be reduced to or explained by a merely formal principle.

1.97 The primary category must be applicable to the contingent as well as to the necessary. *Otherwise it would fail to embody universally applicable principles.*

AGAINST: What applies to the contingent must be other than what applies to the necessary, for the one *might* be false and the other *cannot* be false. If indifferent to this difference it is once again not a category of or for them.

1.98 The primary category must be applicable to the false as well as to the true. *Otherwise either there would not be anything false or nothing could be known to be so.*

AGAINST: What applies to both the false and the true must either be indifferent to their difference or be diversely expressed in each, making it in effect a different category in the two cases.

1.99   The primary category must have at least two parts. *Otherwise it would not utilize the law of contradiction.*

AGAINST: A category is primarily a unity; if it has parts it is divided against itself, and those parts must themselves, if the category is universally applicable, presuppose the category as a unity outside those parts.

1.100   The primary category must inwardly make reference to the content which it organizes. *Otherwise that content would be alien to it and would thus be neither knowable nor real.*

AGAINST: If there be content to which a category refers, it must be outside the category; no inward reference by the category will reach that content. Category and content are distinct, to be united by some power exterior to both.

1.101   The parts of the category and the content for it must already exemplify it. *Otherwise they would not be or would not be known.*

AGAINST: If the parts and the content already exemplify the category, the category must presuppose itself in order to be, for without the parts and the content the category is a category of nothing.

1.102   The category is a unity, representing an external unity in which its parts are embodied. *Otherwise it would not ground a single act of knowing truly.*

AGAINST: A unity is without parts. If it had parts these would be in the category, incapable of being embodied in something other than that category.

1.103   The category has four facets. *Otherwise it would not be embodied in every cognition and being.*

AGAINST: The unity of the category precludes its having parts. When embodied in cognition it must be quite different from what it is in being, since the one is freed from matter, contingency, irrelevancies, whereas the other is submerged in the affairs of a foreign world.

1.104 The relations of the various guises which the category assumes are themselves cases of the category. *Otherwise it would not be universal in range.*

AGAINST: A category which applies to everything whatsoever has no proper negative and thus no definite meaning. And if everything is a case of the category there would seem to be no plurality to relate, since all will so far be alike.

1.105 An Actuality seeks to realize possibilities, and the Actuality which is man seeks to realize an all-inclusive possibility. *Otherwise there would be no coming to be, and no self.*

AGAINST: An Actuality is what it is, seeking nothing. And if it did seek something, this would be true of it only so far as it was alive. But then it would not seek to realize possibilities but would try to satisfy itself, or to act. Coming to be depends on action, process, not on possibilities. And since man is but one of many beings in the universe, whatever possibility is relevant to him would be limited. Man's self is self-contained, presupposed by a sought possibility, not conversely.

1.106 The all-inclusive possibility which man seeks and ought to realize is the Good. *Otherwise it would not be excellent or one.*

AGAINST: A possibility, all-inclusive and one, is not necessarily identical with the Good. Nor does man seek to realize the Good; he seeks to be himself or, rather, to maintain himself, utilizing whatever he can.

1.107 The Good is specified in the form of limited objectives which men sometimes consciously acknowledge and bodily realize. *Otherwise the Good would not be their final, inescapable objective.*

AGAINST: A specification of the Good is other than that Good, and is so far not good. There are, moreover, undesirable objectives. And any objective that a man does not consciously acknowl-edge or bodily realize is not his objective. But man does not often consciously acknowledge the Good, and can never fully realize it bodily.

1.108   Men have a freedom of preference. *Otherwise they would not be able to select one of a number of means to a goal.*

AGAINST: So far as a man prefers he is governed by causes, motives, reasons and is so far not free. If he is free he can select a means only capriciously and is so far no better off than if he were forced to take this alternative or that.

1.109   Men have freedom of choice. *Otherwise they would not be able to select ends which make good the losses in value they in fact produce.*

AGAINST: Values that are lost cannot be recovered. No end can make good a loss; only actions can, and these occur in the present. And if there were more than one end, the choice of one would be capriciously arbitrary or deterministically caused. In neither case would a man be responsible for what he chose; in neither case would he really be free.

1.110   Desire for the Good is good. *Otherwise it would be indifferent or bad to desire the Good.*

AGAINST: Desire is a mark of deficiency, defect. It is good only as affected by its terminus. In itself it lacks the Good, that is why it must terminate in the Good. Since it may have bad effects, it is not only not good in itself, but it may not be good in outcome.

1.111   The Good needs more realization than it gets from preference, choice, or desire. *Otherwise action would be unnecessary for the production of the Good in the concrete.*

AGAINST: Nothing can improve the Good. Also, preference, choice, desire can give the Good no more and no less realization than action does. The Good may be illustrated, but itself remains untouched by what men do or seek to do.

1.112 Men have a free will. *Otherwise they would not be able to reconstitute themselves as minds and bodies for the sake of realizing the Good maximally.*

AGAINST: A free will is a capricious will, and would bring something about without cause, reason, or antecedent conditioning. A will could not, in any case, reconstitute a man, but only other things. Moreover, since a will may be bad, its freedom would in no way entail even the possibility that the Good is realized. A maximal realization of the Good, in any case, is beyond human capacity.

1.113 The values of all beings should be maximized. *Otherwise the Good men ought to promote would not be realized.*

AGAINST: It is questionable whether there are any values except in living beings, or as noticed by living beings. And if the values of all beings should be maximized this would seem to be God's work. Man is a finite, limited being, with limited tasks.

1.114 No one can do only what is right. *Otherwise action would not require the use of some things and the ignoring of others.*

AGAINST: There are purely innocent actions. And if there were none, the more we did, the more wrong we would have to answer for. To do good then would be a way of doing more wrong. But an act can be perfectly good in itself, particularly if it expresses a good will.

1.115 No one can do only what is wrong. *Otherwise subjugation would not be desirable, nor would action involve some desirable exercise of the powers of body or mind.*

AGAINST: There can be acts of unqualified malice; otherwise every act would have some justification or excuse. In itself an act can be perfectly bad, expressing a bad intent.

1.116 Men are necessarily guilty. *Otherwise they would not be obligated to do the Good or would be able to do all the good that needs to be done.*

AGAINST: In themselves men are innocent. They are guilty only for what they can but fail to do. But if they can do it, they are free to do it, and may succeed, thereby precluding a guilt for failure.

1.117   All rewards are undeserved. *Otherwise guilt would not be inescapable.*

AGAINST: Guilt is not inescapable. And were it inescapable, one would nevertheless deserve reward for whatever good he did. To say that all rewards are undeserved is to treat rewards as irrelevant to the rewarded acts. Evil could then be rewarded with as much justification as good.

1.118   Men can do all the good that ought to be done if they can utilize other powers besides their own. *Otherwise the Good would not be that which ought to be realized.*

AGAINST: If be the case that the Good ought to be realized, it does not follow that it can be. If it can be realized, it may not be the case that it can be realized by the utilization of other powers. And if other powers did produce the Good, their achievement cannot be accredited to men. Satisfaction of the Good through other agencies is a satisfaction by what is exterior, and in this sense irrelevant to man's duties. And if men, by utilizing other powers besides their own, could succeed in realizing the Good, guilt would not be inescapable.

CHAPTER 7

A NEGATIVE APPROACH TO
Ideality

2.01   Whatever is possible must be internally coherent. *Otherwise the self-contradictory would be possible.*

AGAINST : Since men can and do contradict themselves, the self-contradictory must be possible. Also, no conditions can be imposed on the possible without making it that which might be excluded, and thus which is no longer possible.

2.02   Some possibilities are ingredient in, i.e., are idealizations of Actualities, Existence, and God. *Otherwise the Actualities etc. would not be possible.*

AGAINST : Possibilities cannot be in or be derived from other modes of being; each mode is ultimately irreducible, self-contained. An idealization of an Actuality yields only the Actuality in an attenuated form.

2.03   A real possibility is what in fact can be. *Otherwise what cannot be would not be impossible.*

AGAINST : To define real possibilities in terms of what can in fact be is to define them in terms outside themselves, and is thus not to say what is true of them. Indeed, many things are possible which cannot in fact be. It is possible for Brown now to run though he cannot now run, since he now in fact walks.

2.04   Real possibilities have a being exterior to Actualities and whatever else there be. *Otherwise the Actualities etc. could not be or become.*

AGAINST : The really possible is what can be. If something is possible for an Actuality or other mode of being it is inseparable from it; otherwise it is a mere "can-be" having no necessary bearing on anything. If possibilities have a being exterior to Actualities or other beings they are not possibilities for them.

2.05   Real possibilities are relevant to other realities. *Otherwise these would not seek to realize just those possibilities.*

A G A I N S T : Real possibilities, as having natures of their own, are not relevant to anything else; they just are. On the other hand, realities seek to maintain themselves; they do not seek to realize possibilities.

2.06   Real possibilities change in the course of time. *Otherwise the Actualities to which they are relevant would not be beings which change in the course of time.*

A G A I N S T : What is merely possible is not in time at all. If something is really possible it is always so. No possibility can change or has any need to change; the adventures of Actualities are irrelevant to what is possible.

2.07   Real possibilities form linkages. *Otherwise the realization of one would not implicate others.*

A G A I N S T : Possibilities are independent one of the other, with distinct natures. Were they to form linkages one possibility would depend on another, and thus would have to be possibly possible before it could be possible, possibly possibly possible before it could be possibly possible and so on. This is a vicious regress. The realization of one possibility has no effect on the others.

2.08   Real possibilities are systematically connected. *Otherwise they would not be relevant to Actualities, or Actualities would not limit one another, or what is possible to one would not limit what is possible to others.*

A G A I N S T : A system of possibilities would in effect be a single possibility in which the supposed subordinate possibilities were organically connected. The realization of possibilities would then be the realization of just the same single possibility in every case, with a stress now on this and then on that. Each possibility is distinct, independent, unaffected by and unaffecting the others.

2.09   Real possibilities are relevant and realizable. *Otherwise what occurs would either be unrealizable or would be independent of what occurred.*

A G A I N S T : So far as possibilities are relevant and realizable they cannot be exterior. But then there is nothing to be realized.

2.10   The Good is a possibility which ought to be realized. *Otherwise what ought to be is not desirable, cannot be, or necessarily is.*

A G A I N S T : The Good is not a possibility but a reality or value in which other beings participate. There is nothing which it ought to be, without it thereby being revealed to be not good. The Good ought not to become anything other than good. But this it is already. What ought to be is the submission of man to the Good.

2.11   Real possibilities are to some extent internally indeterminate. *Otherwise realization would not make a difference to them, giving them a content and career they otherwise would not have.*

A G A I N S T : What is indeterminate is so far amorphous, unintelligible. It cannot in any wise be affected by a realization, for the realization is external to it. A possibility is not altered by being realized or embodied.

2.12   The difference between the possible and the Actual, or any other reality, is not merely possible. *Otherwise realization would not add anything to the possible.*

A G A I N S T : If the difference between the possible and other realities is not merely possible, it would either be impossible or presuppose the possible. If impossible, there would be no relation between the possible and the Actual; if it presupposes the possible, there would have to be a relation to that presupposed possibility, which relation would in turn be merely possible or presuppose a further relation, and so on.

2.13   Real possibilities must be realized somehow and somewhere. *Otherwise realization would be excluded by the universe, and they would therefore not be possibilities for it.*

AGAINST: Since he who sits may possibly stand, and since, while he sits he cannot also stand, there must be possibilities which are not realized. Realizability is not an essential trait of possibilities.

2.14   Normative possibilities must be satisfied by a being outside both them and Actualities. *Otherwise the ought is either not possible or is necessarily realized in this world.*

AGAINST: What ought to be may never be. This world is not perfect; it testifies to the reality of norms not realized. If they are to be realized by a being outside both them and Actualities their satisfaction will never be due to the Actualities. They will therefore never function as pertinent norms for those Actualities.

2.15   The Good is an all-inclusive possibility, or Ideal, as relevant to Actualities. *Otherwise it would not be an all-inclusive objective confronting them all, specialized by each according to its nature.*

AGAINST: Were the Good an all-inclusive possibility it would be a possibility for evil. And since there may be regrettable objectives, these either are not specializations of the Good or the Good is a possibility for what is wrong. Each possibility in fact has its own integrity and is directly relevant to a particular type of being. None specializes the Good.

2.16   The Ideal is incomplete. *Otherwise it would not lack the reality possessed by Actualities, Existence and God.*

AGAINST: If the Ideal is an irreducible final mode of being, it cannot be incomplete, lacking the reality possessed by others. If it lacks their reality it depends on them for its full being, and cannot be ultimate.

2.17   The Ideal presupposes Actualities. *Otherwise it would not be able to assume the form of the Good.*

AGAINST : The Ideal cannot owe its excellence to other beings unless it be dependent on and therefore not prescriptive for them—which is to say, unless it is not the Ideal. The Ideal does not need Actualities either in order to be or in order to have the status of the Good.

2.18   The Ideal presupposes Existence. *Otherwise it would not be able to assume the form of the Future.*

AGAINST : The Ideal is not in time and thus is not identifiable with the Future. Nor does it need Existence in order to be; rather it measures and therefore is presupposed by Existence. Existence cannot seek or carry or produce an unchanging Ideal.

2.19   The Ideal presupposes God. *Otherwise it would not be able to have the role of a Principle of Perfection, answering to a divine intent.*

AGAINST : The Ideal is either not outside God and thus cannot presuppose him, or it is outside him and does not necessarily answer to his intent. God needs no Principle of Perfection; if he did, no exterior possibility would suffice to give it to him. God is complete and needs nothing; the Ideal is what it is and needs no God to sustain it or to use it.

2.20   The Good's attempt to encompass all Actualities is qualified by the Ideal's need to keep abreast of Existence. *Otherwise there would be no attempt to bring Actualities within a single time order.*

AGAINST : The Good is impotent; if it were not, it would when acting on Actualities or Existence, violate the conservation laws of nature. The Ideal has no need to keep abreast of Existence, since it is out of time; if it had such a need this would not be affected by its need to deal with another independent being, the Actual.

2.21   The Good's attempt to encompass all Actualities is qualified by the Ideal's need to accommodate a divine intent. *Otherwise there would not be an attempt to order Actualities hierarchically.*

AGAINST: The Ideal is impotent. And if it were not, it would not seek to accommodate a divine intent. God uses the Ideal for divine purposes, and thus not necessarily in consonance with the needs of the Ideal. Moreover, if the Ideal sought to make the Actual exhibit the Good, it would do this directly without regard for anything else.

2.22   The Ideal's effort to keep abreast of Existence occurs together with its effort to accommodate the intent of God and its effort to encompass all Actualities. *Otherwise it would not face them at the same time.*

AGAINST: The Ideal faces nothing alien to it. As out of time it cannot face things 'at the same time,' or keep abreast of Existence.

2.23   The Good encompasses Actualities to some degree by making them desirous. *Otherwise desire would not determine in part what Actualities will do and be.*

AGAINST: Desire springs from within an Actuality; it needs no prompting from without. If it were determined by the Good, it would presumably be satisfied by that Good, and would then and there cease to be a desire. Also, desires are without necessary bearing on what Actualities do or are; they have their own integrity without necessary external cause or external effect.

2.24   The Good encompasses more of a man when it makes him into a being who prefers than it does when it makes him merely desirous. *Otherwise it would not affect him as one who makes decisions.*

AGAINST: The Good does not affect man as making decisions; if it did it would so far deny him his freedom. Also, preference is a free inward decision of a man, and may stress the bad instead of the good. Nor is a being who prefers necessarily better than a being who desires; the latter might desire the good, the former might prefer the bad.

2.25   The Good encompasses more of a man when it makes him into a being who chooses than it does when it makes him into a being who prefers. *Otherwise it would not make him one who is governed by values.*

AGAINST: A man chooses freely, and not therefore by virtue of any power exerted by the Good or anything else. And as choosing freely he may choose the bad. Since he could prefer the good, it does not follow that as a choosing being he is superior to himself as preferring. Choice in fact is an act not distinct from preference; it occurs inside the self-enclosed psyche and testifies to no governance, good or bad.

2.26   The Good encompasses more when it makes a man into a being who creatively wills than it does when it makes him into one who chooses. *Otherwise it would not make him into one who helps it be more widely distributed.*

AGAINST: A creative will, since it is free, is not produced, governed, or encompassed by an exterior Good. And since one can freely will to do the evil while choosing to do the Good, a free will does not testify necessarily to a determination by the Good, or in fact to any relation to it.

2.27   It is good for the Good to be fulfilled. *Otherwise it would not be good for the Good to encompass all men, working harmoniously on behalf of the Good.*

AGAINST: The Good is already fulfilled, precisely because it is the Good. It needs and can have no further fulfillment. It is neither good nor bad therefore to fulfill the Good, though it may be good for men to recognize that Good.

2.28   Men, as forming a community, can encompass a wider range of goods than is possible in a group. *Otherwise the community would not deserve to encompass and control groups.*

AGAINST: So far as a group lives up to its ideals it need not and ought not to be controlled by any larger whole. Nor does the fact that a community is larger than a group testify to its possession of or even to its capacity to possess more goods than is possible in a group. Indeed, the larger community will more likely include more conflicts than the smaller.

2.29   A class is a group in which the common character controls the activities of the members. *Otherwise it would not be a whole.*

A G A I N S T : Individuals cannot be controlled by characters; characters are but abstractions, derivatives from them. Each individual acts on his own.

2.30   There ought to be classes functioning on behalf of the community. *Otherwise the community would have no representative parts.*

A G A I N S T : No class can represent the whole, since the whole is made up of distinct classes having quite distinct needs and objectives.

2.31   The community should contain a number of classes. *Otherwise needed representative functions would not be performed.*

A G A I N S T : A community should be a unity. Classes divide it into possibly antagonistic parts.

2.32   A class of reasonable men is one whose members' grasp of causal processes and whose adjustments are accepted as representative by the rest. *Otherwise there would be no rationale which was characteristic of a community.*

A G A I N S T : Men are reasonable whether or not their views and responses are accepted by others. Nor does reasonableness involve a grasp of causal processes, for there are no such processes. Nor can any one kind of adjustment, appropriate to one type of man, be representative of the adjustments of others. Nor does the rest of the community take the adjustments of the members of one class to be representative. Each group reacts in its own characteristic independent way.

2.33   A class of prestigious men is one whose members' behavior, values, or standards of what is important are models for the rest. *Otherwise they would not be models for that society.*

AGAINST: Those with the most prestige are not necessarily models. And when they are models, their behavior, values, or standards are not often representative. And where they are representative they are not representative of what others should do, or will do, or are willing to do. Each class of men has its own norms of behavior, its own ideal values, its own standards.

2.34   The members of a class of empowered men have control of the might of a community. *Otherwise they would not be men of power in that community.*

AGAINST: Each man and each class has its own strengths and needs. Each controls only what it has, and thus what must be less than the might of the community.

2.35   A mature community contains at least three harmonized classes of men. *Otherwise essential functions would be neglected.*

AGAINST: Communities are equally mature; they differ only in that they have different structures and bring about different results. So far as a community did harmonize classes it would effectively destroy them, depriving them of their autonomy and independence.

2.36   A model community makes provision for the good of men outside it. *Otherwise it would not be mature.*

AGAINST: Each community has its own tasks and needs; to concern itself with the good of others is on the one side to neglect its own, and on the other is to interfere with what is distinct from it in kind, objective, and need.

2.37   Men are justified in claiming to have their natures preserved or enhanced. *Otherwise their natures would not be good or improvable.*

AGAINST: A claim is made against others, and is so far not justified. Nor has a man a claim to preserve or enhance his nature. Human nature is neither good nor improvable; it just is a nature over against other natures, having no rights and therefore making no claims.

2.38   Each man makes a number of essential claims to have his nature preserved or enhanced. *Otherwise he would not embody a number of distinct values.*
A G A I N S T : So far as a man is a unity he can have only one value. And since a man may with warrant sacrifice himself, he cannot make an essential claim to have his nature preserved or enhanced. Men claim nothing; they just are.

2.39   A native right is an essential claim defined in terms of others as required to satisfy it. *Otherwise there would be rights without corresponding duties.*
A G A I N S T : A right defined in terms of others required to satisfy it is a right which must vanish with the disappearance of those others. But a right follows on an essential claim. Rights are to be defined independently of duties, and can therefore be without corresponding duties.

2.40   A right denied is a right alienated, and entails the insistence on some other right having a stronger case because better able to satisfy a superior claim. *Otherwise just claims could be denied without loss.*
A G A I N S T : Each right is independent of every other; its denial cannot then entail the insistence on some other right. Nor does the fact that a right satisfies a superior claim justify the denial of some other.

2.41   Not all rights can be justifiably alienated at any one time. *Otherwise a man might have no rights at all at a given time.*
A G A I N S T : If a right denied is a right alienated, the killing of a man and with it the extinction of all his rights could never be justified. Rights as integral to a man are justifiably alienable at least to the degree that his destruction is justifiable.

2.42 Men with the same type of right may be in conflict. *Otherwise it might never be the case that they are faced with material adequate to the satisfaction of the right in only some of them.*

A G A I N S T : A right cannot be in conflict with itself, and so far as men have the same right, the men are not in conflict. When there is material adequate to the satisfaction of the right in only some men, a superior right of equitable distribution takes over.

2.43 Men have the privilege of ordering and interrelating their native rights. *Otherwise they would not be able to alter their claims in any way.*

A G A I N S T : The rights of men follow from the claims their very natures and values entitle them to make. If those rights are altered, they are in effect alienated, since what is rightfully claimed will then be denied. No man can have the privilege of denying a legitimate claim.

2.44 Men have the privilege of exercising every one of their rights. *Otherwise some right could be forever denied satisfaction.*

A G A I N S T : The exercise of a right depends on no privilege; it is demanded by the very nature of the right itself. But rights have different times and occasions for exercise, and any one of them can be denied exercise if the occasion is inappropriate. Such a denial of exercise is one with the holding of the right in abeyance, and this is one with having the right be when and where it can.

2.45 There is no privilege to exercise all rights at any one time. *Otherwise there would be no resolution of a conflict of rights.*

A G A I N S T : If the rights of a man could be in conflict the man could be divided against himself. But each right expresses a value which he has as a single unified being. All the rights that constitute him demand exercise, and all of them may demand such exercise at the same time, without in any way coming into conflict. A right is not detachable from a man, but is one with his very being; all the rights together make up a single whole of right answering to his unitary value.

2.46   Men have the privilege of alienating any of their specific rights. *Otherwise they could not adjust themselves to circumstance.*

AGAINST: If men had the privilege of alienating any of their specific rights, those rights would thereby be shown to be no rights at all. A right answers to a value possessed, and cannot be separated from the value without destroying that value's place in the world. No one has the privilege of denying what ought not to be denied; this could be supposed only by one who viewed rights from the outside in terms of alien conditions.

2.47   Men have the privilege of alienating all their specific rights. *Otherwise they could not justly forge a unity of their rights, thereby promoting their eventual satisfaction.*

AGAINST: Since men do not have the privilege of alienating any of their rights, they evidently cannot have the privilege of alienating all of them. And if they had the privilege of alienating some rights, this would be far from warranting their alienating all of them. A man who had alienated all his rights, no matter for what purpose, would be one who had denied the rightful and intrinsic claims of his own essential values.

2.48   Men have the privilege of constituting a single unitary right. *Otherwise they would not be able to promote the satisfaction of all their alienated specific rights.*

AGAINST: A complex being such as man cannot have only a single unitary right. And so far as he could have such a right, it would follow from the value he has as a single being; it would not be constituted by him. The satisfaction of such a single unitary right, since it is quite distinct from whatever specific rights he has, would not provide a satisfaction for those specific rights. Each right demands its own satisfaction; satisfying one is not satisfying another.

2.49   Man's unitary right cannot be justly alienated. *Otherwise the claim of an inclusive right could be denied without wrong.*

A G A I N S T : A unitary right is over against specific rights. When these specific rights justly demand satisfaction, they may preclude the satisfaction of the unitary right, and so far alienate it, set it aside as one whose satisfaction is not then and there propitious. A unitary right that could not rightly be set aside would demand satisfaction everywhere and always, no matter what the circumstances. Such a right presupposes a right to and perhaps also a control of the whole world, which no one in fact has.

2.50   Man's unitary unalienable right is the right to benefit from social existence. *Otherwise there would be no point to his venturing into society.*

A G A I N S T : Men have unalienable rights which transcend society, such as the right to worship or the right to know. Also, they are in society whether they like it or not. They don't venture in to it, nor do they come into it with irresistible demands. They are thrust into it to begin with. Whatever rights they have there are not unalienable. All that is unalienable in society are social duties whose performance may benefit the society but not necessarily the men themselves.

2.51   Society dictates in part which specific rights are to be satisfied, and when they are, and how. *Otherwise it would not rightly include and control men.*

A G A I N S T : A society which dictates what rights should be satisfied dictates what rights a man has. But a society should serve the true interests of man, and these are defined by the rights they have. It is for man, not society, to dictate what rights are to be satisfied. Men should control society, not conversely. They are realities and of value; society is a derivative outcome, more or less useful.

2.52   Society should satisfy a man's unitary right to benefit from social existence. *Otherwise it would fail to do what it ought.*

A G A I N S T : Men are individuals with individual demands and needs. No one can satisfy them from without. The most that a society could do is to provide opportunities for the individual to use in the satisfaction of his rights. To suppose that society should satisfy man's unitary right is to look at man from the outside. He is not a unit to be used, answered, and altered according to society's views and needs, but an individual to be understood from within.

2.53 Society is justified in denying satisfaction to some rights. *Otherwise it would be denied a necessary opportunity to satisfy them and others eventually.*

AGAINST: No denial of a right is ever justified. And if there were such a justification it could not be credited to an external society. Whatever society does to get in the way of the satisfaction of a right is unjustifiable; its work is solely the serving of man, a being who has ingredient rights, imperiously demanding satisfaction.

2.54 Civil rights are correlate with duties in others to do or forbear. *Otherwise they could be rightly ignored or denied by others.*

AGAINST: Since a right expresses a value possessed by man, its definition has nothing to do with the presence of others, their acknowledgment of the right, or their willingness to satisfy it.

2.55 Rights are satisfied with the aid of might outside themselves. *Otherwise they would have power in and of themselves.*

AGAINST: Rights have a power; they insist on themselves. If they did not, no alien power could be expected to act on their behalf.

2.56 Might has the right to be preserved or enhanced. *Otherwise it would not have a value of its own.*

AGAINST: Might is brute, unharnessed force, which compels without reason and without warrant. It has no value of any kind. The attribution of value to might is the result of the effort to deal with it as though it were a kind of being or individual. Dealt with in its own terms, it is naked energy, compelling beings in ways which are alien to those beings' needs and rights. If it had a value that value would not necessarily be one which had to continue or one which had to be enhanced.

2.57   The right of might can be alienated only by might. *Otherwise there would be something more powerful than might.*

A G A I N S T : If might had a right it could not be alienated. If the right could be alienated it could not be alienated by might, for then might would be in opposition to itself. If a might could alienate the right of might, there would be as many kinds and grades of right as there were subdivisions of might. And, finally, the fact that one bit of might was more powerful than another gives it no privileges or rights over that other. Might is the totality of energy available, and can be used well or ill. When used well it is endowed with rights because it continues the expression of an intrinsic right in that being which is using it well.

2.58   The right of might can be justly alienated. *Otherwise it would always have to be satisfied.*

A G A I N S T : If might had a right it could not be justly alienated. A right which might possessed, particularly if it were of the very substance of might, would require satisfaction always and everywhere. Rights can be thought of as deniable only by one who looks at them from a position which cancels out the claim they intrinsically make. And even if might had a right and this could be justly alienated, there is no power which could alienate it.

2.59   Might has rights and duties in relation to men. *Otherwise there would be no opposition to it nor agencies for it.*

A G A I N S T : Nothing could oppose might unless it itself had might, and thus was one with it. Also, nothing can have a right or duty with respect to what is entirely different in kind from it. Might has no rights or duties in relation to men. If it had any rights these would belong to it regardless of whether or not there were men. To ascribe rights and duties to might is in fact to turn it into a kind of man, and thus to ignore what it intrinsically is.

2.60   It is the sovereign duty of might to help man achieve an eventual satisfaction of his alienated rights.

Otherwise it would not have to support man's basic right.

AGAINST: Might has no duty towards men. If might had a duty, this would not be a duty relating to men's rights; it would relate to what might by itself had to do with respect to a good. Nor can a sovereign duty be defined as serving the interests of something weaker or subordinate to it. Finally, if it were the duty of might to support men's rights, it would not know this, and could not be, in fact or in justice, required to perform that duty. Might has its own needs and mode of operation regardless of the nature, needs, and rights of man.

2.61   Might must alienate its right. *Otherwise it would not be able to acquire and fulfill its sovereign duty to constitute a set of distinct powers.*

AGAINST: Nothing can alienate its own right. If it were the duty of might to constitute a set of distinct powers, this would not require it to alienate the right it has as a unity. And, finally, if the might could divide into distinct powers which had rights in place of its own, it would not thereby acquire a duty, unless one could acquire a duty by abandoning one's rights.

2.62   Might should be divided just so far as this promotes the satisfaction of man's rights. *Otherwise there would be no warrant for the division.*

AGAINST: A division of might need not promote the satisfaction of man's rights; it is made independently of those rights. If made by some conscious being who divides it in the light of man's rights, might would be unjustly divided, divided from an exterior standpoint, one not necessarily in accord with might's nature and needs.

2.63   Each of the classes of a mature community satisfies part of man's unitary right. *Otherwise that right would not be fully satisfied.*

AGAINST: A unitary right is all of one piece; it is not possible to have it satisfied only in part. If the three classes in a community satisfy man's unitary right they would so far constitute a single class.

If they were then able to satisfy some one man's unitary right they would not necessarily be able to satisfy that right as resident in other men, going their own independent ways.

2.64   The divisions of might should answer to the needs of three classes of men. *Otherwise those divisions would not help promote the rights of men.*

AGAINST: The three classes of men do not promote the rights of men; often they block their satisfaction. And so far as they do promote the rights of men, they do so in the light of what men are. But the divisions of might are made in independence of what men are or need.

2.65   A political whole correlates self-divided might and the classes of a community. *Otherwise they would not be in harmony.*

AGAINST: To be able to correlate might and a class it would be necessary to have more might than might, and also to be more directly related to men than a class can be. These are impossible objectives. Nor could a correlation of these two disparate realities be possible if each has a rationale different from that of the other. A political whole has its own integrity, and would not have as its task the correlation of independent realities, since this requires it to give up, in part or whole, its own needs, work, rights, and duties.

2.66   A political whole has three essential organs. *Otherwise it would not correlate essential divisions of might with essential classes to constitute executive, legislative, and legal structures.*

AGAINST: There are political wholes without one or the other organ; these organs cannot therefore be essential to the being of a political whole. Moreover, these organs have a nature and being independent of the divisions of might or of the existence of classes, or of the need to correlate the one with the other.

2.67   A state is a persistent political whole forcing classes and institutions into harmony. *Otherwise it would not do good or would not have to exert compulsions in order to do good.*

AGAINST: The better the state the less it compels. It is not therefore of the essence of the state to force classes and institutions into harmony. Nor is it essential to a state that it persist. A state is a state even if it has only a short duration.

2.68   A man ought to acquire the habit of functioning as a man should. *Otherwise he would have no virtues.*

AGAINST: To have a habit of functioning as a man should is not yet to have a virtue. Virtue involves intent and knowledge, deliberation and decision, expressing the very inward substance of a man. It is not an adventitious structure which could be accidentally acquired. Such a structure would tell nothing of what a man is, but only what he might tend to do.

2.69   Men should be taught virtue and be forced to act virtuously. *Otherwise they will be worse than they need be.*

AGAINST: Virtue cannot be taught; it must be inwardly forged. And to force a man to act is precisely to force him not to act virtuously. Virtuous action issues freely from within, and cannot be prescribed or compelled from without.

2.70   There is a natural law. *Otherwise there would be no minimal demands a just society must meet.*

AGAINST: Each society has its own problems; there are no minimal standards applicable to all. And men differ too radically to be brought under a single aegis, subtending all the different societies and their differences. Natural law in fact is a matter of conscience, relating to fundamental rights, some of them nonsocial in nature and import.

2.71   Natural law is germane to all societies. *Otherwise there would be no measure for all societies.*

AGAINST: A universal natural law is a law for all men, and not a law for societies. If it could be made pertinent to societies it would, in order to take account of their vital differences, have to be made so general and flexible that it would be unable to provide a measure for them all. A natural law states what ought to be, and this in independence of the existence of societies or what they might or could do. The ought-to-be is not intrinsically related to what is.

2.72 There ought to be a common law. *Otherwise there would be no test of what a man ought to do inside his society.*

AGAINST: Common law characterizes only one type of legal society; it expresses a traditional type of sanction having no necessary intrinsic merits. It need not serve the interests of virtue, nor need a conformity to it keep a man inside an actual society. The test of what a man ought to do inside a society is in the society itself, in him, or in some ethical standard. In itself the common law is without prescriptive power; it seems to have such power only because we look at it in terms of what societies use and often endorse.

2.73 There ought to be positive laws, public declarations of what is to be done or avoided in a given society. *Otherwise what is expected of a man would not be known or done.*

AGAINST: Positive laws would not be needed if all men were to do what they ought. And men can learn through living together what it is that society expects of them. Also, there are positive laws which work to the injury of a society. None of them need be pertinent to man's welfare.

2.74 Positive laws threaten realizable punishments for violations. *Otherwise they are laws in name only.*

AGAINST: A threat can be expressed only by a man. Punishments are produced only by men. No law can threaten, or threaten a punishment; it is just a set of words. And many positive laws redefine and organize, direct rather than threaten.

2.75 Positive laws are backed by might. *Otherwise they could be violated with impunity.*

AGAINST: Many positive laws are violated with impunity.

Might is employed sometimes to defy the law. In any case the sanction of a law is not in the might that may support it, but in the justice it expresses and promotes.

2.76   Positive laws should be expressed in an official language. *Otherwise they will express a bias.*

AGAINST: The use of an official language does not preclude the expression of a bias. Also, the use of an official language is a temptation to obscure, complicate, and confuse, hiding the prejudices of the ruling class. Such a language puts the positive laws in irrelevant frames. These laws ought to be embodied in habits, and need not be expressed in a language. If they are to be expressed in a language, it should be one that men in fact forge in the course of experience and commonly use, not one which they artifically create.

2.77   Positive laws should be impartial. *Otherwise they will not be laws for all in the community.*

AGAINST: Impartial laws are not directed to specific problems; nor do they take account of specific interests. They are laws abstracted from the concrete setting where they could express the living dispositions of an actual people. Laws should be relevant to power stresses and human needs. They ought not be impartial. Also, no one law is a law for all in the community; only all the laws together constitute one law. This one law is not a law *for* anyone; it is the very structure of the community, reflecting all its prejudices and stresses. An impartial law is a fiction.

2.78   Positive laws ought to define a man's civil rights and duties. *Otherwise they will not express what a good social man should do.*

AGAINST: A good social man should do what is traditional and accepted; this need not be what is right, even civilly, and may go counter to what is his proper duty. And so far as men have civil rights and duties there is no need to refer to positive laws for their definitions; rights and duties are defined in the course of daily living. Positive laws give quite limited injunctions, and often in independence of what is civilly right or obligatory.

2.79   Positive laws require interpretation in relation
to social powers, social expectations, and social values.
*Otherwise they would not be able to vary with
circumstance.*

AGAINST: A positive law is an abstractly formulated demand;
it does not vary with circumstance. Interpretation has nothing to do
with it, but only with the use to which it is being put.

2.80   Judges interpret the law in a threefold way.
*Otherwise the law would not offer neutral, effective
measures of what should be done and avoided.*

AGAINST: No one need be a judge to know what should be
done and avoided; and if one can know this without being a judge then
a judge is not in principle needed. Moreover, judges are fallible and
biased; if they are the only guarantee of the use of neutral, effective
measures, one will not know what is to be done or avoided in fact or
by right. Laws carry their own justification within them.

2.81   A wise, creative judge guides his interpretations
by natural law. *Otherwise he will be unable to guide his
society properly.*

AGAINST: Some of the wisest and most creative of judges deny
that there is a natural law, that they have any knowledge of it, or
that they make any use of it. The wise, creative judge guides his
society by knowing his society, what it has done and what it needs.
A proper guide for society is built in, is intrinsic to it, not exteriorly
imposed.

2.82   In the ideal state citizens are law-abiding and
law-controlled, and guided by the interpretations of
wise, creative judges. *Otherwise it would not be a just
state.*

AGAINST: An ideal state is not necessarily just, but only effective. A just state may be one which is far from ideal; it requires the
existence of laws, the obeying of these, and the wise interpretation
of them by creative judges—and none of these may be perfect. An
ideal state is not a state for real but only for ideal men, ideal judges,
and ideal conditions; a just state is a state for real beings.

2.83   The Good is most completely publicly fulfilled in a perfect state, a state where all are wise, creative judges. *Otherwise some men would be subordinate to others.*

A G A I N S T : Some men ought to be subordinate to others; they are less mature, less healthy, less intelligent, less controlled, less virtuous. And were all men equal in all these respects, none would need to be a creative judge, interpreting laws. All would be as excellent as men should be, and would need to look nowhere beyond themselves for guidance. A perfect state is a fiction peopled by fictitious beings, a misconstrued consequence of the neglect of what states in fact are and require.

2.84   The good in a state fails to encompass the ethical man. *Otherwise the ethical man would not be one who concerned himself with the whole Good.*

A G A I N S T : The good in a state, and particularly an ideal state, must encompass the ethical man without residue. To suppose that the Good falls short of the ethical man is to suppose that he exists outside the state; it is to tear him away from the only place where he in fact is and can be real.

2.85   The good in a state fails to encompass the aesthetic man. *Otherwise he would appreciate only the values contained in or supported by the state.*

A G A I N S T : The aesthetic man is educated in, controlled by, and presented with material in a state; the range of his appreciations is a function of that state, and of its tolerance, control, and encouragements. If the good in a state did not encompass a man he would by that very token be defined to be not in that state. But a state without aesthetic men would not be as good as it could and ought to be. It would be an abstraction, a fiction, a derivate from actual states, and from ideals genuinely relevant to these.

2.86   The good in a state fails to encompass the religious man. *Otherwise there would be no religious interest in what was outside the reach of the state.*

AGAINST: A state should encompass all of a man's interests, and therefore his religious interest no less than others. Even if there were a God outside the state, the fact is that the men are in it, and their religious interest is there too. To deny the religious man place inside a state is to define it as deficient; it is to ignore the way in which religions reflect the training, location and political structures of the states in which men live.

2.87   The good in a state fails to encompass the speculative man. *Otherwise there would be no philosophic criticism and evaluation of the state and other realities.*

AGAINST: What is supposed to stand outside a state is but a projection of occurrences within it, or is something ideal, having nothing to do with what men are or how they behave. One can be wholly inside a state and yet criticize it. The speculative man is a politically conditioned man whose criticisms reflect his training and location, but which nevertheless can be applied to whatever occurs around him. A state which does not encompass the speculative man has been unduly constricted.

2.88   Education is the art of reconstituting individuals so that the Good can be maximally achieved in and by them. *Otherwise it would have only an instrumental social function.*

AGAINST: Education does have only an instrumental social function; it is but another term for the training and disciplining of men so that they can function well within their societies. The Good is not known by educators; those who might know it are not engaged in communicating it or in enabling individuals to realize it. Indeed the Good is good enough, and needs no help from educational systems or from men.

2.89   Education should include discipline, the subordination of the individual to the group. *Otherwise it will fail to satisfy the just demands of the group.*

AGAINST: Education should make men free or well adjusted; to subjugate them to the group is to deny them their rightful being, as well as their rightful freedom to exercise their inherent powers. The just demands of the group do not reach to a rightful subordination of any man. And if they did, discipline would not bring about that result, for it can do nothing more than habituate men, get them ready for certain work. Men in themselves are already loci of the Good, and need no exterior manipulation.

2.90 Education should include training, the mastery of techniques. *Otherwise men will not be enabled to be part of society.*

A G A I N S T : Society needs no help to get men to be part of it. If it did need such help, mere techniques or any other mode of promoting training would not accomplish the desired end.

2.91 Education should include the art of civilizing, the acquisition of professional competence. *Otherwise men will not be enabled to constitute their society.*

A G A I N S T : Civilizing is a process by which men are helped to enjoy the goods of the spirit. Since societies are not necessarily civilized, civilizing is not necessary to enable men to constitute a society. Civilization is an instance of the Ideal, and needs no help. Nor could it obtain help from what in the end must be judged by it.

2.92 Education should include a mastering of values. *Otherwise men will not be enabled to deal with what is of permanent significance.*

A G A I N S T : Man is, by his very nature and the nature of the world, confronted with matters of permanent significance—life and death, virtue and vice, the beautiful and the true. These values reflect the fact that there is an Ideal dictating to but in no way dictated or controlled by what is other than it.

2.93 Education should teach men to engage in the creative, intellectual mastery of the total Good, social and nonsocial. *Otherwise it will not liberate.*

A G A I N S T : Education routinizes, destroys the free spirit of the genuine creative person. And so far as it does not, it should not teach a mastery of the Good, but of what ought to be done here and now. The Good is good enough, and needs no help from man.

2.94   Liberal education should terminate in an understanding of the Ideal. *Otherwise it will not convey the full significance of the Good.*

AGAINST: The Ideal illuminates itself; it is because of what it is that we can know it. No education can lead to an understanding of it; at best it can only eliminate obstacles to our seeing what is so. But a liberal education has nothing to do with such elimination; its task is to make men parts of civilized wholes.

2.95   The Ideal provides testimony to the reality of Actualities. *Otherwise the Ideal would have been able to provide its own occasions for expression.*

AGAINST: The Ideal is not so impotent that it must look to what is not excellent to help it be, or to be effective. Its occasions for expression there are provided by it through its own native "cunning," as Hegel put it. And if it did not make such provision, it surely would not provide testimony for the reality of anything else. Whatever is true of it points to it and not beyond it to something else.

2.96   The Ideal provides testimony that there is a real Existence. *Otherwise it would not be involved in the affairs of the spatiotemporal world.*

AGAINST: The Ideal is outside space and time; Existence is spatiotemporal. Oppositely designatable beings cannot condition one another, particularly if they are independent in being, meaning, and function.

2.97   The Ideal provides testimony that there is a God. *Otherwise the Ideal could provide its own satisfaction.*

AGAINST: The one thing least clear in the realm of speculation is that there is a God. And there is no way of knowing, short of a direct acquaintance, just what his nature is and what he does. The Ideal testifies to nothing.

2.98   The Ideal partly satisfies the needs of Actuality. *Otherwise it would not be one of Actuality's correlatives.*

AGAINST: If Actuality needed the Ideal it would not be able to obtain it, for the Ideal, no less than Actuality, is a self-enclosed reality, just what it is, never moving away from itself. A correlative is always over against.

2.99   The Ideal partly satisfies the needs of Existence.
Otherwise it would not be one of Existence's correlatives.
AGAINST: As a correlative of Existence, the Ideal remains outside and over against Existence; it cannot satisfy the needs of Existence. Indeed, it is questionable whether Existence could have any needs. Existence is an all-inclusive, all-engulfing domain.

2.100   The Ideal partly satisfies the needs of God.
Otherwise it would not be one of his correlatives.
AGAINST: God, above all beings, has no needs. He could not have needs unless he were a finite being over against finite material of a similar sort—and then he would not be God. The Ideal has a nature and an integrity of its own, just as God has, and they neither need nor satisfy one another.

2.101   The Ideal provides Actualities with a desirable permanence. *Otherwise they would be permanent by themselves or because of something else.*
AGAINST: Actualities are not permanent; they are continually coming into being and passing away. And if they needed and could have permanence they would have to look to some substantial being which was eternal. The Ideal is nothing to the Actual; if it were permanent it would not transfer its permanence to Actualities. Nor is there any reason why it should.

2.102   The Ideal provides Existence with a desirable intelligibility. *Otherwise Existence would be fully intelligible in itself or because of something else.*
AGAINST: Existence is not intelligible. To be intelligible because of something other than it, is to be unintelligible in fact. If it were really intelligible, Existence would be intelligible in itself.

2.103   The Ideal provides God with a desirable relevance to what else there be. *Otherwise he would be relevant by himself or through the agency of something else.*

AGAINST: A being as final, powerful, and concerned as God is can make himself relevant to whatever else there be. If he could not, he would not be truly a God. Nor would he be able to achieve the relevance through the aid of anything else. If God is not relevant to the rest of things, there is no reason to suppose that the Ideal is so relevant, and would or could help him. In fact, both are in themselves, apart from all else.

2.104   The Ideal, while guaranteeing the satisfaction of some needs of the other modes, fails to do full justice to any mode. *Otherwise it would not be involved with and yet resist the others.*

AGAINST: If the Ideal could guarantee the satisfaction of some of the needs of the other modes of being, it would thereby reveal those things to be dependent on it, and it necessarily involved with them. They will thereby be revealed to be not final, independent, irreducible. And if the Ideal could go so far as to guarantee satisfaction of some needs, it should be able to guarantee the satisfaction of all needs and of the modes of being to which those needs are integral. There would then be nothing like a need in fact. The Ideal is by itself, needing nothing, guaranteeing nothing, satisfying nothing.

CHAPTER 8

A NEGATIVE APPROACH TO
Existence

3.01 Existence is being, as engaged in the activity of self-division. *Otherwise opposition would not be at once irreducible, over against, and in other modes of being.*

AGAINST : Opposition is dependent on the presence of opposing realities. It has no nature of its own; if it had it would be self-defeating. There is Existence, to be sure, but this is only a domain in which what is intelligible can be placed, and which in itself is nothing more and nothing less than sheer energy, unified and cosmic, not reducible to or explicable in terms derived from other domains. Moreover, to be self-divided is to cease to be one and to cease to be capable of further division. Being cannot divide itself.

3.02 Existence perpetually divides. *Otherwise there would be no production of extensionality.*

AGAINST : Extensionality cannot be produced; it is an irreducible phenomenon. And if it had to be produced it could not be by division, for this is the elimination rather than the making of extensionality. Existence is complete and unified in itself, possessing extensionality as one of its features.

3.03 The endless expansion of energy, towards which Existence tends, is restrained by Actuality, Ideality, and God. *Otherwise there would be no restraining measure for the expansion of energy.*

AGAINST : Energy is not expansive; it is "conservative," always the same in quantity. And if there were a tendency for it to expand, this could not be restrained except by other energy, and thus not by Actuality, Ideality, or God.

3.04 The endless expansion of time, towards which Existence tends, is restrained by Actuality, Ideality, and God. *Otherwise there would be no restraining measure for the expansion of time.*

A G A I N S T : Time does not expand; one moment merely replaces another. And if it did expand, that expansion could not be stopped by something foreign to it. No other mode of being can put a limit on Existence or on any of its features. If it could, its presence or action would provide not a measure but merely a stop to the expansion.

3.05 The endless expansion of space, towards which Existence tends, is restrained by Actuality, Ideality, and God. *Otherwise there would be no restraining measure for the expansion of space.*

A G A I N S T : Space does not expand, though of course some objects in it may. And if it did expand this expansion could not be restrained by any such reality as Actuality, and certainly not by such realities as Ideality or God. Could they restrain it, that would not provide a measure for the expansion. Space no less than time has its own integrity, unaffected by and not affecting anything else.

3.06 Existence as separated from Actualities is their spatial field. *Otherwise Existence would not provide a place for them.*

A G A I N S T : A spatial field is a field for Actualities; it has nothing to do with Existence. Nor does Existence have anything to do with Actualities.

3.07 Existence as separated from the Ideal is its causal ground. *Otherwise there would be no relevant cosmic Future.*

A G A I N S T : The Ideal is not caused. Were it caused, it would not be caused by Existence, for this is essentially in the present, serving to precipitate out or to vitalize Actualities there. Existence and the Ideal are distinct, having nothing to do with one another.

3.08 Existence as separated from God is his cosmic vitality. *Otherwise he would not need to make himself one with it.*

AGAINST: If Existence were God's cosmic vitality, he, as apart from it, would be either noncosmic or nonvital. In either case he would cease to be God. Existence and God are one and the same; if there be a difference between them, it must be a difference between part and whole; if anything more, they would be without any bearing on one another.

3.09 From the perspective of Actualities, Existence is that which makes them contemporaries. *Otherwise contemporaneity would not be an external determination of Actualities.*

AGAINST: Contemporaneity is not a matter of fact; each being exists by itself and comes into relation with others through processes which travel at a finite rate. One Actuality links with others that are past or future for it; it is unrelated to those which are neither the one nor the other.

3.10 From the perspective of the Ideal, Existence is that which adds implications to those derivable from what is merely possible. *Otherwise it would not be at once rational and nonformal.*

AGAINST: The possible has no implications; it is just what it is. And if it had implications, Existence would not add anything to them. Existence is unintelligible, final, over against the possible, neither explaining nor being explained by, neither subtracting from nor adding anything to it.

3.11 From the perspective of God, Existence is the power to make something become, by making others pass away, and conversely. *Otherwise he would not need Existence to enable him to play a role in the spatiotemporal world.*

AGAINST: Existence is not over against God but is God himself, his very essence. And that Existence is forever. Things come to be and pass away because they lack Existence. So far as they have Existence they just are.

3.12   From the perspective of Existence, Actualities are focal points, the Ideal is future, and God is essence. *Otherwise they would not satisfy Existence.*

AGAINST: Existence has no needs. If it did, it could not be satisfied by other modes of being. Nor can it turn these modes into facets or phases or features of itself. Existence might provide a locus for the others, but this would involve no alteration of them or of it. Each is self-contained.

3.13   The failure of Actuality, Ideality, and God to do full justice to one another imposes a burden on Existence. *Otherwise there would be no need and no way to make good these defects.*

AGAINST: If there are defects in any mode of being they are there forever. But, strictly speaking, no mode can in fact have a defect. "Defect" is a relative term, pointing to an exterior standard. Since a mode of being is ultimate and irreducible, it is wrong to judge it in terms of such an external standard. Nor can the failure of one being become the responsibility of another. Existence carries no burden of any sort.

3.14   Existence is unified by the other three modes. *Otherwise they would not together express what it is.*

AGAINST: Nothing can express what Existence is. If anything could, that would show Existence to be something abstract, not a basic mode of being. A basic mode of being does not require reference to other modes of being. Nor could other beings unify Existence, both because Existence is irreducible, and because it generates and sustains whatever we know.

3.15   Existence is intelligible. *Otherwise we would not know what it was to exist rather than not to exist.*

AGAINST: If there be anything constant in the history of thought it is the conviction by the greatest thinkers that Existence is not intelligible. The intelligible is the cognizable, the unified, the stable essence, but these are all antithetical to Existence and its properties. To know that something exists we must encounter it. Such an encounter does not involve a cognition of Existence, but only the acceptance of it as a locus for our ideas or for acknowledged essences.

3.16 "Existence" is a predicate. *Otherwise it would not make sense to say that something exists.*

AGAINST: Grammatically "exist" and "smile" in "some men exist" and "some men smile" have the same role. But this is deceptive. It makes sense to say "some men do not smile," it does not make sense to say "some men do not exist." "Existence" is no predicate; the addition of it or its cognates to any expression gives no further information, adds not a penny to whatever money one might conceive. All predicates are essences, universals, mind-sustained ideas. Existence is where these might be posited or encountered; it is not one of them.

3.17 "Existence" is predicable of every idea and predicate. *Otherwise one could not say of them that they exist.*

AGAINST: Things exist; ideas and predicates do not, except as carried by things. If we say that Existence is predicable of ideas and predicates, we turn the matter upside down, and moreover leave no room for the expression "nonexistent." But what has no contrasting term has no meaning.

3.18 To know an idea is not yet to know the career it has. *Otherwise it would not be an existing idea.*

AGAINST: To know what an idea is, is precisely to know the career it has. Its career is its meaning. We can have a partial grasp of an idea and thus not know just what adventures it will undergo, but this is only to say that we do not altogether understand it.

3.19 The features of beings are involved in careers not identical with those they have as part of a mind. *Otherwise they would not exist apart from a mind.*

AGAINST: If the features of beings had quite distinct careers in and outside a mind, the knowledge of them as in a mind would not be one with them as outside a mind. But this is what is meant by saying that the idea one has of those features is false or inadequate. To know is to grasp what things are. If our ideas are distinct in locus and adventure from those characteristic of the features of beings, they will fail to be true ideas of those features.

3.20 The passage from what is in mind to the object known goes through Existence. *Otherwise what is in mind would not be distinct from what is known through its agency.*

AGAINST: The mind is distinct from the body; there is no passage from one to the other. If there could be such a passage the mind would have to be existent, or the passage would be a kind of leap from an abstract or effete idea to something substantial, different in nature, career, and meaning. No passage is needed; if there were, it would involve an act of faith or belief and thus be irrelevant to knowledge.

3.21 Predication produces a change in the meaning of the predicate. *Otherwise the predicate would not thereby achieve a career other than that which it had in mind.*

AGAINST: A predicate is a self-enclosed idea in no way affected by the world in which it happens to be resident or by the mind which happens to consider it. If predication were to produce a change in the meaning of the predicate, we would not know anything truly or adequately by means of the predicate. The career of the predicate in mind must be, if the predicate is to be predicated correctly, isomorphic with the career it has in the object.

3.22 Attributes are altered by being abstracted from objects. *Otherwise abstraction would not obtain a predicate for the mind.*

AGAINST: If abstraction altered an attribute, then in isolating it we would have that which misrepresented the world. It is questionable, in addition, whether there ever could be an act of abstraction, if by such an act one means a dissection, a breaking up of the object. We take positions with respect to objects and this without dismantling or dividing them.

3.23 The perceived is contemporary with the perceiver. *Otherwise perception could not reach an existent.*

AGAINST: All causation takes time, and the perceiver receives impressions at a time later than that of the object at which they originated. Existence carries the process of causation. The effect of that process is cut off from its cause as a present from its past; it is contemporary then only with what is unrelated to it, and therefore not with the object perceived.

3.24   What is in the mind tests what is in the body, and conversely. *Otherwise these would not exist separately, or would have no bearing on one another.*

AGAINST: So far as mind and body do exist separately, they cannot properly test one another. So far as they have a bearing on one another, they are deprived of the capacity to be just themselves, self-enclosed, judging nothing and judged by nothing. And in any case the test is not reciprocal, because it is only minds and not bodies that could possibly judge.

3.25   A claim to truth is vindicatable if a consequence in mind is abstractable from a consequence in nature in a predesignatable way. *Otherwise all claims to truth would be only surmises which could never be certified.*

AGAINST: The proper vindication of a claim to truth is the demonstration of the adequacy of a report of something exterior and real. To be content with an anticipated consequence abstractable from some later fact is to ignore where one had begun, the route through which one had moved, and the difference between an outcome in the objective world and one in the mind. Since there are fallacious ways of going from premiss to consequence, the fact that the consequence can be obtained from a later object in no way indicates that the idea one originally had in mind is true of the original object.

3.26   A vindicatable claim to know the Ideal, Existence, or God requires a capacity to repeat the methods by which we obtained our initial knowledge of them. *Otherwise we could not vindicate our claim to know them.*

AGAINST: There is no necessity to suppose that a significant claim to know something requires one to be able to use the same method by means of which one had obtained the knowledge initially. If there were such a necessity, our last act of knowing could not significantly claim to yield knowledge.

3.27 A unique characterization is not an attribute. *Otherwise there would be no distinction between an existing and a nonexisting unique entity.*

AGAINST: Nothing can be unique except an individual, and it must be existent. Could there be a unique characterization this would have to be identical with the unique attribute of the individual, or fail to report that individual. The only difference between an existing and a nonexisting entity is that the former is already part of a realm of possible experience.

3.28 A "collective" disjunction is distinct from a "distributive" disjunction. *Otherwise there would be no contingent occurrences.*

AGAINST: There is only one type of disjunction, and this occurs solely between propositions in the mind. The fact that this disjunction is "distributive" does not require the supposition that what occurs is not contingent. The acceptance or selection of one alternative does not destroy the others; their presence makes the one selected have the status of a contingent occurrence.

3.29 An "extensional" conjunction is distinct from an "intensional" conjunction. *Otherwise there would be no difference between an aggregate and an organic whole.*

AGAINST: There is no need to consider more than one type of conjunction. A conjunction, moreover, produces neither an aggregate nor an organic whole, but only a "truth functional" unit.

3.30 A negation in thought is distinct from a rejection in fact. *Otherwise by taking thought things could be destroyed.*

AGAINST: Rejection is not destruction, nor is negation. Rejection and negation are of course distinct, but the distinction is not necessarily relevant either to the nature of Existence or to the function of thought. But it can be made in both domains.

3.31   Formal implications are distinct from material implications. *Otherwise there would be no tendencies in things.*

A G A I N S T : Formal and material implications have to do with the sentences, propositions, or judgments of logic; they have no necessary relation to tendencies either in mind or things. The world of logic is self-enclosed; nothing that is true of it is necessarily relevant to the world beyond.

3.32   Inferences and processes are distinct. *Otherwise a deduction would be a way of experiencing the future.*

A G A I N S T : So far as processes are intelligible they, like inferences, have a logical structure. So far as inferences are matters of psychology, they are cases of processes.

3.33   Inference makes a difference to what is formally implied. *Otherwise nothing would be achieved in inference.*

A G A I N S T : Strictly speaking, nothing is an inference unless it is valid and therefore does nothing at all to what is formally implied. An invalid inference adds to what is formally implied; that is why it is invalid. All other inferences bring in only psychological factors, having no effect on what is implied and thus not really adding to it.

3.34   Inference is an art in which one risks replacing a satisfactory premiss by an unsatisfactory conclusion. *Otherwise it would accomplish nothing.*

A G A I N S T : To accomplish something it is not necessary to risk doing what is unsatisfactory. An inference in fact is a psychological process following the structure of an implication, formally defined and valid eternally. There is no art to it; its work could be performed by a machine.

3.35   Processes add to what is materially implied. *Otherwise there would be no difference between what is predicted and what occurs.*

A G A I N S T : Processes are quite irrelevant to material implications. And in any case, if there were a prediction which gave a result different from what in fact occurs, it would be a mistaken or a partial prediction. An adequate prediction tells us exactly what will occur, and does this precisely because processes do not add anything to what is materially implied.

3.36 Formal implications and processes are not necessarily in accord. *Otherwise experience and vindications would be unnecessary.*

A G A I N S T : There is no disaccord between formal implications and causal processes; they are irrelevant to one another or they are isomorphic. Experience is needed to provide us with factual content, and vindications of judgments are needed because our knowledge is partial and distortive. But a formal implication is a matter of cold logic, and processes are but mathematics exhibited in nature, open to logical examination and thus to an eventual expression in implications.

3.37 Each Actuality has its own Existence. *Otherwise it would not be present, and would not be able to act.*

A G A I N S T : If an Actuality had its own Existence it would be unable to perish. There would be no coming to be. The Actuality would be eternal.

3.38 Existence makes Actualities concordantly effective. *Otherwise Actualities would not have spatiotemporal careers, dictated partly from without.*

A G A I N S T : Actualities are essentially private, in themselves; space and time provide them with only external characterizations. The careers and natures of Actualities are theirs without any aid from Existence. And, on its side, Existence has no need of Actualities and is in no way affected by them.

3.39 Existence makes Actualities determinate. *Otherwise there would be no difference between a possible and a real Actuality.*

A G A I N S T : A possible Actuality is not an Actuality at all. And what is possible is in no way affected by becoming part of the actual world. It is completely determinate as an essence; realization but provides it with another setting. That realization is accomplished not by Existence but either by Actualities themselves, by the Possibilities themselves, or by some divine agency. Existence is not sufficiently well focused to be able to make anything determinate.

3.40. Actualities can lose their Existence. *Otherwise none could pass away.*

A G A I N S T : If Actualities could lose the Existence they have, they would lose what is integral to them, and this means that they would be totally destroyed. Actualities would not be able to pass away, they would just vanish. What occurs in fact is that an Actuality, with whatever Existence or setting it has, is eventually replaced by another.

3.41 Facts are realities de-existentialized. *Otherwise they would not be at once fixed and ineffective.*

A G A I N S T : Facts are not fixed; they change with perspective. They are not ineffective for they make a difference to what comes after. Nor are they de-existentialized realities, for this would be one with saying that they were not at all. They are determinate characterizations of what is real.

3.42 Passing away is the conversion of an Actuality into a fact. *Otherwise past facts would not have been actual.*

A G A I N S T : Nothing can convert an Actuality into anything else. By passing away an Actuality does not become a fact; it becomes nothing at all. Past facts are fictions.

3.43 The past is a tissue of facts. *Otherwise the past would not lack something characteristic of the present.*

A G A I N S T : What was present is what must be past. Everything that is true of this present object is true of it forever. Were there something left out, it would be the case that something occurring in a given moment would, when that moment became past, cease to be in that moment.

3.44   Nothing occurs in the past. *Otherwise a finite bit of energy would continue to be expended, and the amount of energy in the universe would increase endlessly.*

AGAINST: Something occurs in the present, in which case it must also occur when that present is past; or nothing occurs in the past, in which case nothing could have occurred in the present. The past is as rich as the present; it just occupies a different segment of the whole of time.

3.45   Remembering is a present act. *Otherwise it would destroy what it was supposed to report.*

AGAINST: If the act of remembering does not reach into the past it would be an act of imagining, inferring, anticipating, not of remembering. To remember is to terminate in a past occurrence, and this no merely present act can do. Memory has its own integrity, mode of operation, stretch, and is not subject to the divisions characteristic of a time in which the past is separated from the present.

3.46   Subsequent occurrences provide the past with new settings. *Otherwise they would be indifferent to it or change it.*

AGAINST: The past is what it is, and nothing outside it could make a difference to it. There are no new settings for it, but only new ways of thinking or speaking about it.

3.47   The past is necessarily related to the present. *Otherwise it would not be a past for what is now present.*

AGAINST: The past is past, the present is present, each well defined and wholly self-confined. We are in the one; we cannot get into the other.

3.48   To say "x existed" is to say that the Existence which x's fact had co-ordinate with it, is co-ordinate with a present fact. *Otherwise there would be no continuity between past and present.*

AGAINST: Existence is not co-ordinate with facts; it has nothing to do with them. Facts are abstractions, fictions, modes of speaking of things; Existence is a setting, a place for things to be. A present fact does not have an advantage over a past fact in regard to being; as facts both state the eternal structure of whatever there be. To say "x existed" is to say "x at such and such a date" if "x" be the name of something; or it is to say "there is a being in which x was ingredient," if "x" be some feature or character. In neither case do we make reference to a domain of Existence.

3.49   To reach Actualities as they are in themselves, they must be freed from the qualifications produced by Existence and other modes of being. *Otherwise these qualifications would be intrinsic to the Actualities.*

A G A I N S T : The qualifications of Actualities are all intrinsic, being partial or delimited expressions of them. If they were nonintrinsic they would not be the product of other modes of being, but of contingencies. But if they were the product of other modes of being, there would be no way of freeing the Actualities from them. To speak of qualifications is to view Existence from the outside as a mere extraneous factor, rather than as the locus of whatever there be, from which nothing could really be freed or held apart.

3.50   The prescinding of qualities is a desirable dislocation. *Otherwise it would not be desirable to free the qualities from irrelevancies.*

A G A I N S T : Whatever pertains to qualities is not irrelevant to them. Taking anything away from them is but a way of destroying them; each is in fact a simple, a singular, allowing for no dissection or dislocation.

3.51   A dislocation of the natures of Actualities is desirable. *Otherwise it would not be desirable to free them from irrelevancies.*

A G A I N S T : It is impossible to dislocate the natures of Actualities without destroying them; their natures are integral to them. And if such dislocation were possible, it would displace and not remove irrelevancies. But in fact there are no irrelevancies, and there is no possible act of dislocation; there are just Actualities about which we can speak, at a distance, with more or less adequacy.

3.52   The Ideal component in an Actuality should be
dislocated, and conversely. *Otherwise neither would
ever be known as it is in itself.*

AGAINST : There is no Ideal component in an Actuality, nor an
Actual component in the Ideal. Each stands over against the other,
unaffected by it. They are ultimate realities and therefore never are
in a position where they need to be dislocated. If they did have such
need, nothing less than they themselves could be powerful enough
to separate them from one another. But then, if they were so powerful, they would not, in the first place, have become involved with
one another.

3.53   The divine component in an Actuality should be
dislocated, and conversely. *Otherwise neither would
ever be known as it is in itself.*

AGAINST : There is nothing divine in the Actual, nothing Actual
in the divine. The one is local and transitory, the other is cosmic and
eternal. The ultimacy of both requires their independence. If there
were a divine component in Actualities nothing less than God could
extract it; if there were Actualities in God, no power but theirs
could free them from him.

3.54   Knowledge and art provide new carriers for freed
Actualities, their qualities and natures. *Otherwise they
would not be productive.*

AGAINST : Knowledge is not productive; if it were, it would distort what it purports to report. Art is productive, but it makes both
form and content, not carriers for dislocated or freed items. Production is an ongoing, practical sequence of occurrences generating its
products; it is not dependent on prior acts of "freeing."

3.55   Myth provides a new carrier for free Ideals.
Otherwise the Ideal could not be adequately presented.

AGAINST : A myth is a fiction, and distorts whatever Ideal it purports to represent. The Ideal could not be adequately presented in a
myth. Nor does it need myth; its nature is evident to any detached,
calm intellect.

3.56   Sacraments provide new carriers for a freed divine component. *Otherwise they would not be religious objects.*
AGAINST: Sacraments presuppose divine activity and not an act by men. To view them as carriers for some artificially separated item is to look at them from below. It is to deny that they are sacraments. Objects are religious either in themselves, or as part of God, or as expressions of him.

3.57   Criticism is the establishment of the import of freed items as carried by new media. *Otherwise it would not evaluate human production.*
AGAINST: There are no freed transported items for criticism to consider. Criticism is the analysis, dissection, understanding of creative products in their own terms, making evident where alien factors have been introduced.

3.58   Maximal freedom from nonessential qualifications by Existence, objective and human, is achieved through epitomization. *Otherwise limitations in artistic media could not be overcome.*
AGAINST: There are no nonessential qualifications produced by a mode of being. Indeed, neither Existence nor any other mode of being imposes qualifications on anything. If they did, there would be no way of freeing oneself from them. Epitomization is at best a human way of dealing with beings from a distance.

3.59   Existence is made integral to and thus specified by Actualities when and as they change in state and position. *Otherwise they would not have their own Existence.*
AGAINST: If Actualities have their own Existence they need not make it integral to themselves or specify it. If they need to do these things they are so far without Existence; but then they would be impotent. Actualities have an Existence all their own, which no one can give to them or take away.

3.60   Existence imposes a limit on what Actualities and other realities can do, and do with it. *Otherwise it would not be a fundamental mode of being.*

AGAINST: If Existence can limit Actualities and other realities, it can limit the Existence in them, and both of them together will be but facets of some more inclusive being. A fundamental mode of being is self-enclosed.

3.61   At any moment beings are at different stages of typical careers. *Otherwise there would be no beings older than others.*

AGAINST: All beings could conceivably have been created just a moment ago; none need be older than any other. Moreover, as in the present, each is the contemporary of all the rest. Older and younger are comparative terms involving a reference to an external measure.

3.62   Attention has a temporal span. *Otherwise evidence could be given in a flash.*

AGAINST: A span of attention has a psychical extension, it occupies only a "specious" present. It has nothing to do with facts or evidence, but only with a private act of concentration. There are in fact no acts of attention; there is only a single activity of attending which has neither beginning nor end, being one with the possession of a consciousness more or less dim and more or less persistent.

3.63   No evidence can be provided to show that nothing endures. *Otherwise the evidence would not endure.*

AGAINST: One thing evidences to another, without necessarily sharing the traits of that other. Nontemporal evidence in the mind of man or God could be provided to show that nothing endures. Endurance outside these is as a matter of fact impossible, since to be in time is to pass away, to give place to something else that succeeds.

3.64   Evidence that beings are of different ages can be judged untrustworthy only if there is a truth more basic than that some beings are older than others. *Otherwise the historic consciousness would be self-defeating.*

A G A I N S T : That some beings are older than others is a mere contingency, due to the fact that there is more than one Actuality, and that these have persisted for different periods. But there is no evidence that there has been such persistence; we merely infer that there has been. The historic consciousness makes use of the idea of persistence, but does not presuppose it. It could conceivably record the course of development of a single being, whose entire career consisted of simple parts in sequence.

3.65   Knowledge of the past is inferentially derived from present evidence that some Actualities have different ages, and thus had origins at different dates. *Otherwise we would have to penetrate into the past to know it, and would there find what was not relevant to the present.*

A G A I N S T : Knowledge of the past is the outcome of an attempt to understand. It may conclude that beings had different ages, but it cannot start with this, for to know that they have different ages is already to know some truth about their past. We can and must penetrate to the past, for this is where the historic facts lie. History is a distinct mode of knowing, at home in the past, which it represents.

3.66   A history is reconstructive. *Otherwise it would have to report the past or rethink it.*

A G A I N S T : To be reconstructive is to be distortive, not to recount what had happened, and is thus to engage in the creating of a fiction. The past for history must forever be a hard datum. To this history must subject itself. When history knows that past, it recaptures what had been thought or done, and thereby makes it be once more. History reports the past by rethinking it.

3.67   Historic occurrences have significant beginnings and endings. *Otherwise there would be no distinguishable events.*

A G A I N S T : The breaks in history are due to the attention men pay to features which interest them; history like time is a continuum, and divisions in it are exteriorly imposed.

3.68   The beginning of an historic occurrence is relevant to its end. *Otherwise it would not make a unit.*

AGAINST: For a beginning to be relevant to an end, it must continue to be up to the end, or the end must be at the beginning. In the one case the beginning, and in the other the end is destroyed. A beginning is a beginning and an end is an end; to relate the two requires an exterior agent.

3.69   History provides explanations of facts in terms of transformations produced by Existence. *Otherwise there would be no historic explanations.*

AGAINST: Nothing can transform a beginning; it remains as it was. And if Existence transformed it into an end, the beginning would become that end, and cease to provide a means for understanding it.

3.70   Historic occurrences have different temporal spans. *Otherwise history would be made up of aggregates of simple units.*

AGAINST: There are no breaks in time; history is the result of man's arbitrary divisions of the continuous. Were it otherwise there would be present moments of various magnitudes, answering to the rhythms of different occurrences. But then one occurrence could be followed by another in a new moment while some other occurrence was still in the process of coming to be. The world would be divided into temporal layers having nothing to do with one another, despite the fact that each thing directly or indirectly impinges on or has some effect on the rest.

3.71   There are unit measures for the historic past. *Otherwise the shorter sequences would not be as determinate as the longer.*

AGAINST: The past contains the very possibilities which the past objects confronted when they were present. The items in it are all indeterminate, and on a footing, no one serving as a unit for the others.

3.72   There are no determinate historic occurrences in the present. *Otherwise it would not take more than an atomic moment for an historic occurrence to take place.*

AGAINST: Were there no historic occurrences in the present, there would be none in the past, and since there is no future yet, there would be no historic occurrences ever. The only time when historic occurrences can take place is in the present. History is a self-contained domain defining time to be a delimited, abstracted facet, in which a fictional past and future are contrasted with a fictional present. Only the present of history is.

3.73   Incompleted historic occurrences are grounded in the present. *Otherwise there would be no order in what is happening.*

AGAINST: What is incompleted as an historic occurrence is not yet real, and what is not yet real cannot affect what is real. Nothing is effective but the complete real historic occurrence, and this is in the present.

3.74   Every historic occurrence must be at least two moments long. *Otherwise it would not have a span longer than that of a unit physical occurrence.*

AGAINST: If every historic occurrence had to contain subordinate historic occurrences, we would be forced into an infinite regress; if it had to contain subordinate nonhistoric occurrences the integrity of history would be jeopardized.

3.75   An historic field contains a number of occurrences not related in sequence. *Otherwise it would not encompass a number of lines of activity.*

AGAINST: History is essentially temporal; what can be analyzed out of it as nonsequential is, strictly speaking, not historically relevant. A history has a spatial spread of course, but this is unified by virtue of the temporal forward thrust of the unitary history.

3.76   An epoch is a field of works of art, structured by myth, and sacramentally unified. *Otherwise it would not contain embodiments of other modes of being.*

AGAINST : Each mode of being has its own integrity, remaining to and in itself. If it did encroach on other modes it could not be separated off from them. If it could be separated off it could not be re-embodied except by itself. And if it could be re-embodied, it would not take the shape of a work of art, a myth, or a sacrament. These are expressions of human activity and interest, below the level of the modes of being. At best only creatures of history, they cannot be definitory of any part of it.

3.77 A civilization is a field containing great men, given direction by an ethical norm, and unified by a religion. *Otherwise it would leave out vital human values.*

AGAINST : There have been civilizations, such as the Confucian, which have had no religion, or at least have not been unified by one. Religions in fact have more often than not been the cause of dissension in, division of, and the destruction of civilizations. Ethical norms are known to few, and do not offer direction even to these. Great men are matters of contingency. A civilization has a nature, a rationale, a rhythm which need not depend in any way on the exercise of powers by religions, norms, or great men.

3.78 The men of a given civilization constitute a people. *Otherwise they would not express that civilization in their being and actions.*

AGAINST : The men in a civilized community do many things which are outside that community's reach, interest, or power. They live private lives, and at times in their acts and their being oppose their civilizations quite radically. Men have an irreducible being outside civilization.

3.79 A guided people make up the body of a civilization whose nature is defined primarily by great men. *Otherwise there would be no real leaders.*

AGAINST : There are no great men, for all are on a footing. But there are conspicuous men, men who are thrown towards the front of attention. The consequences of some reach further than those of others, and that is all.

3.80	A religious people make up the body of a civilization whose nature is defined primarily by a religion. *Otherwise there would be no religiously dominated civilizations.*

A G A I N S T : A religion has to do with men in relation to God. This is a matter of private belief, devotion, dedication, and cannot be treated as defining the nature of a civilization without making both lose their proper functions.

3.81	An ethical people make up the body of a civilization whose nature is defined primarily by an ethical ideal. *Otherwise there would be no ethical civilizations.*

A G A I N S T : An ethical ideal serves to test a civilization and not to define one; nor can there be an ethical people. There are only ethical men or ethical communities, at rest perhaps for a time within a civilization, but in root always at war with it.

3.82	There are three types of civilization. *Otherwise a civilization would not be Existence epitomized, and characterize an historic people.*

A G A I N S T : There are as many types of civilization as there are ingenious men to classify them. Each civilization has its own individuality, its own history, its own nature; it is a singular, not a member of a class or an illustration of a type.

3.83	A people exhausts its being and meaning in a civilization. *Otherwise it would not be confined within it, passing away when the civilization does.*

A G A I N S T : A people is made up of living men, and these exhaust their being and meaning in the course of life, and not in the course of a civilization. No civilization begins with fresh men; few if any end with just dead ones; the people of one civilization pass imperceptibly into those of others. Also the nature of a civilization changes even while the people remain more or less the same. And if the two were made co-ordinate, each would still retain its own nature and being, and never exhaust itself in the other.

3.84	A people's potentialities are not exhausted in a civilization. *Otherwise it would have no unused potentialities.*

A G A I N S T : To perish with one's civilization is to perish with one's potentialities. If a people could exhaust its being and meaning in a civilization, it would by that very token also exhaust all its potentialities as well.

3.85   A people has a nature not exhausted in a civilization. *Otherwise it would not be linked to what will be.*

A G A I N S T : Anything's nature is where and when it is. When it perishes it perishes with its nature; there is no nature left to be linked with anything else. We have a sequence of natures, with links supplied by men, or we have a single nature with divisions supplied by men—and nothing in between.

3.86   A people has an organic unity not exhausted in a civilization. *Otherwise a people would not contrast with its successor.*

A G A I N S T : What is essential to a being is integral to it, and comes to be and passes away with it. A people's unity is when and where the people is; it has no power or status, since it is only a way of referring to the fact that men are together.

3.87   A people faces a standard not exhausted in a civilization. *Otherwise the people would not be justly criticizable.*

A G A I N S T : It is either civilization or the people that sets and defines the standard. In the first case the standard is exhausted in the civilization; in the second it has no necessary reference to a civilization and is neither exhausted nor not exhausted there.

3.88   Civilizations are comparable because there are principles which apply to all. *Otherwise there would be only biased references from each to each.*

A G A I N S T : To compare civilizations in terms of principles which are not ingredient in them is to use either effete or irrelevant standards. But what is ingredient in one is not necessarily in harmony with what is ingredient in another. Comparisons are made by arbitrarily imposing irrelevant principles on concrete, individual, basically incomparable civilizations.

3.89   Great men provide universal principles measuring the creative energies of a people and a civilization. *Otherwise they would not be epitomizations of Actualities, works of art of the greatest magnitude.*

AGAINST: Great men are largely the accidental products of the pressures of their communities. They reflect rather than provide the principles of their civilization or people. They are no more works of art than is any person, which is but to say they are not works of art at all.

3.90   A religion provides a measure of the purity of a people and a civilization. *Otherwise it would not offer an epitomization of a divine element.*

AGAINST: A religion can be practiced by peoples and in civilizations which are far from pure. It has to do with man and his God, and this regardless of what peoples and civilizations want or do.

3.91   Ethical ideals provide a measure of the moral worth of a people and a civilization. *Otherwise peoples and civilizations could not be evaluated.*

AGAINST: There is no ethics which stands outside a civilization; each civilization has its own code. And if there were an ethics outside, it would not measure the civilization; it would state principles applicable to individual men, the only beings who can act ethically, and therefore who ought to be judged ethically.

3.92   Peoples and civilizations have hovering natures, unities, and values, exhausted only in a longer history. *Otherwise they would not be integral parts of that history.*

AGAINST: A hovering nature, unity or value is one not yet embodied. As not yet embodied it does not belong to the people or the civilization. And since what is in the past cannot be affected by what is in the future, nothing that happens to that subsequent nature has any relevance to the people or the civilization.

3.93   The whole of history, and derivatively any people, may be unfulfilled, fail to be actualized maximally. *Otherwise it would not be possible for the whole of history to fail to measure up to some standard of excellence.*

AGAINST: What the whole of history exhibits is real, and what it fails to exhibit is nothing at all, except perhaps a mistaken anticipation of what history would in fact do. There is no place and no function for a standard of excellence which should apply to all history, granted that history could ever constitute such a whole. Standards of excellence are but phases of the whole of history, or stand outside it as independent and irrelevant.

3.94 The whole of history, and derivatively any people, may be incoherent, fail to be unified maximally. *Otherwise it could not be a persistent locus of conflicts.*

AGAINST: A unity is nothing apart from what it in fact unifies. The unity of history has whatever degree of cohesion the events in history in fact exhibit. What is other than that unity is an effete, irrelevant abstraction, or characterizes what is independent of history and its unity.

3.95 The whole of history, and derivately any people, may not be wholly good, because it fails to be idealized maximally. *Otherwise there could be no residual evil in the universe.*

AGAINST: Evil is a relative matter, and disappears with the disappearance of men, or with a shift in their standards. History is never to be idealized; it is through and through concrete, to be taken as it occurs. If in any sense there is evil in its parts or throughout the whole that will be a brute and unalterable fact. It will in no way warrant the judgment that history is not wholly good, for that evil helps constitute the only good that has any meaning in history—the good which history in fact exhibits.

3.96 From the perspective of Actuality, the whole of Existence is only potentially excellent. *Otherwise it would be individualized throughout.*

AGAINST: If an Actuality is to make a proper evaluation of Existence it must deal with Existence in relevant terms. But in its own terms Existence is not unfulfilled; if unfulfilled in other terms this has nothing to do with it, its nature or its functioning.

3.97   From the perspective of the Ideal, the whole of Existence is not wholly rational. *Otherwise Existence would not have a being independent of the Ideal.*

A G A I N S T : Nothing should be judged except in terms appropriate to it. The whole of Existence can have no other rationale but that which it in fact does have as just that whole. To evaluate it from the outside in terms of the Ideal is to deal with it in alien terms.

3.98   From the perspective of God, the whole of Existence is incoherent. *Otherwise it would not be the domain of becoming.*

A G A I N S T : Since God is the source of unity there is nothing which can remain incoherent from his perspective. Moreover, if he were the cause of Existence he would make it coherent when he made it be. Existence, just so far as it is, is coherent in itself, and this regardless of what God does.

3.99   Actuality, the Ideal, and God are deficient from the perspective of Existence. *Otherwise they would not lack desirable features, characteristic of Existence.*

A G A I N S T : A being is not deficient if it fails to exhibit features which are appropriate to some other mode of being. The perspective of Existence either does not terminate in other modes, or it gets to them as in no way deficient.

3.100   Existence provides testimony to the reality of Actualities. *Otherwise all its features could be accounted for without making a reference to real individuals.*

A G A I N S T : No mode of being can provide testimony to any other, for each remains in itself, apart from all else. Existence has a structure and a rhythm all its own, in no way to be accounted for by the presence of individuals.

3.101   Existence provides testimony to the reality of the Ideal. *Otherwise Existence would not be present in relation to a future.*

A G A I N S T : The Ideal is not involved in the affairs of Existence;

and so far as it could be involved, it would be ingredient in Existence, pointing to nothing outside that Existence.

3.102   Existence provides testimony to the reality of God. *Otherwise Existence would not be united with its own essence.*

AGAINST: God alone could provide testimony to his own reality. And an Existence which was not united with its essence would have no nature at all, and no being. Existence has an essence apart from God, and God has a being apart from Existence. Neither needs nor refers to the other.

3.103   Existence partly satisfies the needs of Actualities. *Otherwise they would not have energy and flexibility.*

AGAINST: An Actuality without energy or flexibility would be only a possibility or a fiction. If an Actuality has needs, they are for other Actualities, which alone could make up the deficiencies that the Actuality may have.

3.104   Existence partly satisfies the needs of the Ideal. *Otherwise the Ideal would not have a status in space and time.*

AGAINST: The Ideal remains forever outside space and time; nothing that Existence could do affects it. Existence neither satisfies nor frustrates it, neither spatializes it nor temporalizes it. Each has its own nature, function, status, uncompromised by the other.

3.105   Existence partly satisfies the needs of God. *Otherwise he would not need or get a field for action.*

AGAINST: God has no needs; he is a perfect being, dependent on nothing else. And if he had needs he could not be satisfied by Existence, self-divisive and unorganized.

3.106   Existence supplements the contributions other modes make to one another. *Otherwise something that ought to be could not be.*

AGAINST: Whatever work is possible to one mode of being could not be transferred to a different mode of being. And if it could be transferred, the former would not be freed from the onus of a failure to do what it ought, nor would it be benefited by the quite distinct activity of the other. Each being has its own tasks, and fulfills them according to its powers and on the occasions when it can.

3.107   The Ideal relates Existence and Actuality.
Otherwise they could not be together in harmony.

A G A I N S T : Real relations must be appropriate to the objects related. But an Ideal is of an entirely different order of being from Existence and Actuality. Its relations have no extensionality, and can have no power to bridge the radical difference in kind which separates Existence and Actuality.

3.108   Actuality relates Existence and the Ideal.
Otherwise their efforts would not be harmonized.

A G A I N S T : If Existence and the Ideal encroach on one another, the outcome is determined by their interplay. They need no Actuality to mediate them. If it could mediate them it would transform them. Each in fact stands outside the other, indifferent to its being, unaffected by its activity.

3.109   Existence relates the Ideal and Actualities.
Otherwise they would not be mutually relevant.

A G A I N S T : If the Ideal and Actualities could act on one another they would be directly relevant to one another, needing no other agency to unite them. But since they are independent modes of being, they are not at all related; they are just different.

3.110   A "proof" of a mode of being involves the use of the other three modes. *Otherwise a proof would not require premiss, rule, and inference.*

A G A I N S T : No mode of being can be proved; proof relates only to conceptualized objects. Not even a truth regarding a mode of being can be proved, without compromising the independence of the being to which that truth applies. A mode of being is too independent, too substantial, too self-enclosed to be the object of a proof.

CHAPTER 9

A NEGATIVE APPROACH TO

God

4.01 Each mode of being is ingredient in the others. *Otherwise it would not qualify to the being of those others.*

AGAINST: An ultimate, irreducible mode of being stands over against all else. If any being is ingredient in any other it is by that token a dependent reality, not a genuine mode of being.

4.02 Each mode of being needs the others. *Otherwise those others would not have a reality which it lacks.*

AGAINST: A need which must be satisfied in order that a being have reality never could be at a stage where it was unsatisfied. It could never therefore be at the stage where it was a need. But a need which cannot in principle be unsatisfied is no need at all. An ultimate mode of being is self-contained, final, irreducible, in no way affected or determined by any other mode of being. Independent beings have no need of one another.

4.03 Each mode of being seeks to adjust itself to others. *Otherwise they would make no effort to overcome vital limitations.*

AGAINST: The independence of the modes of being requires that each function apart from and without reference to the others. If they sought to adjust themselves to one another they would strain to behave with respect to what they do not know and in ways which would not necessarily be appropriate.

4.04   Each mode of being partly satisfies the others. *Otherwise they would not be supplementary modes of being.*

A G A I N S T : Each mode of being is complete in itself, needing nothing. If it had any needs these could not be satisfied by beings which were as irreducible as itself, and existed in total independence of it. If those beings could satisfy it they would satisfy it completely and at once by their mere presence.

4.05   Each mode of being imposes a burden on every other. *Otherwise each would be required to do what could not possibly be done.*

A G A I N S T : Whatever task one mode of being might have is peculiar to it; if it fails to engage in it or to fulfill it, this can have no bearing on what other distinct modes of being can or must do. And if a mode of being did part of the work some other should have done, the benefits or virtue for doing it do not accrue to that other.

4.06   Each mode of being provides testimony to the reality of the others. *Otherwise there would be no nonessential features.*

A G A I N S T : Each being is self-enclosed; it provides no testimony to any others. If it did provide testimony it could be only of itself (through the agency of some appearance or facet of itself), in which case the acknowledgment of the testimony would be question-begging.

4.07   Each mode of being provides both direct and indirect testimony to the reality of others. *Otherwise there would not be features instancing the being who imposes them, as well as features which instance beings that do not impose them.*

A G A I N S T : The features of a mode of being are integral to it; they are not imposed on it by any other. And if they were imposed they would be revelatory of that other in the guise of a power. All testimony is direct so far as it is testimony, since it then is a sign of some relevant object; all is indirect so far as it requires someone to

acknowledge it and relate it to something else in accordance with
rules of interpretation, causation, evidence, and so on.

4.08   Each mode of being relates two other modes of
being. *Otherwise they would be disconnected and
could not together help constitute reality.*
   A G A I N S T : Each mode of being is other than the others, and as
such has no relation to them. If it needed a relation this could not be
provided for by a mode of being distinct from it and its correlate.

4.09   A being is related to another by a third in a
primary and a secondary way. *Otherwise there would
be no relations to objective duplicates and to sources.*
   A G A I N S T : If fundamental modes of being were related to anything the relation would either be real or merely conceived; in the one
case it would be primary no matter to what it was related; in the other
case it would not be related in fact. There are no secondary relations.
But the modes, because they are ultimate beings, are unrelated.

4.10   Each mode of being enables one to hold any
other apart from the rest. *Otherwise there would be
no terminating in a mode of being.*
   A G A I N S T : Modes of being stand apart from one another by the
very fact that they are diverse; they need nothing to separate them
from one another. If they did need something to separate them it
would have to be by some power greater than the force in the
modes which are together. But this power must then be as other than
a mode of being, has and can therefore have no reality.

4.11   Each mode of being permits of the detachment
of a directly or indirectly originative being. *Otherwise
one could not arrive at that being, starting from any other.*
   A G A I N S T : Modes of being are already detached, and need no
power to detach them. And if there were such a detaching agency it
could not itself be detached except by some higher power, and so on
endlessly.

4.12   A "proof" of a mode of being begins with testimony, acknowledges a relation, and terminates in the being. *Otherwise it would not be valid.*

A G A I N S T : Beings cannot be proved. And what can be proved does not begin with testimony but with premisses, is not ruled by a relation but by an implication, and does not terminate in a being but in a conclusion.

4.13   There are three basic and six subordinate testimonies for, relations to, and terminations in God. *Otherwise there would not be four basic modes of being.*

A G A I N S T : God is not testified to by anything but himself; there are no relations which could connect him with other beings without making him into a mere correlate; there can be no terminations in him, for he is not an outcome. He is an irreducible beginning and a source of all else.

4.14   Teleological testimony offers evidence requiring God for its explanation. *Otherwise it would not originate with nonessential features which owe their presence to a cosmic unitary being.*

A G A I N S T : So far as one is in the presence of God no testimony is necessary. So far as one is not in his presence no testimony is possible.

4.15   A substantival teleology begins with primary Actualities offering direct testimony to the reality of God as their Absolute Other. *Otherwise they could persistently be others by themselves, or in relation to some being less than God.*

A G A I N S T : No Actuality has the role of an other. If it did it would not need anything outside itself; just by being in itself it would be potentially opposed to anything else. And if it needs something else as a correlate, this role can be played by the cosmos as a whole, for this has the endurance and the distinction to enable any Actuality to be over against it as an other.

4.16   A rationalistic teleology begins with universals offering indirect testimony to a God concerned with the Ideal. *Otherwise Actualities would not be at once individuals and members of classes.*

AGAINST: Whatever features characterize Actualities are ingredient in them. Classification approaches them from without in terms which have no relevance to their being. It reflects man's interest or knowledge; its universals testify to nothing.

4.17   An historical teleology begins with facts offering indirect testimony to a God concerned with Existence. *Otherwise the existence of the past would not be descriptive of it.*

AGAINST: The existence which the past has is ingredient in it. Since it must be produced when and as the past is, it is evidently essential to that past.

4.18   A moralistic teleology begins with normative possibilities, directly testifying to an evaluating God. *Otherwise there would be no exterior relevant norm measuring the worth of the universe.*

AGAINST: What is outside the universe is nothing. If there could be anything outside it, it would be irrelevant. And if the irrelevant measure could be applied to the universe, it would not be able to measure the worth of the universe, for the universe as a whole has no value. Values have to do with the parts of the universe in relation to one another.

4.19   A directional teleology begins with realizable possibilities which indirectly testify to a temporally oriented God. *Otherwise the realizable would not be relevant.*

AGAINST: Possibilities have their own integrity and need not be exemplified in anything else. If they are realizable they must be relevant, for to be realizable means to be related to what could in fact realize them.

4.20   A providential teleology begins with a cosmic possibility which indirectly testifies to a purposing God. *Otherwise the Future would not be exhausted by Existence.*

AGAINST: It is of the very essence of the Future to remain outside the present. No power could make that Future exhausted by Existence without thereby radically altering both.

4.21   An architectural teleology begins with unified Existence as providing direct testimony to the reality of an effective God. *Otherwise Existence would not possess its own essence.*

AGAINST: Existence without its essence is a surd; to impose an essence on it is to give it something alien. And if its essence were imposed on it, that would not testify to a God but at best only to a blind power forcing realities together.

4.22   A mathematical teleology begins with phenomenalized Existence as offering indirect testimony to the reality of a cosmic God. *Otherwise Existence would not have a variable geometry.*

AGAINST: The scientific world is self-enclosed, requiring no reference to God in order to be, or in order to be understood. The geometry of Existence is determined by the laws of the cosmos and the distribution of the matter in it. Existence, without any help from God, has just the structure which the criss-crossing of the relations between Actualities in fact now provides.

4.23   A structuralized teleology begins with idealized Existence as providing indirect testimony to the reality of an ordering God. *Otherwise Existence would not be in the present.*

AGAINST: The present alone is. The future is but an intellectualized extension of it in one direction, the past is but an intellectualized extension of it in the other. Existence does not need any power to be in the present; if it did, that power would not be God's, for he is outside time altogether; if concerned with time at all he is concerned with abrogating rather than with producing it.

4.24   There can be no teleological proofs of God. *Otherwise there would be no distinction between premiss, rule, and conclusion.*

AGAINST: The only possible satisfactory proof of God is one which expresses his purpose or intent; what proves less than this proves only the reality of a cosmic principle, a prime mover, or some such philosophic abstraction.

4.25   There are three primary and six secondary cosmological approaches to God. *Otherwise the various modes could not mediate one another and God.*

AGAINST: A plurality of proofs testifies to the inadequacy of each. There is either only one proof or none. And what is true of proofs is true of cosmological approaches; there is a single relation connecting Actualities with God, and that is all-sufficient, or there are no satisfactory cosmological approaches to him.

4.26   A formal cosmological approach to God relates some mode of being to him by means of the formal structure of possibility. *Otherwise there would be no logically certifiable proof.*

AGAINST: A logically certifiable proof is precisely one which can arrive only at an attenuation or concept of God, and not at God himself. A formal cosmological proof must relate a mode of being to God himself, and then express this in a formal way. To do less is to deal with God and his relations externally, in irrelevant terms.

4.27   A devotional cosmological approach to God relates some mode of being to him by means of an individualized structure of possibility. *Otherwise there would be no personalizing of a formal proof.*

AGAINST: So far as a logical proof is personalized it is corrupted; so far as devotion is a proper means of being related to God, formality is either swept away or is subjected to such transformation as to make references to the structure of possibility irrelevant.

4.28   A naturalistic cosmological approach to God relates some mode of being to him by means of an existentialized structure of possibility. *Otherwise the laws of nature would have no theological import.*

AGAINST: The laws of nature are integral to nature and do not involve a reference to any being outside. And if there is to be a reference to a being outside, it will not be mediated by a mere structure but by something more concrete, more adequate to the being from which it begins and to the being at which it ends.

4.29   An individualized cosmological approach to God relates some mode of being to him by means of the structure of Actuality. *Otherwise reverence would not be an agency for reaching God.*

AGAINST: An Actuality is a finite being, caught inside a space-time world. No use of the structure of such a being could possibly relate a mode of being to God. It is the category of Actuality, not Actualities, which is on a par with other modes of being and can relate one to the other. But such a category does not have God, but only the category of God as a terminus.

4.30   An institutionalized cosmological approach to God relates some mode of being to him by means of the structure of Actuality when qualified by Ideality. *Otherwise churches and religious communities would not provide opportunities for reaching God.*

AGAINST: Churches and religious communities offer only occasions or ways for regulating the activity of religious men. They constrict, distort, and conventionalize whatever relation there might be between individuals and God.

4.31   A worshipful cosmological approach to God relates some mode of being to him by means of the structure of Actuality when qualified by Existence. *Otherwise an acceptance of the cosmos would not have religious value.*

AGAINST: Existence nails Actualities to this world; it forces them away from divinity. So far as Existence qualifies Actualities it precludes their being related to God.

4.32 A materialistic cosmological approach to God relates some mode of being to him by means of the structure of Existence. *Otherwise there would be no genuine cosmological relation to God.*

AGAINST : Existence, as self-divisive, is the antithesis of God, the supreme unity. Existence cannot therefore serve to relate any one to him. Moreover, it is without genuine structure, and thus cannot yield any relation. And, finally, as a self-enclosed domain, it can relate only items within it, not something outside itself to something beyond.

4.33 An idealized cosmological approach to God relates some mode of being to him by means of the structure of Existence when qualified by Ideality. *Otherwise immanent laws would not have religious import.*

AGAINST : Ideality does not qualify Existence. If it did, it would not have anything to do with a relation of a mode of being to God, for it concerns only possibility, what is not yet.

4.34 An historical cosmological approach to God relates some mode of being to him by means of the structure of Existence when qualified by Actualities. *Otherwise the fact that men are involved in a cosmological proof would have no relevance.*

AGAINST : Actualities do not qualify Existence, but are at best subject to it. And if they did qualify it, they would not have anything to do with a structure relating a mode of being to God, but only with Existence as the field in which those Actualities are contemporaries.

4.35 There can be no cosmological proofs of God. *Otherwise one could go from the finite to the infinite without begging the question.*

AGAINST : Since the universe is a contingent one, which might not have been, an adequate account of it requires a reference to God as its cosmological cause. No other proof is adequate but one which has a cosmological import; only this relates to God, the being who is over against all else.

4.36   Teleological and cosmological approaches to God are supplementary. *Otherwise one would not need both a beginning and a relation to ground a proof.*

A G A I N S T : Since each approach acknowledges different data, and terminates in a different facet of God, these approaches cannot supplement one another, as premiss and relation, but at best only as coordinated arguments.

4.37   A conjunction of teleological and cosmological approaches cannot provide a proof of God. *Otherwise no inferential act would be necessary.*

A G A I N S T : Inference is a psychological matter. If the cosmological and teleological approaches provide adequate grounds for the conclusion that God exists, they provide all that is necessary and possible for a proof of God. To ask for more is to depart from the conditions of a proof.

4.38   A proof of God requires an act of ontological detachment of him from the structure of the proof. *Otherwise there would be no concluding to God.*

A G A I N S T : An act adequate to the detaching of God would be a divine act, not possible to anyone but God. If there is to be a concluding to God it is an act outside of and uncontrolled by any formal conditions of a proof.

4.39   There can be no ontological proofs of God. *Otherwise it would be possible to move with warrant from predicates to Existence, or from Existence to the divine.*

A G A I N S T : The only proof adequate to God is one which attends to his unique perfection and relates this and an appropriate existence. Such a proof is offered in the ontological argument. This is the argument, as Kant observed, to which the others finally come in order to be sure to reach God and not a mere philosophical principle.

4.40   There are three pure and six qualified modes of detaching God from a cosmological rule which begins with testimony to his existence. *Otherwise the various modes would not have the same ultimacy.*

AGAINST: God is not attached to any rule. And if he were he could not be detached except by means of divine power. And if there were such a divine power of detaching, it would be single, simple, not threefold or ninefold. God is not a being arrived at; he is a being who is beyond all proof.

4.41 The existence of God can be logically inferred. *Otherwise it would not be possible to conclude to a warranted conclusion.*

AGAINST: The existence of God is beyond the reach of any proof, firstly because all Existence is outside the reach of proof, and secondly because God's existence is entirely distinct in locus and nature from that of the premiss and activity of a proof. No Existence is open to logical derivation; it is available only in an encounter.

4.42 The existence of God can be accepted through an intellectual assent qualified by the self. *Otherwise it would not be the self which infers.*

AGAINST: So far as the self enters into a proof, the proof is distorted, deprived of its pristine objective validity. To go beyond the formal conditions is to spoil the argument.

4.43 The existence of God can be acknowledged through an intellectual assent qualified by Existence. *Otherwise there would be no sacrificial approach to God.*

AGAINST: Sacrifice is an offering, and in no way guarantees an acceptance. And it occurs entirely outside the area where proofs are made and can be vindicated. Moreover, a qualification by Existence presupposes God, the being who most perfectly exists.

4.44 God can be reached through faith. *Otherwise there would be no facing God as one's Absolute Other.*

AGAINST: Faith leaves reason behind; it moves into the emptiness where no reason can enter. It terminates in nothing and cannot therefore be said to reach to God. If it did reach to him it would no longer be faith but possession, and he, by virtue of being reached, would not be an Absolute Other.

4.45 God can be reached through prayer, a faith qualified by possibility. *Otherwise God would not be one who answers to fear or wish.*

A G A I N S T : A petition need not be granted; a prayer remains a prayer though unanswered. And if one prayer may be unanswered, so may they all. And since an answer to a prayer can be given only by God, it cannot be qualified by possibility, without limiting God's answer. Prayer can reach God only so far as God reaches down to him who prays.

4.46 God can be reached through humility, a faith qualified by Existence. *Otherwise faith could not be modified by an environing cosmos.*

A G A I N S T : Humility is a retreat, not an advance. And in any case it is essentially a private matter, in no way affected by the Existence which environs one. And so far as it involves a recognition that there is a universe larger than oneself it remains a this-worldly attitude. God alone is able to make humility a way of getting to him, and this by reaching down to those who have a simple faith in him, a faith unaffected by the environing cosmos.

4.47 God can be reached through work. *Otherwise getting to him would not require the energy of Existence.*

A G A I N S T : All work is this-worldly; it begins and ends in this world and in no way takes us out of it. And even if in some way it could serve to move one away from the world, it would, because finite, restricted, imperfect, fail to reach God. No activity begun by man nor even any which made use of the whole of Existence could be equal to the task of reaching to God.

4.48 God can be reached through good works. *Otherwise an ethical life would not be theologically effective.*

A G A I N S T : No matter how good works may be, they are limited, finite, this-worldly, and thus incapable of enabling one to reach God. Also "good works" is a metaphor, expressing the fact that there is good will or good results before or after the works; works in themselves are indifferent. If there is to be a reaching to God through "good works" it will be in fact a reaching by means of our wills, or by virtue of his acceptance of the results, and not by virtue of the works themselves. No work can compromise, obligate, compel God.

4.49   God can be reached through dedicated work. *Otherwise religious work would be without efficacy.*
A G A I N S T : Work can be dedicated to God, but this does not assure one's reaching him. To reach him by these means would either compromise God, forcing his action, or it would presuppose him as one who has already accepted the work and thus who allows or helps a man to reach him.

4.50   Teleological and ontological approaches to God are supplementary. *Otherwise an argument would not require both a beginning and an end.*
A G A I N S T : Neither approach is adequate. Since they are concerned with quite different matters, the one with exhibitions of God's purpose or efficacy, and the other with his being or perfection, they are independent of one another, and are in no way supplementary.

4.51   Cosmological and ontological approaches to God are supplementary. *Otherwise an argument would not require both a rule and a conclusion.*
A G A I N S T : Neither approach is adequate. The one is concerned with the universe as presumably unstable or not self-sufficient; the other is concerned with God as he is in himself. The one if adequate, would reach to God as a cause, the other to God as a necessary being. They are quite independent, adding nothing to one another.

4.52   A proof of God begins teleologically, is validated cosmologically, and terminates ontologically. *Otherwise it would not have a proper beginning, rule, and ending.*
A G A I N S T : No teleological beginning could be satisfactory, since it is rooted entirely in this world. No such beginning could be mediated by a cosmological approach, for that connects any Existence with a cause which is not necessarily purposive. And no ontological terminating could end with God without having already begun with

him, unless real beings could be extracted from thoughts, and a supreme being could be produced by finite acts.

4.53 There are nine basic ways of proving God's existence through faith. *Otherwise there would not be three distinct testimonies relatable in three distinct ways to a God who is to be reached by means of a proper attitude.*

AGAINST: If one could prove the existence of God, a single proof would suffice. If there were nine proofs, all carried by faith, they would reduce to one, or faith would be divided in a ninefold way, and reach a ninefold God.

4.54 There are nine basic ways of proving God's existence through a logical inference. *Otherwise there would not be three distinct premisses and three distinct rules of inference terminating in God, who is to be reached through an intellectual act.*

AGAINST: No one has ever proved God logically. If there were one proof the others would be unnecessary. A logical inference, moreover, never gets to anything but a proposition or a sentence. If it could get to an object, that object would have to be graspable by man; its essence would be known. Since God's essence is one with his existence, he who could logically infer to God would have him, the infinite being, within a finite grip. A logical proof of God is a mistaken idea based on the neglect of the truth that God is a self-contained being. It looks at him exteriorly and tries to reach him by exterior manipulations.

4.55 There are nine basic ways of proving God's existence through work. *Otherwise there would not be three distinct types of structure terminating in God, to be reached through an effective detaching of him from the structures.*

AGAINST: No more than one proof is ever necessary. No man's activity, moreover, can be adequate to the work of having a real God stand over against him. And no matter how effective a work, it cannot extract a real God out of a God treated as the terminus of some structure, particularly if it is a structure of a being whose beginning and ending are distant from God.

4.56 All proofs of God are circular and question-begging. *Otherwise the evidence, the structure, and the terminating would not be adequate to him.*

A G A I N S T : To suppose that a proof is circular or question-begging is to suppose that one in fact has had the answer in advance. But this supposes that there is a God. None of the "proofs" here given reaches the level of being circular or question-begging; none proves anything at all. If there is a God, he is beyond the reach of our devices.

4.57 A proof of God is satisfying only so far as God is encountered in other ways as well. *Otherwise one would not need to be confronted by him as well as to confront him.*

A G A I N S T : If a proof were satisfactory there is no need to look outside it. And if there is need to look outside it the evidence that is then provided will not improve the proof. Moreover, an encounter with God as outside the proof must be made to harmonize with him as revealed in a proof. But this would require either another proof or another encounter.

4.58 God's nature, as apart from proof, includes all that has been truly testified regarding him. *Otherwise the proof would be mistaken in beginning, in structure, or in concluding.*

A G A I N S T : To say that God's nature includes all that has been truly testified regarding him is either to speak tautologically or is to point up the irrelevance or incompleteness of the proof or the testimony. An adequate proof of God encompasses all that and only that which is demanded by evidences of him.

4.59 God's nature, as apart from proof, includes whatever is known of him through the agency of a systematic dialectic. *Otherwise he would not be one of four independent but interlocked modes of being.*

A G A I N S T : If God could be known without recourse to any testimony or evidences, he would have been known before this. And if a systematic dialectic arrives at him it can do so only by going through something like a proof. There is no other way of reaching him than by means of a proof—unless it be revelation. No being can be reached through dialectic; at most this can be a way of showing what is incomplete in what we in fact know. But the completing of what we know requires more than mental or verbal juggling.

4.60   Our most adequate idea of God is self-engendered. *Otherwise it would not have its root in a longing, solitary self, pointing to its absolute Other.*

A G A I N S T : An idea engendered by man is conceivably delusory. It is moreover finite, exterior to whatever object it purports to characterize. No idea of God could be adequate which was not bestowed by God and which therefore did not reflect something of his majesty, self-completeness, and self-containedness.

4.61   Theoanalysis is the art of dealing with other realities in theological terms. *Otherwise these other realities would not be "images" of God.*

A G A I N S T : To deal with things in terms inappropriate to them is to distort them. To deal with them in theological terms is to distort them on the basis of what is less well known than themselves. If there were such a subject as theoanalysis it would involve an obscuring and falsification of whatever there be to know.

4.62   In theoanalytic terms, Actualities are God's self-identity endlessly multiplied and combined. *Otherwise Actualities would not be self-identical through and through.*

A G A I N S T : Actualities change. Often in internal disharmony and in external conflict, they are entirely other in being, range, value, or power than God, and cannot be understood in terms appropriate to him. It is questionable whether any one is self-identical; so far as it is, it stands over against all its features as the permanent and nonextended over against the transient and extended, dividing the being in two.

4.63   In theoanalytic terms, the Ideal is all-encompassing. *Otherwise it would not express God's essence.*

A G A I N S T : God's essence is one with his existence. Were the Ideal to express his essence it would express it in irrelevant terms and at a distance from his being. Moreover, the Ideal, by virtue of its lack of power, its lack of extensionality, its lack of individuality, is incapable of encompassing Existence or Actualities, and thus cannot be all-encompassing.

4.64   In theoanalytic terms, Existence is creativity. *Otherwise God would not make himself manifest everywhere.*

AGAINST: God alone is creative because he alone fully is. And what he creates he makes be. Existence is either himself or what he has brought about; creativity is at best the connection between these two. Since this is a world of sin, vice, folly, and ugliness, it is evident that God is not everywhere.

4.65   God's nature, mind, and expression are one with the being, knowledge, and creation of all there is. *Otherwise he would not be self-contained while encompassing all.*

AGAINST: The identification of God's nature, mind, and expression with the being, knowledge, and creation of all else involves a reduction of God's being to the being of others. This involves a pantheistic blurring of the truths of both religion and cosmology. God is not the Actual, the Ideal, or Existence. God is God, no more and no less.

4.66   God internally reproduces other modes of being. *Otherwise he would not do justice to the natures they have apart from him.*

AGAINST: No beings can be reproduced without being doubled. And as doubled they will occupy different domains, and therefore will have distinctive careers which will immediately destroy the supposed duplication—or God will turn out to be the universe all over again. Each being has its own integrity and stands over against all others. The thesis confounds a possible representation with an actual reproduction.

4.67   God has a direct awareness of exterior Actualities. *Otherwise he would not know how to reproduce them.*

AGAINST: If God has a direct awareness of exterior Actualities, he is not altogether confined within himself. And if he does actually grasp what they are, he has no need to reproduce them. God is self-contained, exterior to and independent of all other beings.

4.68 God has an indirect awareness of Actualities in relation to the Ideal. *Otherwise he would not know them as occupied with the Ideal.*

A G A I N S T : If God could be aware of Actualities he would be directly aware of them. And if his awareness were accurate it would involve a direct grasp of the fact that Actualities are occupied with the Ideal. An indirect awareness is in effect no awareness at all. What God knows, he knows without mediation.

4.69 God has an indirect awareness of Actualities in relation to Existence. *Otherwise he would not make the past be.*

A G A I N S T : The past has no being at all. If it had any being it would have it apart from God, for it can be made up only of what has been in the present, over against God. Granted though that God endows the past with an "existence," it does not follow that he thereby achieves an awareness, direct or indirect, of Actualities. The space-time world of Actualities stands over against an unextended God, and he stands over against it. Neither depends for its being or functioning on the other.

4.70 God has a direct awareness of a normative Ideal. *Otherwise he would not know himself to be perfect, or know others as valuable.*

A G A I N S T : If God were perfect there would be nothing outside him. Nor would he need to look outside himself to know his own excellencies. And if he did look outside himself to the Ideal this would not give him a principle of value measuring other beings, but just some other mode of being over against himself, as fundamental and irreducible and self-contained as he is.

4.71 God has an indirect awareness of the Ideal in relation to Actualities. *Otherwise he would not know it either in*

its normative role with respect to them, or as exhausted by
them in the course of time.

AGAINST: A divine awareness is direct. If God had an awareness of the Ideal he would have an awareness of it as independent of
Actualities. But he knows and needs know only himself.

4.72   God has an indirect awareness of the Ideal in relation
to Existence. *Otherwise he would not know it as a cosmic*
Future.

AGAINST: An awareness of the Ideal, if adequate, is a direct
awareness of it as exercising whatever functions it does exercise in independence of Existence.

4.73   God has a direct awareness of an extensive Existence.
Otherwise he would not be able to guide his self-analysis
by the nature of what it is intended to reproduce.

AGAINST: God is simple. And because he is simple he is entirely
distinct and over against whatever is extended. He does not analyze
himself, does not reproduce Existence. If he did, he would not have to
look outside himself to know what it is he must do.

4.74   God has an indirect awareness of Existence in relation
to Actualities. *Otherwise he would not know the variable*
geometry of the world.

AGAINST: God's awareness is direct and accurate. If he has an
awareness of Existence it must be of it as it is, with whatever features
it may possess. The awareness does not have to be mediated by Actualities.

4.75   God has an indirect awareness of Existence in
relation to the Ideal. *Otherwise he would not know it to be*
temporal.

AGAINST: Existence is temporal in and of itself. To have an
awareness of it at all is to have an awareness of it directly and as possessed of temporality. But God is eternal, altogether other than, directed away from that which is temporal.

4.76   God is omnipotently omniscient, providential, and self-expressive. *Otherwise he would not reproduce Actualities, Ideality, and Existence.*

A G A I N S T : Since there are modes of being other than God, going their own way, sometimes in defiance of him or his supposed commands, God cannot be omnipotent. Since he cannot know the future (for this is not yet), he is not omniscient. Since there is evil in this world he is not providential. And since his nature is not manifest, he is not self-expressive.

4.77   Actualities relate God's reproductions to the objects of his awareness. *Otherwise he would not have them to encounter.*

A G A I N S T : God needs no help. If he did he would be unable to get it, for God is an independent being, outside all else. If he were not outside all else he would already be at, or with, or in other objects, and would not need Actualities to mediate him and them. But if God reproduces Ideals and Existence, Actualities would not be able to help him become aware of them, for the reach of Actualities is less than cosmic, whereas these have a cosmic range. Also, if he reproduces these others, and is aware of them, there would evidently be no need for him to use Actualities to relate himself to them.

4.78   The Ideal relates God's reproductions to the objects of his awareness. *Otherwise he would not follow the structure of logic.*

A G A I N S T : One need not look outside oneself in order to reason logically. And if one had to look outside one would not be able to reach an individual Actuality or an extended Existence through the agency of an Ideal. Nor does God subject himself to anything, including logic; if he did, he would not be a perfect sovereign being.

4.79   Existence relates God's reproductions to the objects of his awareness. *Otherwise he would not follow the structure governing all activity.*

A G A I N S T : God's acts are not determined, restricted, defined by anything else. Whatever activity he engages in is free. Whatever structure that activity has is there and then produced. If he had to act in consonance with the structure of Existence, he would be subject to alien conditions, and nevertheless would fail to reach an individual Actuality, or a genuine Ideal, or a distinct dynamic Existence, for these are irreducible, ineluctable realities.

4.80   God arrives at the other three modes of being through the agency of love. *Otherwise he would never encounter them in an individual act.*

A G A I N S T : God's love is a gift, a benefaction. It does no relating, serves no purpose for God; it is not an instrument, an agency, a power. But if it were, it would not be directed towards the detaching of possible outcomes, but towards the enjoyment of real beings and the promotion of their good.

4.81   God arrives at the other three modes of being through the agency of divine understanding. *Otherwise it would not be the case that he assents to the reality of purified, ennobled modes.*

A G A I N S T : Granted that divine understanding is distinct from love, it is also quite distinct from the reciprocal of an inferential act. In any case, it occurs freely and is not subject to limitation by any exterior structure or object.

4.82   God arrives at the other three modes of being through the agency of grace. *Otherwise he would never encounter other modes by an act of will.*

A G A I N S T : God's will is a creative will, not a will which seeks merely to encounter an object. His will, also, is not the source of grace alone, but of love and understanding as well. God gives himself and thereby makes other beings better than they were, or he remains within himself and allows them to be unchanged. In neither case does he arrive at other beings or detach them from a relational structure.

4.83   Beginning with God, there are nine primary ways of proving the existence of each mode of being. *Otherwise the modes would not be equally basic and necessary.*

A G A I N S T : If a mode of being could be proved, one proof would suffice. If it had to be proved, it would not have to be proved by God. He needs none of the devices of discovery which men require in the light of their limited vision and knowledge.

4.84 God needs and makes use of Actualities. *Otherwise he would not need and make use of individual avenues for the expression of his nature, intent, and demands.*

AGAINST : God has no need of Actualities, being sufficient to himself. And if he needed them he could not obtain them, for each is self-centered, an ultimate being, other than he. And if he could obtain them he would not make use of them, for being finite and corrupt, they cannot do anything but distort him. God is everywhere; he may be manifest through Actualities, not because he needs or makes use of them, but because he thereby makes them be.

4.85 God needs and makes use of the Ideal. *Otherwise he would not be evaluated; nor could he judge others.*

AGAINST : God's evaluations are made in his own terms and in his own way. He needs no exterior Ideal to enable him to judge. But if he did need the Ideal, he could not make use of it, for it has its own integrity, rationale, being, standing forever outside him.

4.86 God needs and makes use of Existence. *Otherwise he could not have an historic, cosmic role.*

AGAINST : So far as Existence is distinct from God it is characterized by features which God does not have, does not need and cannot use—extensionality, transience, divisiveness. If God needed Existence he would, as other than it, have no power to get it. And if he could get it, he could not use it except by destroying it or himself.

4.87 God preserves Actualities. *Otherwise they would not enable him to be an Other who knows the Good, and who uses transient Existence.*

AGAINST : Actualities pass away, and never are or could be preserved. If God preserves anything it must be a shadow of what is really Actual, not Actualities themselves. And such preservation, precisely because it is his work, will not provide him with what he needs in order to be a distinct Other, to know an independent Good, or to use an Existence which is over against him.

4.88 God preserves whatever excellencies can be obtained from Actualities. *Otherwise he would not be concerned with them as at their best.*

AGAINST: The values of things are ingredient in them; to isolate their excellencies is to destroy them. The preservation of excellencies in God is but a way of God remaining himself; it occurs outside, apart from, in abstraction from Actualities as they really are.

4.89 God establishes the Ideal as a perpetual standard of value. *Otherwise there would be no evaluating of others and no evaluating of himself.*

AGAINST: The Ideal provides a standard of value which makes demands on all. It cannot therefore be the creature of any. God's evaluations in any case are made without reference to an exterior standard; he is the judge of all else, and in his own terms.

4.90 God provides the Ideal with satisfying Actualities and Existence. *Otherwise the Ideal would not be fulfilled; what ought to be will not be done.*

AGAINST: Actualities and Existence are outside both God and the Ideal. If they fail to satisfy the Ideal that is the end of the matter. Were God to help out the Ideal by means of them, they would evidently not themselves satisfy it. Whatever guilt or defect they might have had, because they had failed to do what they ought, would belong to them still.

4.91 God unifies Existence. *Otherwise it would not have an essence.*

AGAINST: If Existence had no essence it would not be at all; it would be indistinguishable from Nothing. Existence has its own unity, and what unification it lacks it lacks without remedy. If God gives Existence its essence, he also makes it be. But he could not do this without existentially acting, and that act would have an essence inseparable from its existence, terminating in an Existence inseparable from the essence of Existence.

4.92   God eternalizes Existence as his private extensionality. *Otherwise he would not reproduce it.*

A G A I N S T : To eternalize Existence is to deprive it of its essential
transiency. And to give God an extensionality is to convert him from
a simple into a complex being, and is therefore to make him into the
opposite of himself. God and Existence are independent. Neither
transforms the other. Each has the other as a counterweight.

4.93   God supplements the work performed by any pair
of modes on behalf of a third. *Otherwise there would be
cases where what ought to be would never be.*

A G A I N S T : God does not depend on other beings for tasks. He
has his own nature, and his activities are dictated solely by himself. But
if in fact he does supplement, complete the work of other modes, what
they ought to do will still not be done by them.

4.94   Each mode completes work God should do on behalf
of other modes. *Otherwise there would be cases where
what ought to be would never be.*

A G A I N S T : Each mode is as complete as it could be. Any addition would come from another mode of being, and would either distort it or make no genuine difference to it. But if it needed an addition
and could get it from God, God could give it this without limitation.
There would then be no need to refer to other modes to complete
the work of God who, after all, is omnipotent.

4.95   All the modes of being merge with the being which
is God. *Otherwise there would be no reaching him.*

A G A I N S T : God is self-enclosed, merging with nothing else. To
be apart from him is to have no grasp of him. And if one merged
with him one would lose either oneself or him, thereby destroying the
integrity of the one or the other.

4.96   A religious man seeks God as apart from him,
convinced that the search will be successful. *Otherwise
his claim would not be: seek and you shall find.*

A G A I N S T : If one is really convinced that the search will be successful, there is no genuine risk involved in religion. To those who do

not make the attempt we can then say only that they avoid a perfectly assured venture. The religious man does not make a search; he is a man who is found by God and sustained by him. All the religious man can himself do is to hope or petition for God's love and forgiveness.

4.97   The search for God is provoked by evil, tragedy, sorrow, pain. *Otherwise he would not be sought as the great preserver.*

AGAINST: So far as a search occurs in this world we may be able to learn something of the temporal causes and effects of what occurs. All else is irrelevance or confusion. It is a particularly poignant mistake to look to God for an explanation of evil, tragedy, and the like, for these are the very antithesis of God, owing nothing to him. Could we begin a search for him, we would be provoked to it not by the bad but by the good things in this world, which alone are like him and express his loving-kindness.

4.98   God can be sought and found anywhere. *Otherwise something would be entirely cut off from him.*

AGAINST: If God could be sought anywhere, he could be sought in dirt, filth, ugliness, vice, and folly. And if he could be found anywhere, one would expect him to have already been found at some place and time. Yet who really has found him? God is not to be sought but to be awaited, and then at an infinite distance. To suppose otherwise is to blur his nature and boundaries, mix him up with what is distinct from, unworthy of, or subject to him. God is in and to himself; to find him one must go where he is, apart from everything else. But one cannot get to him unless he first makes this possible.

4.99   The search for God cannot come to an absolute end. *Otherwise his center would not be inviolable.*

AGAINST: A search for God that never comes to an end does not terminate in God. But then he is not known, and one does not know whether he exists or not.

4.100   God reaches to and finds every other being. *Otherwise he would not insist on himself everywhere.*

AGAINST: Each being has its own rationale and separateness,

and cannot be reached by any other. If God reached to and found other beings he could not be resisted by them. But there are those who oppose him in speech and act, and everything else opposes him in rhythm and career.

4.101 God and men are related in a common field. *Otherwise they would not be together in the same cosmos.*
AGAINST: A field which is inclusive of God and other modes of being is a new mode of being, requiring still another mode to enable it to be together with the rest, and so on without end. Also, if there were a field including him and anything else, he would so far be subordinate to that field, and would thereby cease to be God. God is subordinate to nothing.

4.102 The mystic traverses the field he constitutes with God. *Otherwise he would not reach God.*
AGAINST: The mystic undergoes a private experience; there is no traversal by him to any other realm, for all the while he remains rooted in our space and time, with ideas of the same finite sort the rest of us have, though offered as expressing an experience of God. No one could reach God except by God's aid, but that aid is not forthcoming. God remains forever self-enclosed, a being over against all other beings.

4.103 God completes the work of man. *Otherwise possibilities that must and ought to be would be beyond fulfillment.*
AGAINST: Whatever tasks man has are his own; they cannot be transferred. If they could be, they would not be assumed by God, for he and man have different sets of interests and abilities. Nothing subsequent can wipe out the past, and nothing in another domain can alter what occurs in this. Any performance by God of what men should have done would not change their guilt at all. And they would have to be identical with him—which is impossible—if they are to benefit from what he does.

4.104 Trust is the belief that what man takes to be good is good in God's sight. *Otherwise God would not be faced as deserving man's submission.*

AGAINST: A religious man trusts in God, without conditions. If he insists on conditions he subtracts from God's independence, and from his status as a being who is subject to no external restrictions.

4.105   Ethics and peremptory religion make independent demands. *Otherwise there would be no atheistic ethical men and no wicked religious ones.*

AGAINST: Ethics and religion are both concerned with ultimate values and with what men ought to do about them. They differ at most as part and whole. If they were really independent, two basic equally legitimate enterprises having to do with man's undivided being could be in conflict.

4.106   Scientific and religious claims are independent. *Otherwise they would not be perpetually opposed in method, claim, and discourse.*

AGAINST: Truth is one, and cannot be divided amongst different enterprises in such a way as to permit them to conflict. There are conflicts between partial and inadequate sciences and religions; no conflict between them when fully mature, for they are then occupied with the same ultimate truth in supplementary ways.

4.107   Psychology and religion are grounded in independent attitudes. *Otherwise they would not be directed towards quite distinct types of salvation.*

AGAINST: Attitudes ought to be rectified until they do justice to what is the case. The fact that psychology and religion emphasize different realities, with respect to which attitudes should be rectified, cannot compromise the fact that man's good is one, emphasized in this place by one discipline and in that place by another.

4.108   A proper adjudication requires neutrality. *Otherwise there would be no final reconciliation possible.*

AGAINST: Neutrality is cold, indifferent, too external to make a genuine difference. And if it did make a difference it would add a third party which in an act of adjudication would necessarily distort each claim. No opposition can be overcome by going outside it.

4.109   A genuinely neutral treatment of what is the case is at once prescriptive and descriptive of all the modes. *Otherwise oppositions would not ever be really overcome.*

AGAINST: Each mode of being stands over against all others; each deals with the others from its own perspective. There are no other perspectives to be had. To suppose there are is to endlessly add modes to the accepted modes.

PART III

The Modes Together

CHAPTER 10

Being:

THE TOGETHERNESS OF THE MODES

I   THE PROBLEM AND SOME ANSWERS

HE WHO would like to affirm that there is no more than one entity is faced with serious difficulties. To say nothing more than "One" is not yet, as Plato long ago observed, to say anything significant. Yet to say "One is" is already to have said two things, and in fact to have made a distinction between Unity and Being. An intelligible acknowledgment of a One involves an encounter with a Many.

Yet if there be a Many there must be a number of units somehow together. Were items entirely separate from one another, related in no way at all, they could not add up, make a plurality. A radical atomism offers not a Many but just a One, and then a One, and then a One, and so on, and thus has no way of ever knowing that there is more than one entity. To know that there is a Many it is necessary to have them all brought together under the aegis of a common or comprehensive One.

The problem of the One and the Many is not simply a problem of knowing or saying that there is a One or a Many without somehow knowing or saying the other as well. It is also a problem of how a plurality of entities can be together without the very fact of their togetherness adding another member to the totality of things, which in turn must be brought together with the original set, and so on. This problem haunts every view, for every view acknowledges many entities, if not in the shape of realities, then in the shape of illusions, elements, conditions, words, or beliefs.

To this problem five great answers have been offered in the past. They may be conveniently characterized as (A) Synthesis, (B) Concurrence, (C) Self-Diremption, (D) Dualism, (E) Identity in Difference. Each does, I think, provide some answer to the problem. But each is also faced with embarrassments which cannot, I believe, be avoided unless we take up a new, sixth approach to the problem of the One and the Many.

A. *Synthesis*

Synthesis is a process (of being or of knowing) by means of which disparate elements are forged into a unity in such a way that each of the elements completes the others, offering them the additions they need in order to be as excellent as possible. It is thus a process by which a One for a Many is brought into existence, and the Many is thereby enriched. Taken at its thickest, as maximally engulfing the elements, leaving out either none or little of them so as to constitute a new being which is richer and more substantial than they are, synthesis is a source of novelty in thought or in being, the cause of the emergence of new values and new events in the universe of discourse or fact. Taken at its thinnest, as merely joining the elements with little or no effect on their being or natures, synthesis is a mode of sheer addition, of tying things together in an external way. Thick or thin, synthesis starts with entities which are unstable, incomplete, inadequate taken severally, to bring about a One of all of them, a One in which they achieve supplementation from one another. There are of course many different theories of the nature and need for synthesis, but perhaps all can be treated as variations on Kant's brilliant attempt to explain how what is in fact diverse can be understood and exist in a single irreducible unitary whole. Hegel more resolutely and systematically exploited the idea of synthesis, but the principles and the problems involved in it do not seem to be for him really much different from what they were for Kant. I find four difficulties with the idea.

1. The doctrine of synthesis holds that Many ones are brought together through some act. But then it is evident that synthesis presupposes someone or something to do the synthesizing. And since synthesizing is a real occurrence, it also presupposes, in addition to its Many, an activity affecting that Many. Whatever number of entities there be, if synthesis is the agency by which they are together, there will always be one more entity than those which are synthe-sized, since the synthesizer is another, and there will always be one other fact to take account of, the synthesizing, since this encompasses and is therefore not included in the original Many. Synthesis thus precludes us from saying that such and such make up the Many of the universe of thought or being; no matter how few or how many entities are acknowledged to begin with, the synthesizer and the synthesizing must be added to them to make a larger Many.

2. Synthesis produces a One out of a Many. That One is a func-tion of the Many, and of the method by which they are united. Such a One is only a One *from* a Many; it is not yet a One *for* a Many. A One for a Many must have a Many over against it, which it somehow relates. But a One which is merely produced out of a Many has as yet no significance for that Many. A synthesis somehow must cut back on itself, push aside the very items which it is bringing together, in order to have a Many for the One which it produces.

3. Synthesis operates on a Many. But before it can operate, the various items in the Many must somehow constitute a single Many. If they are entirely cut off from one another, there would be no Many to be synthesized. But if synthesis is the only agency by which a Many is to be brought together, every synthesis must presuppose a prior synthesis. Only because a Many already has a One for it, en-abling it to be a single Many, is it possible to have a synthesis. But then the synthesis is no longer necessary.

4. A successful synthesis yields a new entity. That new entity must be related to the original Many. It must be a One among a Many, make up with the original Many a larger Many consisting of that original Many and itself. It will then require a further synthesis to bring it together with that Many. Every synthesis thus requires a subsequent synthesis to relate its outcome to the material with which it began. No synthesis can ever be more than partial, incomplete, re-quiring ever more syntheses to deal with the problems raised by earlier ones. But unless the problem of the togetherness of the Many were solved to begin with, these subsequent syntheses could not take place.

B. *Concurrence*

Some of the difficulties that beset the theory of synthesis are avoided in the theory of concurrence. On this view too we start with a Many. But instead of invoking a synthesizer and ending with a One which must apparently be synthesized with the original Many, the Many ones are acknowledged to produce a One by the mere concurrence of the Many ones outside themselves at some common point. To my knowledge, no one has urged this as the account of how there can be a One and a Many, though perhaps this idea is at the root of Hobbes's theory of the origin of a state and his justification of sovereignty. In any case the One is here a derivative, which presumably does not add an additional element to the entities with which one starts and which were assumed to exhaust the furniture of the universe. The position takes the Many seriously, seems to account for the One in a way that is intelligible and plausible, and does not, as synthesis seems to do, both require and make unnecessary prior and subsequent acts of bringing the Many together. I find three difficulties with the idea.

1. A concurrence happens either by chance or by necessity. If by chance, there can be no guarantee that the various items in the Many will have a common convergence. A chance production of a One is a production which could conceivably fail. A One is necessary to the Many; it is impossible for there to be a Many without a One; the presence of the One cannot therefore be the outcome of chance. Yet if the One comes about through a necessary convergence of the Many, the Many must act in concert, and in order to do this they must make up a singular totality, presuppose a One. But if a One is presupposed, the need for the convergence disappears. Thus, if a convergence does not presuppose a One it may never attain it, and cannot in any case take place without miracle, for its Many has to be together from the very start.

2. The One at which the Many is supposed to converge is a part of that Many or stands apart from it. It is the former if it is produced by the Many through their convergence; it is the latter if it makes the convergence possible. But if it is the former it is not yet a One for that Many; if it is the latter it is presupposed by and is not the product of the convergence.

3. A One which is produced through a convergence, and which somehow manages to stand apart from the Many, must dominate, encompass, bring the Many together. The Many ones out of which it issued through convergence must lose something of their original separateness or freedom, to constitute that One which dominates them, for otherwise the One would be a new entity adding to the original Many. The Many must engage in an act of self-diremption, self-denial in order that the One be, and yet not be something added to the Many. But self-diremption is a different solution to the problem of the One and the Many—it is, in fact, the third of the suggested solutions.

c. *Self-Diremption*

Instead of starting with a Many, out of which a One is to be generated, it might be thought desirable to start instead with a One, and generate a Many out of it by a process of self-alienation, exfoliation, exteriorization. This is the alternative to which monists eventually resort in order to account for their acknowledged plurality of appearances, errors, or subordinate realities. The most persistent effort in this direction has perhaps been made by Plotinus, although it would be difficult to term him a monist, since he grants that the generated items have a status apart from the generating One. Both his view and the view of the monists, east and west, who minimize the reality of the Many, have the great merit of recognizing the ultimacy and power of the One, and the fact that in some sense the Many is subordinate to and depends on it for its being and its intelligibility. I find six difficulties with this idea.

1. The One by itself is unintelligible. What is without division, without complexity, allowing no distinction—in short, containing no Many—cannot be thought or known. The theory of self-diremption must begin with what it cannot understand, proceed by principles it cannot grasp, and end with what it affirms is not altogether true or real.

2. A One which does not act remains undivided, but in that case it surely does not engage in a self-diremption. To produce a Many the One must act. If it and its act are identical, there is no Many produced. But if it and its act are distinct, they already constitute a Many. The production of a Many by the One already presupposes a Many in the shape of the pair of the One and its act of diversification.

3. The One allows the Many to be over against it—or it fails to produce a Many. But then it must minimize itself in order to give some being or meaning to that Many. This requires it to presuppose a One which is more real than its self-dirempted being and the Many with which it is together. It will become a One in a Many, presupposing a One for itself and the rest of that Many.

4. The One engages in a single act or in many. If the latter, there must paradoxically be a radical plurality before the Many has been generated. If the former, there will be only two things in the universe unless the product of that first act of generation generates a sub-ordinate one, and so on, for a series of steps. This alternative has no beings on the same level of reality or excellence; only beings of different orders. It has a sheer Many without a One, and presupposes a distinction between that One and its act. Consequently, both at the beginning and at the end there will be only a Many.

5. The One, before it gives rise to a Many, is distinct from the One as originating a Many. But then before the Many has been produced we have Many Ones. Yet if the generating of the Many was of the very essence of the One and instantly produced its Many, there would be no act of self-diremption. A One which was always faced with a Many could be said to require that Many, but not to have generated it, and surely not by first being a mere One and then becoming a generating source of whatever else there be. A self-diremptive One must not only be a source of a Many but must continue to encompass it; it must have two roles, and thus itself be a Many from the very start.

6. A generated Many is thrust away from the One or is confined within it. If the former, the Many and the One constitute a larger Many which needs a more inclusive One to encompass it. If the latter, there is no real Many, a Many collected or connected by means of a One. There is only a One. This pair of alternatives touches the core of the doctrine of creation in classical theology. If God creates a universe, he gives it its own existence and the universe no longer needs God in order to be; if the universe does not really stand apart, over against God, there is in fact no universe that he creates.

The problem of the One and the Many cannot hope for solution in any account which starts with one side and tries to get the other out of it; each side has some standing, some being, some meaning apart from and over against the other.

D. *Dualism*

In the end most thinkers are perhaps pluralists; most of them end their thinking or their writing, with a number of items which they tacitly or explicitly grant to be separate, irreducible, merely over against one another. The dualist is a pluralist restricting himself to but two items, one of which may, as in the case of the problem of the One and the Many, itself be a plurality. The dualist says flatly and finally, there is a One and a Many, and that is the end of the matter. Neither generates the other, neither grounds the other, neither owns the other. There is strength in the doctrine; it refuses to minimize the value or meaning of either item. Although it was one of his primary objectives to overcome dualisms of every type, perhaps Aristotle ought to be seen as a persistent dualist, particularly when account is taken of his contrasting views of God and nature, the active and the human reason, form and matter, substance and accident. Those who like Descartes deliberately set themselves to oppose the Aristotelian outlook usually do so without overcoming the basic dualism which defines the Aristotelian view. I find four difficulties with this idea.

1. A One and a Many is a Many. Dualism sides with one of the positions—that which starts and ends with a Many. And yet it confesses that a One is needed, for the One is the necessary correlate of the Many, never to be reduced to it or placed alongside it.

2. A One and a Many form a pair. They must be together in some way, and thus be under the aegis of a One. That One is and must be distinct from the One which is paired with the Many. A dualism thus proliferates endlessly, pairing opposites only by turning the result into a single item to be paired with a One in terms of which the original pairing occurred, then pairing the new pair with a new One, and so on.

3. To form a pair, the One and the Many must be related. That relation is neither the initial One nor the initial Many. It is a third item which somehow must be paired with the supposedly original and exhausting pair. Once again a dualism proliferates without end.

4. A dualism has two final items on a level. If it is to avoid an infinite production of new items to pair, it must refuse to acknowledge anything more than the items with which it begins. These must be thought of as irreducible, final, unrelated. But then to know or grasp or become acquainted with one of them is to be cut off from the other. How then, knowing or having one half of the duality can it be possible to know the other? And if we do not know or have the other, what warrant is there for supposing there is anything more than the original side with which we begin? A dualist, to know his two items, must somehow be above or in both, and in any case must acknowledge something other than and additional to the items with which he originally tried to remain content.

E. *Identity in Difference*

Identity in difference is the doctrine that the final items are in a sense the same: the One is the Many, the Many is the One. Each of the two components is seen to need the other before it can have the status of a full reality. That other is in fact itself from another side; the two sides as together, as one despite their being two, alone constitute a reality. Starting with the Many it acknowledges a One, but not as another item to be added to the Many; starting with the One it acknowledges a Many, but not as a further reality somehow generated out of and standing over against the One. The doctrine is subtle, perhaps too subtle for a noninitiate to grasp, perpetually seeming to disappear as it does into self-contradiction. This is true even in the case of the master of this view, that resolute dialectician and existentialistic rationalist, Hegel.

No one of the Hegelian school seems to have taken the One and the Many with equal seriousness. All tend to favor the One over the Many. They remark that the One exteriorizes itself as and yet continues to possess the Many, differentiating itself from while identifying itself with that Many. There are similar statements to be found faintly urging somewhat similar feats on the part of the Many, but on the whole the Many is taken to be a product of the One, subordinate to it in reality and in meaning. But only a view which takes the Many as seriously as it does the One does justice to the thesis of identity in difference. Such justice will, however, preclude the desire of the school to move from a world of heterogeneous items to a single absolute within which whatever Many there be is somehow absorbed. Taken this boldly the thesis of the identity in difference of the One and the Many seems to accommodate the contentions of the dualists without falling into the characteristic embarrassments of that view. It grants the One and the Many equal status, but it does not cut them off from one another. The other is held on to while it stands apart. To be with either the One or the Many, it holds, is not to be cut off but instead is to have the Many or the One as well. I find three difficulties with this idea.

1. It is not clear whether the Identity is supposed to be identical with or different from the Difference. If it is identical with it, we have nothing more than sheer Identity; if it is different from it we have a radical dualism inside the initial Identity in Difference.

2. Each basic reality is supposed to have another with which it is identifiable. But then Identity in Difference should have an other. The basic reality will, as a consequence, not be expressed as an Identity in Difference but rather as an Identity in Difference connected by an Identity in Difference with its other. This last in turn will need an other of its own, and so on.

3. If the One is in any sense an other of the Many it must have features which the Many does not have, or lack features which the Many has. If this were not the case we would have nothing more than just a One or just a Many. Yet if the One and the Many are genuinely distinct, the acknowledgment of both will inevitably lead to the acknowledgment of one more entity, another One, a One for both. This, because distinct from the original One and Many, will require the acknowledgment of another One, and so on.

II   ON BEING TOGETHER

EACH OF THESE five answers has considerable power. No solution to the problem of the One and the Many which neglects their insights will eventually do. A satisfactory account must, like the theory of synthesis, recognize that if we start with a Many, a One must be an emergent of some sort and yet not add to the total number of entities in the universe. It must recognize, with the theory of concurrence, that the various members of the Many must have a common One, but must avoid thereby compromising the status of that One as a One for that Many. With the theory of self-diremption it must acknowledge that the One is presupposed by the Many as that which allows many items to be together and thus make a Many, at the same time that it recognizes, without compromising the fact that the One is as basic and as real as the Many, that this Many is an inevitable referent of that One. With the dualist it must affirm that the One and the Many are on a par, each irreducible and final, but related in such a way as to make possible a knowledge of them both. And finally it must, with the defenders of the doctrine of Identity in Difference, recognize the fact that, despite their diversity, the One and the Many are not alien to one another in meaning or in being; but this recognition must not lead to the abrogation of the law of contradiction, nor prompt the forging of irresponsible paradoxes. This is a formidable array of demands; yet one cannot avoid trying to meet them except by giving up a claim to be self-critical and systematic beyond any preassignable limit.

For simplicity's sake let us begin with a consideration of only two entities, x and y, making up a Many. Let these be all the beings that there are in the universe; let them be viewed as irreducible, final realities, two independent basic dimensions or modes of being. Let us once again use the symbols "x,y" and "x.y". "x,y" expresses the demand that x and y be together. It presents x and y as simply over against one another. They cannot of course be in this state unless they are united by the ","; the "," is a unity *of* them as separate from one another, and demanding that there be another unity *for* them. That other unity is symbolized by the "." There will be an "x,y" only so far as the x and y together constitute the ".". The "." is x and y as merged, as terminating in each other; the merging of x and y is what constitutes the togetherness of them both. Like a point which is the outcome of the intersection of two lines, a border which is the limit of two figures, a standing erect which is the outcome of opposite stresses, the "." exists only as something constituted by the very items it serves to sustain. It has a nature of its own but only so far as x and y continue to stand over against it as distinct, in "x,y". The "," is also constituted by x and y; it also has a nature of its own, but only so far as x and y stand over against it as merged in "x.y".

Each of the elements, x and y, acts on and is blocked by the counterthrust of the other. Neither the "," nor the "." is an entity additional to the x and y; each expresses their togetherness, the one so far as they are distinct, the other so far as they are intermingled. For each of the elements, x and y, however, the "," and the ".", which it constitutes with the help of the other, is something over against it. As partly constituted by the x, the "," and "." belong to that x, and the x, in order that the part of its being which it contributes to make the "," or the "." should not be in the control of y, is driven to try to possess them entirely. It tries to make them part of itself. Could it succeed it would then possess the y by virtue of its possession of that part of the "," and "." which is continuous with the y. It never wholly possesses these; it can never manage to do more than to deal with them from its own angle. As a consequence it never gets to the y entirely, but ends only with an abstract of it, what y is when approached by x through the agency of a biased mastery of the "," or the ".".

No matter how much of x is comprehended by y, or how much of y is comprehended by x, the x and the y will continue to be as they were. The mastery of each by the other occurs within the area defined by "," and ".", the one expressing the fact that there are *two* entities together, the other the fact that the two are *together*. Each says what the other does, but in a different way The "." has the x and y together but at the price of their distinctness; "," can have the two so far apart that there is only a minimal connection between them. We can say, if we like, that "." is one mode of togetherness of which "," is the other, the first having a minimum of the being of a togetherness while the second has any degree above that minimum. Or we can say with equal justification that "." is x and y in one guise, of which "," offers a complementary other, the first distinguishing them in a variable degree, the second in a steady, maximum way. In either way of speaking the "." will represent a *de facto* descriptive togetherness while the "," will represent a required prescriptive togetherness; both are always exhibited.

There is always a difference between the "." and ",". That difference we can characterize in a "." way or in a "," way, the one stressing the togetherness of the "." and the ",", the other their distinctness. And these two characterizations can themselves be characterized in two ways and so on without end. This is a harmless progression, for it is a progression in analysis and not one towards presuppositions which have to be settled before there can be the situation with which we in fact began. We always have both a "." and a ",". And when we try to say how they are one we must continue to keep

them distinct as a many. From the standpoint of "." the "," is a whole
set of "." which never make a single whole; from the standpoint of
",", the ".", is the unreachable limit of more and more intimate relations between x and y. Each standpoint expresses what the other is.
If we wish to avoid either standpoint, we but take the standpoint of
an abstract mind. We then first assume something like the position of
the "," and go on to treat the "." as a manifold in which "." is a kind
of "," but lacking the separativeness of the ",", which we have in
mind.

Granted that there are only two beings, x and y, there must then
be two forms of togetherness, represented by the "." and the ",".
Each of these requires that the other be. They are polarities of togetherness, correlatives which exist by virtue of the fact that each
being approaches the other in a double way. If a unity could be made
of the "." and the ",", each member of the Many, the "x" and the "y",
would be divided against itself. But each of these is a unity. And because it is a unity, a genuine being, it provides a needed One for the
two ways in which it is related to the other.

The two forms of togetherness refer to one another, the one demanding a separateness, the other a merging of the items they relate.
But one of them, the ",", can be said to be primarily normative for
the other, since it states the minimum which any togetherness must
exhibit or the maximum it ought to exhibit. However, it exerts no
compulsion on the other, for a compulsion can be imposed only by a
real being. It just states an inviolable, perpetually fulfilled condition.

There are then two Manys in which the x and y are members, "x,y"
and "x.y". Each of these Manys has a distinctive type of togetherness.
The two Manys, as are the two types of togetherness, "," and ".", are
not directly related to one another but via the unitary beings, "x" and
"y". Each being offers a distinctive One for both the forms of togetherness, and therefore for the two Manys in which that being can be
a constituent.

Any single mode of being would be radically indeterminate were
it not over against some other. To be determinate is to be opposed to
and opposed by. What is completely indeterminate is indistinguishable
from Nothing. But Nothing is an indeterminate which is determinately what it is, and thus is either a plurality with an indeterminate
and a determinate member, or is an impossibility. But if there are two

beings, they must be somehow together, and kept together. They must be united by an effective agency. If this did not have a counteracting agency connecting the original two beings in an opposing way, the two beings would be absorbed within the agency which unites them. To be two beings which retain their being when and as they are united, they must be united in effective oppositional ways. These oppositional ways are what a pair of beings appear to be from the vantage point of the beings they relate; from the perspective of these oppositional ways, the original two beings are agencies for keeping these ways merged as well as distinct. The relating of the ways of togetherness is via the items which are related; they mediate these ways just as these ways relate the beings to one another.

The One and the Many are related by a kind of *identity in difference*, for the "." and the "," articulate one another, restate one another in different terms. The one presents in a united way what the others has as separate. But the relation of these two is not a paradoxical selfsameness which is different; each is the continuation of the other, the extreme limit of what the other exhibits. They can be said to form a *duality*, but not as a pair of items characterizable in the same terms. The full being of the "." requires the distinguishing of its items by ","; the being of "," requires their merging as ".". Both the distinguishing and the merging are necessary. Nor does the existence of "x" and "y" involve the production of another entity "," or ".", which together with them make a new Many. The x and y exist as "x.y" and as "x,y". These Manys are inseparable; if we start with either, we must express ourselves through the use of the other. They can be had as distinct, but only by our standing over against them in a neutral position. But then it is evident that their status as distinct is but a way of articulating the fact that we have them together, not directly but via the unities, "x" and "y". Starting with "x.y", the "," is the product of a *convergence;* starting with "x,y", the "." is the product of a *self-diremption.* But in neither case do we get a being separated from its origin, a genuine other adding another fact to the universe, additional to that with which we began. And finally the "," and the "." can each be viewed as a product of a *synthesis* of the x and the y, but a synthesis which never had to be performed. The synthesis of "x,y" is completed in the ".", and of the "x.y" in ","; the "." and the "," exist when and as "x,y" and "x.y" do.

We started with x and y. They make one Many by virtue of a togetherness ",", and another Many by virtue of a togetherness ".". These two, "," and "." are not new entities; they are x and y together, in a prescriptive and in a descriptive way.

III   THE FOUR MODES TOGETHER

THERE ARE not two, but four basic modes of being, four irreducible realities, each needing the others in order to be a constituent of the cosmos. The foregoing analysis must be extended so as to apply to them. The four of them are and must be over against one another and yet together.

The forms of togetherness of the four modes of being are distinct from the kinds of togetherness possible to any pair or triplet of modes. The forms of togetherness of the four are complete, ineffective, without power of being, and thus are incapable of actually interplaying with the four. The four modes cannot make a single whole and cannot therefore have a unity over against which they can stand. They cannot be made subordinate to some neutral mode of unifying them all; they are related to one another by virtue of those powers which they themselves exert. The togetherness of beings is the being of them together.

The being of the four modes together is the four of them together. Such a togetherness is not a new, distinct entity; it is a fact constituted by the demands or thrusts of each to the others as met by their counter demands and counterthrusts. Each of the modes is, from its own position, together with the others in a way in which they are not together with it. There are then four ways in which the modes are together. These four ways can be represented by ",", ".", "⊃" and ".·.". The first expresses an eternal condition, the second an actual way in which beings can be with one another, the third the fact that the modes are structurally involved with one another, and the fourth an existential area of their interplay. Each of these requires the others; each defines a different kind of Many; each stands apart from the others.

The four modes of being constitute four sets of Many, each with its distinctive form of togetherness. The four modes of being are thus in four Manys, and each of these Manys has its own distinctive way of being together. The four modes also offer the four Manys (and their ways of being together) distinctive ways of being united; each provides the four Manys with a distinctive type of One, enabling those Manys to be together in one of four ways. The Manys never make one single neutral concrete Many. Could they do so, they would by that very fact require the dissolution of all the modes of being, break them up into an inside and an outside, a process and a terminal point.

We can get genuine full neutrality only when we can get to the position where we have the four modes together in such a way that no one of them is functioning as a relation or One for the others. Such a position transcends, wholly escapes the bias of the different modes of being. One never can, however, escape some reference to them. As a consequence there can never be less than four types of neutrality, four ways of speaking of all of the beings. There is the neutrality of knowledge achieved by the Actuality which is man; the neutrality of appreciation which is exercised by God; the neutrality of subjugation characteristic of the Ideal; and finally the neutrality of ubiquitous manifestation characteristic of Existence. Each is the outcome of an effort, inside the area of some one mode, to overcome its own bias by abstracting from itself as a concrete interrelated mode of being. There is no way of amalgamating these four efforts, no way of being neutral in all four ways at once except so far as a mode not only abstracts from itself in its concreteness but takes full account of the others—or what is the same thing, except so far as one of these forms of neutrality is recognized to have a fourfold structure in which each of the others has a characteristic role to play.

IV   BEING AND THE MODES

IF WE TRY to make a unity of the various types of togetherness, we will have to make each of the beings into a plurality. Togetherness can be said to be polarized into a plurality of togetherness by each of the Many to the extent that this maintains itself as a unity. The plurality of unified beings requires a plurality of Manys, which in turn requires a plurality of ways of being together. We can stress any one of these beings and make it into a supreme One having the rest as a Many for it. But we cannot make a genuine all-encompassing One out of them all. We can bring beings together only in a correlative set of ways. We cannot therefore ever get to the stage where we have only one being, one Many or one One. But we can abstract from the characteristic bias of any being, any Many or any One, and grasp what the others are. We will then lose the Ones which in fact govern the different Manys, and in their place will put a distillate of them which is neutral to them all only to the extent that it lacks their power and concreteness.

Each mode of being is what it is only because the others are. May not the same thing be said with respect to the various Actualities there happen to be in this world? May not these be only so far as and because they are opposed to one another? Is it not the case that each, precisely because it is the other of all the rest, dialectically requires and is required by them? Actualities would then, instead of being so many different instances of one mode of being, be so many different modes of being. Instead of there being just four modes, there would be at least as many as there were Actualities, and whatever these entailed. A number of difficulties stand in the way of such an idea.

Firstly, Actualities have something in common; they have common characters, needs, and objectives. But the modes of being exhaust being, and do it in diverse and opposed ways. There are no features which they share, no needs they have in common, no terminus at which they together point. Secondly, there is a real space connecting the Actualities, but there is no such space between the various modes. Even if one were to view space as a kind of dialectical agent which precipitated itself out as distinct Actualities, this would not yet make those Actualities into the dialectical termini of mere being, and thus would not define them as real modes of being. Thirdly, Actualities come to be and pass away, whereas the modes of being do not. What the latter require must be, and is. If Actualities required one another, what must be might not be. Fourthly, the modes of being oppose one another without residue, because they are beings which leave over no being to connect them. But Actualities, precisely because they do not exhaust being, can be connected. The space, time, objectives, unity which encompass them owe part of their being to what is other than Actuality. A plurality of Actualities is together in an area made possible by other modes of being.

Each mode of being possesses three nonessential features, pointing to the reality of three distinct and effective modes over against it. Each mode of being also possesses three nonessential features pointing to a reality of a mode of being in the guise of a relation between the given mode and another mode of being; it also possesses three nonessential features pointing to the correlate of this relating mode. To hold that there are less than four modes of being is to hold that there are less than nine nonessential features in some mode of being. To hold that there are more than four modes is to hold that there are nonessential features in addition to these.

We know that there must be a position outside the four modes taken severally, for we do speak of them together, from a position not implicated in the being of any of them. It is a neutral position which we reach by an abstractive act in which we balance the bias of one mode by the others, thereby revealing the position to be without efficacy with respect to any of them. We know, by virtue of the very way we get to it, and by virtue of its constitution, that the togetherness of the four modes is not a fifth mode of being. But might there not be a fifth mode alongside the other four, for which we have been unable to obtain any evidence as yet? If there were, the togetherness of all the modes should have a nonessential feature pointing to the reality of this fifth. Either then the forms of togetherness we now know are not forms of the togetherness of all the modes, or there is a nonessential feature of a togetherness of which we know nothing, or there is no fifth mode. In short, the warrant for the supposition that there is a fifth mode is that there might be a form of togetherness or some feature of which we know nothing. But ignorance provides no warrant of any sort.

Unless, however, one can show that the fifth mode is impossible one is left with the result that though there are in fact only four modes, there might be five. But for there to be five modes, a togetherness of the four modes must (*1*) be identical with that fifth, or (*2*) be over against the fifth. (*1*) If the togetherness of four were like the togetherness of two or three, it would have to be identical with a fifth mode of being. This would require it to be effective, to be ingredient in each of the remaining four and they in it. But this it is not. And the five of them would have to be together in a new way, so that there would be a sixth mode which was the togetherness of the five, and so on and on. A togetherness of the four modes is too ineffective and indifferent to be a fifth mode. (2) Nor could the four modes as together be over against a fifth, for then the togetherness of the four would have a being of its own requiring that the fifth mode be in fact a sixth—which is a self-contradiction. There cannot be a fifth mode of being without a togetherness of four modes becoming a mode additional to the four, but yet one which is distinct from the fifth, and so on.

There are no more and no less than four modes of being. To be is to be one of four beings. What is less than all four is an imperfect being; what is more than all four is self-contradictory; what is just four is being as exhausted in four modes together.

As one passes from one mode to another one brings into focus a different way in which they are together. Just as the modes exhaust the meaning of being, so these four ways exhaust the meaning of togetherness. To be is to be one of four distinct modes; these constitute four distinct ways of being together. He who was primarily interested in the fact of togetherness can with justice treat all the modes as products of the juncture of the four ways of being together, but then he must go on to affirm that these products themselves produce the different ways in which they themselves are together. For him the world would be a tissue of "ands," the thickest being identified as a primary togetherness. For us the modes are primary and constitute the bare fact of their togetherness. Only the latter way of speaking does justice to the truth that we never can entirely free ourselves from the fact that we at least are, and thus ground and are not functions of a number of states of togetherness.

Understanding:

THE ACCEPTANCE OF THE MODES

I THE PROBLEM AND SOME ANSWERS

WE UNDERSTAND an object just so far as we can follow its adventures —before, after, or while they take place—in a context other than that which we as knowers provide. We understand something when we treat it as having one significance in the context provided by us as knowers and another in a context which it has apart from us as knowers. Despite the fact that the object is approached from an individual perspective, it can be known so far as we are aware of it as also facing away, as having a nature and consequences outside the apprehension of it. To understand that this before me is a pencil is to confront it as having a status apart from that confrontation, as capable of being used, of being seen from another side, and so on. To understand that this before me is brown is to confront it as being sustained by some object and thus as subjected to a career which cannot be deduced from a mere consideration of it as a sheer color. To understand that one and one is two is to confront it as that which can be entertained by another, or by myself at another time. To know is to respect the other, to deal with it in other terms as well as in ours.

While confronting an object, he who would know it must see it as having a status apart from that confrontation. Not to confront the object at all is not to have it as an object to be known. To have it only in relation to himself is to experience it, to live with it, as something undergone or encountered, but it is not yet to have it as something for a mind. But if understanding requires us to be aware of an object as apart from our act of apprehending it, we would seem, while confronting an object, to occupy another point of view at the same time. How is this possible? How can we grasp what something is from a perspective which we do not in fact occupy? The question becomes most acute when we reflect on the fact that it is of the essence of the work of historians, sociologists, and psychologists to try to deal with times, places, customs, and outlooks not their own. And the question is particularly acute for anyone who holds that there is more than one mode of being. Where is it that we stand when we speak of another mode? Where do we stand when we speak of all of the modes?

There are at least nine different approaches to this problem which seem to offer hope for a solution: (A) the theory of adumbration; (B) the affirmation of the Nothing; (C) the doctrine of the Golden Rule; (D) the bifocal view of knowledge; (E) the principle of analogy; (F) the act of sacrifice; (G) the idea of adoption; (H) the power of rejection; and (I) the hypothesis of the microcosm.

A. *Adumbration*

In all perception we divide and abstract from what we encounter, synthesizing the result in a perceptual judgment. But when and as we do this we directly adumbrate, reach into the shadow cast by what we have isolated, and make immediate contact with the being over against us, as other than ourselves, and as other than the content that we obtained from it and accepted in our judgment.

Knowledge never exhausts what is the case, for all knowledge is knowledge of that which is not yet caught in knowledge. Since for pure empiricists all that is significant is gathered from experience, and since for them this can yield only probable knowledge, there is no alternative for them other than to say that it is only probable that their knowledge at each moment fails to exhaust all there is and can be known and that it is conceivable that they might be ignorant no longer and thus are in fact omniscient. We know that we are now ignorant. This cannot be a consequence of the discovery that we were ignorant in the past—for then it would be only probable that we are still ignorant—but of the fact that here and now, while perceiving this or that, we adumbratively apprehend that there is still something lying beyond our knowledge. To deny the act of adumbration is to deny the very grounds of a "contrite fallibilism."

Strictly speaking, adumbration occurs only in perception; it reaches to other beings only in an act having reference to what those beings are then also cognitively being judged to be. Adumbration therefore is not adequate to account for our nonperceptual grasp of other modes of being, though the distinctions it involves must evidently be carried over into a more comprehensive account. More important perhaps is the fact that adumbration approaches objects through the veil of ex-teriorly employed terms, judgments, meanings. But what is needed is an understanding of objects from their side. Adumbration tells us that there is such a side, but it does not tell us that this is at least as in-telligible and basic as that which we embrace in judgment or dis-course.

B. *The Nothing*

Whatever is apprehended is comprehended, held within the orbit of the apprehending being. What terminates its apprehension is, *for it,* a Nothing. But in fact it is another being with a counterthrust, a being whose direction and efforts are opposite to that of the apprehending being. That is why the apprehending being has something at which to terminate. But he knows it, one can claim, as only a Nothing.

A Nothing is empty, devoid of content. If all we know of what is in fact beyond us is that it is a Nothing, we will not know anything about the nature of what is not yet caught inside our perspective. Also, if that which lies outside our apprehension is a Nothing, we, the knowers, must be no less Nothings than the beings we apprehend. The two Nothings would be opposed to one another, the one sustaining, the other terminating the act of apprehension. We would then know a Nothing as over against a counteracting Nothing, or we would not know we were knowers and that there was an object to know. In either case, knowledge of something positive would stretch between two presupposed points outside its reach, which alone were supposed to be real. Positive knowledge would be knowledge only of what was not real.

A Nothing is a being in opposition to our own. This truth enables us to recognize that the content of our knowledge is encompassed in knowledge, and that the object to know is exterior to and as real as ourselves. But it does not yet tell us just what is there for us to know, nor enable us to know it.

c. *The Golden Rule*

The Golden Rule commands us to do to others as we would have them do to us. Given epistemic use, it says that we are to recognize that others have a meaning, being, ontic need, and satisfaction just as we have. It enables us to affirm that what lies beyond us is on a footing with ourselves. Through the use of the Golden Rule in an epistemic guise we can say, as we ought, that the mode of being we enjoy is co-ordinate with other modes of being.

The Golden Rule stresses the ethical component in knowledge, asking us to respect others as much as we respect ourselves. But this rule is effective only so far as we already know something of the others; it does not tell us how to know this. And so far as the others are different in nature and need from ourselves the rule can serve to distort and frustrate rather than to help or illuminate. No use of the Golden Rule tells us how the other modes of being differ from our own; no use of that rule tells us in what sense these are on a footing with us, or how they are to be understood.

The Golden Rule rightly urges us to do justice to others, but this justice may require that they also be treated in terms altogether other than those that pertain to ourselves. We must make use of the Golden Rule in order to take account of the fact that the other modes have a claim to be understood from their own point of view. But it does not tell us how to evaluate that claim, or even how to satisfy it.

d. *Bifocality*

To be affected by others we must maintain ourselves, repulse them when and as we yield to them. To affect others we must be met by them, accommodate ourselves to them when and as we impose ourselves on them. Every act includes a retreat as well as an advance, an imposition as well as an accommodation. The act of knowledge exhibits this duality in the form of a reference to the knower, inseparable from a reference to what lies beyond; nothing less than the double acknowledgment is adequate to the content had in knowledge. On this view we need not, in order to be able to take account of what is other than ourselves, suppose an act of adumbration in addition to that of analysis or judgmental synthesis, acknowledge a Nothing over against ourselves, or assume an attitude, towards what lies beyond, similar to that

which we assume towards ourselves. The very act of knowing is bifocal, pointing in two directions at once. We are self-conscious when
we are conscious of; conscious of when we are self-conscious. What
we know points at once to ourselves and to what is other than ourselves. This bifocality, however, is only referential; it does not tell
us the nature of what lies beyond.

E. *Analogy*

Analogy is a mode of reasoning by which we attribute to a new
case a comparable or proportionate power or feature of an old. It has
been thought at times to be the only available device for dealing with
beings which are ultimately diverse, not subject to a common genus.
Thus for Thomists there is no idea which can encompass both God
and the world; yet both are real and intelligible. The principle of
analogy enables them to speak now of God and then of the world in
terms proportionate to their different excellencies. If God is a father
his relation to his children is analogous to the relation that a human
father has to his children. But since God is infinite in power and wisdom we must recognize that his concern for his children will be cor-
respondingly more effective and wise than that characteristic of a
man.

The four modes of being, because final and exhaustive, are incapable
of being encompassed in some more inclusive genus, or in some other
being. Analogy would seem therefore to be the only appropriate way
of dealing with them. To be sure there are analogous features in all
four. But analogical reasoning begs the question one seeks to answer
with respect to them—how do we know these others with their analogous features?

Analogy starts all over again, taking up its stand with each being in
turn. But the initial question is how we are to get to the others, how
we are to know what they in themselves demand, and thus just what
concepts are appropriate to them. It surely is right to say that all
things are to be understood in appropriate terms; but this is not too
helpful so long as we do not occupy the positions of the others but
know them only from our own. Analogy tells us rightly that we ought
to take up the position of others if we are to understand them correctly. But it does not tell us how to do this. Instead it presupposes the
achievement which it is intended to promote.

f. *Sacrifice*

If sacrifice is not to be an act of self-purgation, a denial of oneself, a submission to the judgment of another, or a futile gesture involving the giving up of something needed to one who does not need it at all, it should give a disadvantaged being the opportunity to achieve its proper status. Now, whenever we know something, we disadvantage the object known by placing it in our perspective. To allow it to have the content which we have mastered, we must sacrifice to it what we have mastered, give to the disadvantaged thing the very content we took from it. This is not a mere repayment, a redressing of a balance; the content which we have isolated and which does not exist except by virtue of our act of cognition, is offered to the object as its meaning. Knowledge is a referential as well as a possessive act; it refers to the object what we have in fact taken from it, though in a form which bears the mark of ourselves as well as of it. Sacrifice in this sense is indispensable to all knowing; but it does not of itself enable us to know other modes of being, for it is only so far as we already know them that we can know just what and how much is to be given to them.

g. *Adoption*

A mere knowledge is without extent and without localization in fact. To know something is to impose what we have in mind on what we do not have in mind; it is to prescribe the very structure, the meaning, which the object that lies outside us is to have. To know is to adopt an object, frame it in terms provided by us. Those terms, instead of being alien to the object, are terms which give it whatever meanings and values it has. From this approach other modes of being have only the natures which we in knowing endow them with; all that the modes, as apart from us, can do is to sustain what we say of them.

This position has been well exploited by Kant, though to be sure in connection with a somewhat different problem. Any account of things must, if it is not to be distortive, express a structure or meaning of what exists outside the knower. But since knowledge idealizes, has meaning apart from the dross of actual existence, the structure or meaning which the knower imposes must, before the imposition, be somewhat distinct from that on which it is imposed. The imposition of it must in a way structuralize, make it become the very meaning of that on which it is imposed. Since it is imposed from the mind, from a perspective other than that on which it is imposed, the imposition must involve some degree of construction of the object known.

This solution entrains almost as many difficulties as it resolves. If the object known is without structure of its own any imposition would be as good as any other. And if there are four modes of being, from the angle of each there would be no way of distinguishing among the other three, except arbitrarily through an arbitrary use of indifferent, irrelevant structures.

H. *Rejection*

Every being is opposed by and opposes every other. Each is the reject of all else; it is of its essence to be not this, not that, and so on. And the others in turn offer ways of rejecting it, of not being it. Whatever beings there are, are divided off from one another; each holds itself away from the others. This truth is in no way compromised by the fact that each also imposes itself on and even adjusts itself to the others.

To reject is, as it were, to place a "not" before all else. This placing of the "not" is a way of imposing oneself on it, of adjusting oneself to its nature. Each mode of being can thus be said to reject the others, and to be in turn the unity of the triple rejection which begins with the other three. Yet if each is necessarily rejected, there is nothing left to do the rejecting; mere opposition makes no provision for something to engage in the opposition. If each is to be over against the others, it must have a positive nature of its own. The rejected rides on the surface of what is positive; it neither suffices to make the four modes possible nor to enable us to know just what they are and how they differ.

I. *Microcosm*

The understanding of oneself involves a reference to others as well as to oneself. The knowledge of oneself is a categorial knowledge of which one part is substantialized as oneself and the other parts are substantialized as other modes of being. He who knows himself knows that there are the others, and knows, just to the very extent that he knows himself, just what they are.

A man knows by means of a category in which he functions as one mode of being over against three other modes. As a being he answers to that portion of the category which characterizes the Actual, and when and as he does this, the other modes of being answer to the other portions. To the degree then that he knows the nature of his own being, he knows the nature of other beings; they are contained in meaning and in principle within him as dimensions of the category in terms of which all knowing occurs. He is a microcosm containing the meaning of all the modes of being in the guise of a principle which is illustrated by whatever there be.

It is hard to see how this consequence can be avoided. But it has little use unless we are able to know ourselves, and unless we are able to understand how the category is illustrated in other beings. Each being must have the category as its meaning; but since the modes differ, they must have the category in diverse ways. A knowledge of the category as requiring the being of other modes does not yet tell us what these modes are like.

II   THE CONDITIONS FOR KNOWING

LET US SAY to begin with, that there are only two modes of being, or only two parts to an ultimate category. Let us say that each mode is ultimate, that together they exhaust the universe, and that each provides a perspective in terms of which the other can be apprehended. Then we must say, I think: (A) Since both modes are known, they must be in relation to a mind or a knower. (B) Since there are no other positions besides these two, the knower must occupy one of them. (c) Since both modes are known, both must have a status apart from him, as knower. (D) Since knowledge requires a grasp of what things are like from a position occupied by the knower and also from a position not occupied by him, he must be able to approach the two modes in two ways. He must be able to confront them and to have them as not so confronted; while in one perspective he must somehow make use of the other perspective.

These considerations require us to distinguish (1) an absolute indispensable perspective, I, in which the knower confronts what is known; (2) the two modes, X and Y, as distinct and exclusive, occupying a status apart from the act of knowing; (3) the modes in the guise of data for knowledge, x and y; (4) the knowing perspective, I, as related to X and Y, the modes of being; (5) X and Y each as related to x and y, i.e., the modes of being as having each other and themselves as data; (6) the knowing perspective, I, as related to x and y, the data.

Let us identify the X with the being who knows, and with what can be known of him; let us identify Y with some other mode of being, and y with the guise it has as a datum for a knower. Unless knowledge is to be distortive, the absolute perspective, I, must be pure, translucent, grasping the modes of being, X and Y, when it possesses them in the guise of the data, x and y. x and y are X and Y respectively, viewed in relation to I. They are abstract versions of X and of Y nondistortively possessed by I. The I in possessing y knows Y. Since the knower is one with himself as knowing, I and X must be one when and as I knows Y through y.

The mode of being, Y, is on a par with the mode of being X. It offers a perspective on that X. For the I to have the X as an object of knowledge is the same thing as for it to have the datum x from the standpoint of Y, since the difference between x and X is the difference which Y makes to X. If the I could not grasp what Y encompassed of X, that is to say, x, the I would not know what it was to know. To know what knowing is the I must have some grasp of both X and x from the position Y outside them.

I and X are one and the same position, but it takes the guise of an I in confronting the data, x and y, and the guise of an X when enjoying the role of a mode alongside the mode Y. In self-consciousness, the X is identified with the I. But for the I to know X it must adopt the standpoint Y, face X in the shape of an x. When the knower is self-conscious he knows himself to be an X, but as mediated by x. He thus gets to himself only by first taking the position of an X dealt with from position Y. He knows himself therefore when and as he knows the import of the Y, i.e., what he himself is from the standpoint of Y. Y x-izes X, and when I knows itself it must have itself as a datum, see itself as x-ized. It thereby is able to know the difference Y makes and therefore what it means to occupy the standpoint Y.

X deals with the Y through the mediation of y; reciprocally, Y deals with X through the agency of x. X-y, X as facing and possessing the datum y, is related to Y, as a form to a content; Y-x is similarly related to X. This means that X-y and Y are reciprocals, each exhausting the import of the other, allowing nothing over but the fact that there is an X which is imposing the X-y on the Y, and that there is a Y sustaining the X-y. The form, X-y, both in reality and in knowledge, together with the content, Y, of which it is the form, constitutes the being of Y as that which is over against X. The content Y is the content for just that particular form, X-y, the form which X imposes.

The form and content make a single entity, the Y as related to the X. When held apart, the form X-y is made more abstract than it was, and the content, Y, is allowed to become more brute. Taken by itself each will be at once too large and too alien to be appropriate to the other. If we start with one we will have to search for, inquire for the other, and will often miss it and end in error.

Statically viewed, from the perspective of X, y is Y as made abstract, and Y is y as made concrete. Dynamically viewed, X approaches Y as that which is to be formalized as X-y; Y accepts X-y as that which Y is to actualize. To know that Y is to be formalized as X-y is to hold on to Y while approaching it from the standpoint of X.

There is nothing more to the knowing I as over against X and Y but the capacity of each to refer to the other; there is nothing more to the factuality of the knowing I than the fact of their mutuality of reference. Because the I expresses itself exhaustively in both X and Y, they become known reciprocals of one another. X and Y exhaust the knowing I just by being together, and the I in turn formally exhausts them as the meaning of their togetherness.

The I is not a third thing. There is only X and Y together. "It is meaningless to ask," said wise old Aristotle, "whether the matter of a thing and that of which it is the matter are one"; X-y is one with Y; it is Y "X-ized," Y as subject to a condition imposed by X. The I by taking up the role of X-y distinguishes itself from X and thereby recognizes that there is a Y; its grasp of the difference between itself as X-y and the X is identical with its grasp of Y as other than X.

There are then two senses of knowledge. There is knowledge as rooted in the primary perspective I. It is in terms of this that we

look at everything, X as well as Y, and in which we possess the data
x and y, and assume the roles of X-y and Y-x. And there is the knowledge that is carried out under limitation, which deals with x and y as
enjoyed from the position of Y or of X. In one sense we as knowers
never enter into the being of X or Y, for we remain always an I
in terms of which we isolate data, x and y. But in another sense we occupy both X and Y at once. We never know except by being identical
with one of them and then confronting all else as material to be used
by us while it is being grounded by something else.

III   KNOWLEDGE   OF   THE   MODES

WHEN WE CARRY OUT the above distinctions and multiply them to accommodate the problem of knowing the four modes of being, we
must distinguish the I, the indispensable perspective, from W, X, Y,
Z, the four modes, and must distinguish these from w, x, y, z, respectively the data which each provides for the others. The discussion
in Chapters 1 through 4 were primarily concerned with W, X, Y, and
Z, as having bearing on one another, and thus as providing the data,
w, x, y, z. Actuality, for example, was dealt with as referring to the
Good (1.106), to Existence (3.09), and to God (4.15), and was in
turn looked at from the vantage point of all three (2.17, 3.12, 4.84).
   Each of the four, W, X, Y, Z, offers a content articulated by the
other three. In three ways a datum is abstracted from each, expressing
what that mode is as envisaged from the standpoint of some other
mode of being. To know what X is is to know what the others need
for their integrity, for they, in relation to it are just three different
demands for X. The knowledge of X is a grasp of it from the position
of W, Y, and Z. Such knowledge is the outcome of the fact that the
I sees each as confronting the others. This the I can do, for the I is
only their togetherness, which assumes the shape of a category of
cognition in an Actuality and other forms of categorization in the
other modes. Because the I is the togetherness of all, it can be in all
four modes; so far as it is a cognizing perspective it is biased towards

one of the modes, X. But by virtue of its abstractness the I can compensate for that bias, transcend the limitations of that cognized mode in its concreteness, as alongside and over against the others.

W, X, Y, Z are modes of being whose togetherness is expressed formally as I. That I is translucent when made abstract in four different ways. Translucent as a category of knowledge for an Actuality, it is also translucent as a category of appreciation for God, a category of relatedness for Existence, and a category of evaluation for the Ideal.

All four modes analyze the I in characteristic ways. Conversely, it is each of them in a different guise. For each mode the I has a concrete illustration as just that mode, and an abstract and translucent status as a formal category for which the various other modes are content. Since an actual knower is in one and not all four modes of being, a knower cannot have the I, as a neutral position, or the togetherness of all modes, except as an abstract category of knowledge. This category differs from other abstract versions of other modes of being in the fact that it is sustained only by Actuality, that it deals with w, x, y, z only in an X way.

The I then can assume four different *functions*, be in the four modes in different guises. And when exercising each function it assumes any one of four distinct *positions*. It can have the position of a form apart from all the modes, allowing them to stand apart from it and from one another; it can be in contact with them as having a bearing on one another; it can blend with them while stressing one of them to make it the perspective in terms of which content is apprehended; and finally it can be submerged in them so that its distinctive nature is in no way manifest in them, to permit of the grasp of content from one perspective as that which is also in the other perspectives. As standing apart, the I is the Actuality of man in his most private recesses; as in contact with the modes it is man in the guise of Existence, as at once one with and over against what is other than himself; as blending with the modes while stressing one of them, it is man in the guise of the Ideal, as taking a position of the possible in terms of which all else is to be understood; and finally, as submerged in the modes, it is man in the guise of an eternal unity in which the knower has lost his individuality and sees only what is to be seen in fact.

A man is at once actual, existential, ideal, and divine; as the first he is primarily appetitive, as the second he is primarily active, as the third he is primarily a value, and as the fourth he is primarily a unity. All four states are his at the same time, not because he is chaotic or confused, but because he is a being who, while maintaining an absolute and translucent perspective, can also stand outside it by allowing it to be limited in various ways, and can confront himself, as in those limited ways, with what he encounters in other limited ways. For him, as for everything else, to be is to be the category in concreto. The I is diversified fourfold in him, at the same time that it is quadruply exhibited in each of the other modes of being.

There is no surd in the universe. Yet there is more to the universe than ideas or knowledge. The insistence with which a cognizing I approaches a mode of being has its reciprocal in a submission to that other as something to know. What the one demands the other provides both in content and in meaning. It could not be otherwise without making knowledge just a way of hoping and an encounter just a way of suffering, both forever without reason and without answer.

Knowledge makes use of all the nine approaches that were passed in review in the first section of this chapter. Each of these approaches was found to be wanting, but this was because they were dealt with separately. The act of knowing is a single act whose nature can be properly expressed only by taking account of all of them. Knowing requires a moment of adumbration, the reality of a Nothing, an exemplification of the Golden Rule, a two-way movement, a use of analogy, an act of sacrifice, a genuine adoption, an effective rejection, and a role as microcosm. In knowledge we adumbrate, but the nothing at which this stops is experienced in a counterthrust whose value is appreciated through the use of the Golden Rule. That rule is employed in the very act of knowing as at once an advance and a retreat, which comes to rest in the object in a way analogous to that in which it comes to rest in the knower. The knower can grasp the object as his other only so far as he endows it with what has been abstracted from it in the act of knowing.

Knowledge is a strategy, open only to Actualities. It enables them to replace their "horizontal" concrete approach to others by a "vertical," one which is capable of encompassing them without distortion. It is Actuality as having attained the state of neutrality, as having become the togetherness of all, though at the price of an abstraction from its concreteness. Knowledge is possible because the category of knowledge is the cosmos in miniature, desiccated, located within us, and within the very beings which our knowledge abstractly possesses. Or, to express this same truth from another side, knowledge is possible because an Actuality is engaged in activities which exhibit in a truncated, impure form the very needs, drives, and structures characteristic of knowledge. We are Actualities who can know, and what we know is what is so, for knowledge is the world as distorted by our being but recovered in an abstract form by our minds.

What is true of Actualities is true also of the other modes; they too, in order to do completely what they cannot adequately do in the concrete, must engage in a strategy. They must endeavor to attain the stage of neutrality, the position of a togetherness of them all, by abstracting from their own characteristic concrete, but biased efforts. What knowledge is for Actualities, correct evaluation is for Ideality, universal co-ordination is for Existence, and appreciation is for God. But whereas Actuality can only sometimes, in the guise of men, in fact exercise a power to know, these other modes of being (since they are primarily singular) always exercise a universal, neutral, and abstract, as well as limited, biased, and concrete powers for dealing with others.

An actual mind and body, an ideal value and intelligibility, existent indivisibles and extensions, a divine appreciation and self-satisfaction are extremes in the different beings enabling them to grasp the nature of the rest. These extremes are inseparable from an inward region, capable of endless nuance. What emotion is for that Actuality which is man, structure is for the Ideal, restlessness is for Existence, and self-assertion is for God—the middle between their extremes, revelatory of their inward beings, i.e., of the self, of reason, of divisiveness, and of unity, and open to endless variation. This middle is the counterweight of a single, unanalyzed concern reaching towards the others. All the modes are biased, are strategic, are in themselves, and are concerned with the others.

Knowledge, at once articulate and experiential, is rooted inwardly in the emotions and outwardly in what is adumbratively encountered. It does not offer a superior way of getting to others; it is just the best way that is open to Actualities.

CHAPTER 12

The Cosmos:

THE INTERPLAY OF THE MODES

I   THE NEEDS OF ACTUALITY

THE FOUR IRREDUCIBLE, distinct, but interrelated modes of being—
Actuality, Ideality, Existence, and God—have much in common with
Plato's motion, rest, other, and the same; with Aristotle's efficient,
final, material, and formal causes; with the scholastic's substance, form,
matter, and being; with Kant's quantity, quality, relation, and modality;
with Hegel's thesis, synthesis, antithesis, and Absolute; with Croce's
ethical, logical, economic, and aesthetic moments of the spirit; with
Whitehead's actual occasions, eternal objects, creativity, and God.
And if one were to add a fourth category of individuality to Peirce's
original three, they correspond somewhat to a Peircean fourth, first,
second, and third. There are, however, striking differences, not the
least of which is the fact that each mode has a finality of its own, and
has systematic and dialectic relations to the other three modes. A
schematic account of the ways in which the various modes affect and
complete one another may make it possible to see this most readily.

From the perspective of the Ideal, an Actuality has the status of an
occasion (see 2.17); from that of Existence it is a focal point (see
3.12), and from the perspective of God, it is himself multiplied (see
4.62). The Actuality in turn affects these in different ways; it makes
the Ideal germane to this world in the guise of The Good (see 2.15);
it converts Existence into a field of relations of contemporaneity (see
3.09), and turns towards God as an eternal judge (see 4.88).

An Actuality exists, in itself and on its own. Its Existence is not borrowed. Still, at every moment it must make an effort to hold on to its portion of Existence (see 3.59); if it fails, it ceases to be present. It is supported in this effort by God; he in fact infects the Actuality with Existence in such a way that, despite the loss of Existence, a simulacrum of it pertains to the Actuality as past (see 4.17). To have Existence properly one with it in the present, the Actuality also needs the help of the Ideal, so far as this keeps abreast of what is happening (see 2.20).

An Actuality has a nature (see 1.07); that nature is its own. But it does not wholly possess it, thus making it possible and plausible always to speak of it as though it were a universal instead of a singular being. It is because it is supported by God that it is able to own the nature while singular (see 4.16). It is God's insistence on the realization of the possible in an Actuality that justifies one in saying that an Actuality, despite its singularity, is one of a kind, an individual in a class. To have the universal one with itself to the maximum degree, the Actuality also needs the help of Existence. This makes it have the meaning as part of its being as present, so that when the Actuality is in fact past it has a determinate nature, a being which is to be understood as that which was once present (see 3.43).

Finally, an Actuality is a substance, distinct and separate from other Actualities and other modes of being (see 1.08). To be fully over against all else it must have the status of an Other. Since otherness is a symmetrical relation, to be a genuine Other, the Actuality must be over against an Absolute Other (see 4.15). This is God. By virtue of its contrast with God, an Actuality is a genuine being in itself. But the separation of the Actuality as an individual from God as individual can never be carried out fully without the aid of Existence and Ideality. Existence is a divisive force. That in which it is integral is cut away from the rest of things, but without precluding its continuity and contemporaneity with them. Existence intensifies the otherness of Actuality to such a degree as to make the Actuality a being involved in a sequence of effects in time (see 3.13). Ideality supplements this consequence of Existence. Because of the pressure of the Ideal in the direction of an Actuality, the Actuality's possibility stands out over against other conceivable divisions in the Ideal (see 2.23), and the Actuality as a consequence is distinguished from others in its promise.

Each of the other modes helps out the Actuality to be fully what it seeks to be. God gives it an otherness by virtue of which it is an individual; he also helps it with its Existence as is manifest from the fact that it can be past, and helps it with its meaning as is manifest from the fact that it is intelligible. Existence gives it vitality in the present; it also helps it have a determinate meaning which it can retain in the past, and to be an individual with a future. The Ideal provides it with the objective which enables it to be one of a kind and helps it to exist as that which is intelligible though individual.

II　THE NEEDS OF IDEALITY

FROM THE PERSPECTIVE of Actuality, the Ideal is the Good (see 1.106); from that of Existence it is the Future (see 3.12), and from that of God it is the Principle of Perfection (see 4.85). The Ideal in turn affects these in different ways; it ennobles the Actual (see 2.98), gives Existence a desirable direction (see 2.99) and provides God with a desirable value (see 2.100).

The Ideal is an ideal for others; it is determinable, specializable, possible. These are designations which require it to be related to these others. It is the function of Actualities to make the Ideal into a possible Good for this world (see 2.15). But there is no guarantee that an Actuality can actualize what is possible for it. Since a possibility that is never realized is not in a world which allows it to be realized, the realization of the possibility must be assured by what is neither Actual nor Ideal. This assurance is given by God (see 2.14) who provides whatever supplement is needed to fulfill whatever in fact is possible. This assurance would be precipitate were it not limited by Existence. Existence gives possibilities a needed space-time import (see 3.104).

The Ideal has being; it is independent of, exterior to all others. But it must also be relevant to the beings that would realize it. God sees to it that the Ideal is realized in Actualities and Existence in such a way as to have its historical meaning exhausted in time (see 3.92). If he did not do this, the Ideal would not really be relevant to what in fact occurs. This work on God's part is, however, qualified by Actualities who deal with that divinely guaranteed possibility in the guise of The Good (see 1.106). It is also qualified by Existence which limits the work of God to what can be accommodated in a moving present (see 2.22).

Finally, the Ideal provides a standard of the excellent. This standard is given cosmic status by Existence, which offers it a causal ground (see 3.07). Actualities impose limitations on this work on the part of Existence, transforming the Ideal into a Good that ought to be realized in substantial, limited beings (see 2.15). It is a standard, however, which serves to measure all realizations in Existence or Actualities, and must therefore transcend these. It is one of God's functions to provide the Ideal with the status of a perpetual standard in terms of which all beings, including himself, can be evaluated (see 4.89).

Each of the other modes enables the Ideal to be fully what it should be. God directly gives it an essential historical relevance, and helps it both to be fully realized and to function as a standard for all. Existence directly gives it a cosmic vital role, and helps it have a space-time import and to be pertinent to the present. Actuality, finally, makes the Ideal something possible for this world and helps it attain the status of the Good and to be realized in the world of things.

III   THE NEEDS OF EXISTENCE

FROM THE PERSPECTIVE of Actuality, Existence is the domain of contemporaneity (see 3.09), from that of the Ideal it is the domain of the logically underivable (see 3.10), from that of God it is a power governing all becoming (see 3.11). Existence in turn makes things into present concordantly effective Actualities (see 3.38), turns the Ideal into a Future (see 3.12), and makes God have the status of an essence (see 3.99).

Existence is in a perpetual process of spatial division (see 3.05). Still it has being and thus some unity. To be able to be fully it must be fully integrated, united to constitute a single being. This unity it acquires from God (see 4.21). Such a unity is only of Existence as by itself. But Existence is also part of Actualities. If the unity of Existence which God provides is to be continuous with the Existence in Actualities, those Actualities must constitute a consonant spatial whole (see 3.06). In addition to the unity it acquires as a spatial field, Existence needs a unity in time. Temporally self-divisive, it needs the help of the Ideal, which hovers before it as its single meaning, to enable it to be a single being while in time (see 3.04).

Existence is expansive (see 3.02). This expansiveness needs limitation, a boundary. Such a boundary is given by Actualities; these offer it so many different terminal points (see 3.03). They do not suffice to bound Existence enough—or more correctly, they bind it too much. Each tends to separate off parts of Existence, holding on to its own portion over against the rest. For Existence to have a unified meaning the help of the Ideal is necessary (see 2.102). But the Ideal remains external to it. Existence needs a more integrated unifying boundary. This is what God enables it to have. He helps out the limiting of Existence by the Actual and the Ideal, thereby giving Existence an appropriate essence (see 4.21).

Existence, finally, has a lawful nature, and needs this in order to continue to be selfsame despite its divisiveness. It must point to the Ideal as that which gives it direction, thereby making its course more than a surge of temporal activity (see 3.101). But the Ideal does not suffice to make it entirely law-abiding, since it is something pointed at, guiding it from the outside as it were. God is needed to help impose that Ideal on Existence (see 4.23), making it in fact, and not merely in aspiration and by virtue of the manner in which it strives, have an order of its own. But neither an Ideal nor a divine order reaches to the core of Existence as the dynamic surge of the world. The aid of the Actual is required. Actualities by virtue of their possession of Existence infect it with their individual rhythms (see 1.27); the way in which they habitually behave determines just what laws prevail in Existence. The harmonious habitual activities of existent Actualities complete the work of the Ideal and the divine in giving Existence its needed law-abiding nature, without which it would be a surd incapable of being understood, or of being effectively productive.

Each of the modes helps Existence to be fully what it should be. God directly endows Existence with a unity restraining its divisiveness, and he helps it have a rationally apprehendable boundary as well as an order of its own. The Ideal directly gives Existence the direction it must have to be law-abiding and helps it to have a unity, as well as a boundary preventing it from expanding endlessly. Actualities, finally, directly limit the endless expansiveness of Existence, and, through their concordant activities help to give it a unity, and by virtue of their habits help to give it a law-abiding career.

IV THE NEEDS OF GOD

AS ONE ONLY of the modes of being, God is inevitably limited by, and needs the help of the others. He has virtues and powers they do not have. But the converse is also true; they have virtues and powers he does not. God is a being in and of himself, as are the other modes. From the perspective of Actuality, he is the preserver (see 4.87); from the perspective of Ideality, he is one who guarantees a final, completing satisfaction (see 4.90); and from the perspective of Existence he provides a needed unity (see 4.91). In turn God treats Actualities as data (see 4.67), accepts the Ideal as an avenue for expression (see 4.70), and confronts Existence as extended (see 4.73).

God makes a difference to what else there is. He is a being of power, effective everywhere. But he is not as effective as he can be, except so far as he makes use of Actualities as so many different channels through which he can make himself manifest (see 4.84). No one or no set of Actualities, however, is altogether adequate to his full majesty. No one or no set of Actualities is excellent enough to be able to do full justice to God's need to make his power effective. The contribution that Actualities make to the exhibition of God's power must therefore be supplemented by that made by the Ideal. This helps him to achieve a more satisfactory expression by making him relevant to the Actualities (see 2.103). But unless Actualities in fact move to that Ideal, they will continue to offer so many different inadequate channels over against one another. Existence must help out both the Actual and the Ideal by providing an inclusive unifying third avenue for the omnipresent exhibition of God's power (see 4.86). God is manifest in cosmic space and time under limitations imposed by Actuality and Ideality.

God is a being, but only one of four basic kinds. To be as excellent as possible he must make his own the kind of excellence which each of the others contribute to the universe. Excellent in himself, he is nevertheless not good in terms appropriate to other realities unless he adopts and adapts the principle of value expressed in the Ideal (see 4.85). But this principle of value is thin, not actualized, not very good. Value must be expressed throughout the whole range of space and time if it is to be a value worthy of God. It is the function of Existence to help out Ideality's effort to provide God with a needed excellence; it makes his adoption of the Ideal not an adoption of an ideal hope, but one relevant to the very structure of historical peoples and civilizations (see 3.92). But unless the Ideal be also exhibited in Actualities possessing a unity and individuality of their own (see 4.84), it will prove too homogeneous and yet too unlimited to do justice to God's richness of being. God must adopt and adapt them as well as the Ideal, if he is to enjoy the multiple facets of individuality which the multiple Actualities provide. God is completely God only when he has made his own the standard of value given by the Ideal, the temporality provided by Existence, and the individuality provided by Actualities.

God is a unity, but a unity which, despite its simplicity, its lack of divisions, is endlessly articulatable, capable of diversification without limit. By himself he has neither occasion nor opportunity to diversify himself cosmically. But Existence gives him both. It is self-divisive, and by accepting it he becomes explicitly what he is implicitly, a being capable of distinguishing himself from himself (see 4.86). A diversification which is not exhibited in Actualities will, however, fail to do full justice to God's self-identity, the self-identity of a substantial, active, individual being. Actualities multiply God concretely, for they are so many different ways of being self-identical (see 4.62). But since Actualities perpetually struggle and are in conflict, only so far as they are under the aegis of relevant possibilities will they be capable of doing justice to God's nature and need (see 4.68). The diversification in space and time which Existence provides, the ethical diversification which Actualities provide, and the rational diversification which the Ideal provides, are all needed if the interior richness of God is to be given occasion to fully be.

Actualities directly provide God with channels for effective action, and help God be more effectively expressed and to become significantly diversified. The Ideal directly provides God with a principle of value and helps him be historically significant and to be diversified in excellent ways. Existence, finally, directly gives God the opportunity and occasion to be endlessly diversified, and helps him be omnipresent spatially and temporally.

These different references to the different modes from angles provided by the others fulfill the injunction that we ought always to respect what is not ourselves. The other modes have virtues, limitations, and supplements as basic and as important as our own. Wherever we are and with whatever we deal, we ought, if only to do justice to ourselves and what interests us, to take seriously whatever else there be, recognizing that it has its own virtues, limitations, and supplements.

V THE FOUR STAGES

THE DIFFERENT MODES, because they have a finality of their own, offer justifiable perspectives on one another. This fact contains a whole nest of issues.

Each of the modes, for example, offers a norm for the others. The Ideal presents a norm in the guise of a value, the Actual one in the guise of individuals, Existence one in the guise of activity, and God one in the guise of unity. Severally they say that the others are more or less good, more or less individual, more or less vital, more or less unified. Conversely, each mode endeavors to realize that single norm which is constituted by the three norms represented by the others. The Actual should be at once good, one, and dynamic; the Ideal should be at once individual, dynamic, and one; Existence should be at once one, rational, and individual; and God should be at once dynamic, individual, and excellent (see 2.21, 2.104, 3.12–14, 3.106, 4.05, 4.90, 4.93).

No being fully realizes the norm offered by some other. The nature of the failure differs from being to being. The Good is too universal to be wholly attainable; individuality is too private to be fully assimilable by another; activity is not exhaustible in any series of beings or occurrences; unity is too simple to permit of full embodiment outside of God.

Each of the modes of being has characteristic ways in which it seeks to satisfy its characteristic norms, leading it to engage in a distinctive process of mastery. The Actual adjusts, the Ideal subjugates, Existence permeates, and God sympathizes. This means that time itself must have four forms, answering to these four different types of process: it is primarily material for the Actual, a structure for the Ideal, a process for Existence, and a datum for God. All four are of course together in the very sense that the four modes of being are together.

Each mode as it attempts to satisfy its norm goes through a process in which it approximates the natures and rhythms of the others. In its characteristic way each insists on itself, offering a *condition* to the others. In this stage it is outside them and merely presents them with something they ought to meet. In the second stage it urges itself, *demands* a conformity to itself. In the third stage it accommodates the others, *adjusts* itself to their presence. And in the fourth and final stage it is one with them, *receptive* to what they in fact are. But since the others remain in and of themselves, engaging in activities not geared to theirs, the last stage is inevitably preliminary to an initiation of a new first stage.

In its full being each mode is receptive to the others, but since those others have their own needs, and in fact can never be accommodated by the others, the receptiveness is not answered appropriately. The receptiveness consequently gives way to the condition, this to the demand, this to the adjustment, this to a receptiveness, and so on, the stages differing from time to time in quality, in strength, in duration, and success. Each mode imposes itself on the others, and because each imposes in ways that reflect its own nature and ultimacy, they together preclude the achievement of a final equilibrium in which one dominates over all the others, or where all are at rest. They are always together, always concordant in being, but the nature of their common togetherness is biased now this way and then that, through four stages.

In ordinary inquiry we start with one of the modes, but do not stay with it long. Instead of keeping constantly in one direction, we accept one standpoint for only a short while, and then move on from there to another. Instead of examining, for example, how God gives guidance to the Good, we soon take up, say, the standpoint of the Good and then perhaps proceed to look at Actuality as material for that Good to use in its effort to become fulfilled. The result is that in the ordinary course of events we soon become acquainted with each of the modes for a while, and perhaps even for a time may note how all of them appear from the position of each. But since we then do not stay with any one standpoint for long we cannot help but have a rather confused body of principles and an inadequate grasp of the four modes, and therefore of the universe and of ourselves.

The reflective mind should be both flexible and disciplined. Starting from one mode it should persistently deal with a second. Not until it has made the second a matter of systematic examination should it deal with the way in which the second faces the first and the others. But because life is short, we cannot remain too long with any one mode. Our reflections must be cut short by the need to take seriously what reflection reveals—that there are other modes of being than our own, and more than one way of encountering them. Each of us must be at home with all four of the modes of being for some time, if only to know who we are and what else must be. And this we fortunately can be, even in our most common-sense conventional moments.

VI   THE   LIMITS   OF   PHILOSOPHY

THE MOST ORDINARY assertion, such as "this is a hand," does not express merely what the speaker believes. Nor does it hold just for this or that moment. It confronts us with what is supposed to be true for any man and for all time. To be sure, it is stated by some one man and relates to some particular matter of fact occurring in some limited region. But it claims to present an objective truth, open and available to all. Anyone who would exercise ordinary powers and bring to bear that minimal body of knowledge characteristic of an ordinary man would, it claims, make the same assertion in these circumstances. Anyone who makes the assertion takes himself, at least implicitly, to be a man like every other, exercising a typical degree of competence in observation, exhibiting a normal intent or purpose to communicate, and having the same degree of honesty and about the same knowledge, language and experience that any other has. To make the assertion is to maintain that one is qualified to speak for all, precisely because one is making a normal use of power daily used by all. If the assertion is mistaken it may be due to a distortion possible to any man; it could be the result of a kind of tribal error to which all are subject under those circumstances. Unless the speaker is one who has not functioned as he himself in the asserting claimed that any man would, he offers an assertion—whether correct or not—on behalf of every one of us.

An ordinary assertion claims to say nothing more than what might in fact have been said by anyone using the very powers he exercises daily. Those who present themselves as spokesmen for ordinary men go further. They claim to say what any man would say had he fully exercised the powers which he now uses only in part. The philosopher, artist, mystic, and mathematician or scientist go still further. They say what anyone in principle could, but in fact now cannot and most likely will never say. Daring though ordinary assertions are, then, they are more moderate than those made in philosophy, art, religion, mathematics, and the sciences. These require for their discovery and therefore claim the support of a more radical kind of honesty, a greater technical competence, a longer-ranged purpose, and a wider body of information than daily existence demands. These exceptional powers, though achieved and exercised by individuals, are attributable to a man only if he exercises them as a representative of all. The powers that he uses the others do not; but they are powers that in root are resident in all. What he therefore comes to know and say expresses what all the rest in principle could have known and said. Were the individual philosopher, artist, mystic, or mathematician to puff himself up as one who is superior to the rest, he would cancel out the very virtues which fed his pride, give up the exercise of the very powers which carried him to this point, for he would then and there make them serve his ego instead of using them impersonally, on behalf of all. And when he errs he can no longer take comfort in the view that his error is perhaps tribal, for he does not claim to exercise only the powers daily used by any man, but rather to exercise powers which, while resident in all, are exercised by only a self-chosen few. Both as an individual and as a member of a special group, the erring philosopher exposes himself as one who has taken on a task too big for himself, thereby misrepresenting the unarticulated wisdom of mankind which he had made it his task to express, free from the distortion which undisciplined mankind necessarily incorporates into any exercise of the wisdom which is native to it.

We tend to overlook the fact that as ordinary men we speak in absolute terms, offering a truth for all and always, because we do not usually question our daily assertions, particularly if we can make some rough tests then and there, or can find some occurrence in daily experience which it was reasonable to expect might ensue. But there is no matter of fact which can logically substantiate the claim to have asserted an absolute truth, a truth holding for all men and all times; consequently, none of the disciplines, even the most practical, is ever content with the slipshod absolutism of daily life. Every assertion made in a discipline is supposed to be capable of being approached from many angles and of withstanding a long and arduous examination. A philosophy even goes so far as to subject itself to radical self-criticism; it drives itself by means of dialectic and speculation to consider extreme and hard, even challenging cases; it asks all to judge it for nothing less than its competence to give an ordered account of whatever there be. It claims that anyone starting with the same facts, studying them with the same degree of intelligence and with the same submissiveness to the evidence, sustained by the same sense of importance, and exhibiting the same need to bring all basic truths together, will not only come to the same result that the philosopher did—which of course is inevitable—but will in fact offer a true and adequate system, since the powers that he will exercise will be those which are productive of the truth. It maintains that the system will be found wanting only so far as the philosopher failed to function as the representative man he was supposed to be, and therefore only when he did not use the intelligence, sensitivity, and persistence which a true, impersonal, and adequate account requires. What the system says may go counter to what men expressly assert and even counter to what they presuppose, but it cannot go counter to the wisdom of men incorporated in their common being, unless the powers used are not common human powers latent in everyone—in which case the philosopher is so far not a man among men—or are not appropriate to the achievement of knowledge—in which case philosophy at least and other disciplines perhaps are unnecessary or foolish, despite the fact that they do clarify what is otherwise left obscure, do enhance and purify what is dull and incoherent, and do criticize and test what is otherwise accepted or ignored.

The philosopher, artist, mystic, and mathematician cut beneath the distinctions which mark the judgments of ordinary men, busy about practical and local affairs. Since they try to dislocate parts of the daily world and to exhibit them in more appropriate media, they seem to the practically minded to be engaged in little more than the production of fancies, folly, and nonsense. But as a matter of fact they are all quite realistic, presenting their objects at their purest, as no longer unduly restrained and improperly qualified. To know what the color white is, we ought to look away from snow and paper and skin to white as isolated by the artist and allowed to have being as a mere, sheer white, a white no longer arbitrarily limited by and adventitiously related to other quite alien beings. Snow is too stupid, too insensitive to offer a good lodgement for white—this Berkeley saw but Aristotle did not. But snow does offer it a lodgement of some kind—which is what Aristotle saw but Berkeley did not. It seems wise with Aristotle to affirm that snow gives lodgement to white, and wise with Berkeley to affirm that white needs a different type of carrier than snow if full justice is to be done to its nature.

No mode of being or part of one can be adequately grasped except so far as it has been freed from the guise it usually has for us in daily experience, where an alien punctuation has been imposed on it by the other modes. The freeing of Existence from alien constraints is best achieved by art. Art, to be sure, never concerns itself with pure Existence. What it does is to separate off some portions of Existence—sounds, colors, words, acts—from the restrictive limits which other modes and particularly Actualities impose on them. It is a primary task—seen most clearly by such moderns as James Joyce, Josef Albers, Gertrude Stein, and perhaps Frank Lloyd Wright—to let these freed items exhibit their characteristic rhythms by giving them no other context but Existence itself. Pure Existence thus, though not directly apprehended or enjoyed in art, becomes a primary medium for the fragmentary cases which the artist isolates in common experience. A similar work is performed by mystics with respect to the divine. They purge the divinely grounded unity of themselves and some other things of the qualifications which were imposed on them by Actualities and other modes. They then let these freed items exhibit themselves as carried directly by God or his representatives. Mathematicians engage in analogous work with respect to the Ideal; they separate instances of the Ideal from the limitations imposed on them by other modes, and attempt to place the resultant isolated quantities, shapes, and so on in revelatory relations to one another inside the Ideal. These efforts presuppose an ability to use and even to know the natures of the different modes of being.

To deal with other modes properly it is necessary to sacrifice concreteness for universality, effectiveness for neutrality. Philosophical knowledge is the outcome of one such sacrifice, enabling an Actuality to master what would otherwise be beyond anything but a biased grasp. In a similar way appreciation is the outcome of a sacrifice on the part of God, just as co-ordination is a strategy exercised by one who represents Existence, and evaluation by one who represents the Ideal. To be successful each of these approaches must provide a place for the kind of apprehension achieved by means of the others. Genuine knowledge contains within it moments or facets of appreciation, co-ordination, and evaluation. Only such knowledge is proper to philosophy. Only so far as he possesses it has a philosopher a right to speak for all men and therefore to present us with assertions which should say what all in principle could but none otherwise would in fact say or know. When he finds that his characterizations are not in consonance with what the modes reveal themselves to be, he knows that he has spoken as an isolated individual who has failed to make proper use of an opportunity to utilize available powers, and who therefore can do little more than express himself in irresponsible paradoxes or repeat uncritically both the truths and errors of common sense.

Philosophy is at once bolder than common sense and more restrained than art, religion, or mathematics usually allow themselves to be. This is because the philosopher is not content to grasp just one mode or parts of it in a purified form, but seeks to know all four modes. His venture is similar to that which occupies God, and which would be duplicated by any one who sought to apprehend the four modes from the standpoint either of Existence or of the Ideal. A concern for all the modes restrains the philosopher's speculative flight by qualifying it with the recognition that he is to think as a representative of all men in their full unexpressed being. Though the artist, religious man, or mathematician is also sustained by and representatively expresses powers possessed but not used by the rest, he does not use powers which express more than a facet of the being of man. The philosopher in contrast seeks to express the whole of human wisdom, which is to say to make himself not only represent the rest but to express them and thereby express what it is they, by virtue of their being, in principle know. This effort of his is one with his effort to know himself. To know who he is he must know what he represents; to know what he represents he must know what it is for man to be; and to know what it is for man to be he must know the modes of being, since these and their subdivisions are all that there is and can be.

The philosopher must, through the agency of speculation, attempt to articulate the substance of the common being which he shares with all. If his system is to be dialectical and categorial, i.e., if it is to offer root characterizations of whatever there be, it must reflect mankind's being in a world which is partially and superficially encountered every day. But what mankind basically grasps is unfortunately much overlaid with and partly obscured in daily life by conventional common sense; a little later than most, but still quite soon even a philosopher will forge explanations which reflect little more than what has been conventionally accepted and which often ought to be summarily rejected. For self-protection, and therefore to fulfill his duty as one who seeks to know what is in fact the case, it is desirable for him to pay more attention to other creative enterprises than has hitherto been the custom. He needs their help if he is to correct an almost irresistible tendency to settle for the conventional, and thereby spoil what should be a representative systematic, speculative account of an encountered world.

Philosophy provides those fundamental characterizations which always apply to the real. Cosmic in reach, it is incurably abstract. With justice it criticizes every other enterprise as too narrow and unsystematic, and they with equal justice criticize it as too pallid and general. It can explain, account for them, and they can account for it—just as it provides an explanation for its several parts while they in turn provide an explanation for it as a whole. Taken as a single, organic, articulated system, comprising an interlocked set of parts with distinctive functions and meaning, philosophy explicates rather than explains. At its best it offers a highly general, neutral statement of the whole of being as exhausted in four distinctive irreducible modes. But since it is primarily an expression only of an attempt to know, it will even then fall short of doing all that can or ought to be done if all that is is to be encompassed. What is can be adequately apprehended by nothing less than a complete philosophy, supporting and supported by a comprehensive system of values working through all time and effective in eternity.

Recapitulation

The Topical Headings

Actuality

1.01   An Actuality is a being in space. (*See 4.62*)

1.02   Some Actualities are active. (*See 1.44*)

1.03   "Some Actualities are active" is necessarily true. (*See 1.02*)

1.04   Some Actualities cannot act. (*See 1.02*)

1.05   There are two types of primary, or active, Actuality: simple and complex (*See 1.01, 1.03*)

1.06   Actualities are temporal beings. (*See 1.05*)

1.07   Actualities have characteristic natures which enable them to be known and distinguished. (*See 1.01*)

1.08   Primary Actualities are distinctive, persistent, resistant, insistent beings in space and time. (*See 1.01, 1.04, 1.06*)

1.09   There are primary beings which are not Actualities. (*See 1.05*)

1.10   There are derivative modes of being. (*See 1.01, 1.08, 1.09*)

1.11   There must be possibilities. (*See 1.09*)

1.12   There must be a field. (*See 1.01, 1.09*)

1.13   There must be an eternal being. (*See 1.09*)

1.14   No Actuality can be absolutely perfect. (*See 1.01, 1.11, 1.12, 1.13*)

1.15 Beings condition one another. (*See 1.14*)

1.16 Each Actuality is unified. (*See 1.05*)

1.17 Actualities engage in acts of self-adjustment. (*See 1.15, 1.16*)

1.18 Actualities affect other beings. (*See 1.15, 1.17*)

1.19 To be at its best an Actuality must adjust itself to others. (*See 1.18*)

1.20 Each Actuality attempts to subordinate and accommodate others. (*See 1.08, 1.19*)

1.21 An Actuality seeks to adjust itself to possibilities. (*See 1.11, 1.19, 1.20*)

1.22 An Actuality seeks to make the field integral to itself, and to submit to it. (*See 1.12, 1.20*)

1.23 An Actuality strives to adjust itself to eternity. (*See 1.13, 1.20*)

1.24 An Actuality engages in all efforts at adjustment together. (*See 1.20–23*)

1.25 All four efforts qualify one another. (*See 1.15, 1.20, 1.24*)

1.26 An Actuality's attempt to deal with other Actualities is qualified by its attempt to deal with possibility. (*See 1.21, 1.25*)

1.27 The attempt of an Actuality to deal with other Actualities is qualified by its attempt to deal with the field. (*See 1.20, 1.22*)

1.28 The attempt of an Actuality to deal with other Actualities is qualified by its attempt to deal with eternity. (*See 1.20, 1.23*)

1.29 Each Actuality attempts to turn all other Actualities into concordant beings under the common aegis of a possibility, a field, and an eternity. (*See 1.26–28*)

1.30 Each Actuality uses other Actualities. (*See 1.26–28*)

1.31 Some Actualities can change without losing identity. (*See 1.16, 1.17, 1.18*)

1.32 It is not of the essence of an Actuality to occupy a particular region of space. (*See 1.01, 1.08*)

1.33 Not everything is eternal. (*See 1.06*)

1.34 There is causality. (*See 1.02, 1.33*)

1.35 The category of causality is an inexpugnable, unrejectable way of ordering what occurs and what we encounter. (*See 1.02, 1.03, 1.34*)

1.36   When a cause is actual, its effect is only possible. (*See 1.02, 1.11*)

1.37   To know a possible effect we must infer to it from its cause. (*See 1.35, 1.36*)

1.38   At least some effects are deducible from their causes. (*See 1.37*)

1.39   An actual effect occurs subsequent to its cause. (*See 1.36*)

1.40   A possible effect is distinct from itself as actualized. (*See 1.36, 1.39*)

1.41   What explains a possible effect does not suffice to explain an actual effect. (*See 1.40*)

1.42   Production is intelligible but not deducible. (*See 1.02, 1.40, 1.41*)

1.43   An actual effect is produced by that which transcends, is outside the cause. (*See 1.41, 1.42*)

1.44   An actual effect is necessitated. (*See 1.36, 1.37, 1.41, 1.42, 1.43*)

1.45   An Actuality makes an effort to change in the face of insuperable obstacles. (*See 1.17, 1.18, 1.31*)

1.46   Man is the product of evolution. (*See 1.45*)

1.47   A man has self-identity. (*See 1.31*)

1.48   A man can discipline himself. (*See 1.47*)

1.49   A man can evaluate himself in terms not exemplified by him. (*See 1.47*)

1.50   A man has a self. (*See 1.47, 1.48, 1.49*)

1.51   A self is expressed as a life of a body. (*See 1.50*)

1.52   The self is immortal. (*See 1.48, 1.49, 1.50*)

1.53   Sometimes the self expresses itself as a mind. (*See 1.48, 1.49*)

1.54   The mind is not a body. (*See 1.53*)

1.55   The mind is not a function of the body. (*See 1.05, 1.51, 1.53, 1.54*)

1.56   The mind can encounter sensuous content. (*See 1.55*)

1.57 Perception yields content, which is in part sensuous, is judged and accepted, and may be believed. (*See 1.55, 1.56*)

1.58 Through perception an external world can be truly known. (*See 1.57*)

1.59 Perception involves the use of nonsensuous content. (*See 1.58*)

1.60 A perceived Actuality has a location, to be pointed to, indicated, not sensuously undergone. (*See 1.01, 1.58, 1.59*)

1.61 Perception involves the contemplation of a universal, distinct from but not alien to the sensuous. (*See 1.59*)

1.62 Indicateds and contemplateds are had as independent, but also as mutually pertinent. (*See 1.60, 1.61*)

1.63 The indicated and contemplated are aspects of the object veridically perceived. (*See 1.58, 1.62*)

1.64 Perception provides knowledge through a union of indicated and contemplated. (*See 1.62, 1.63*)

1.65 A perception is not identical with its object. (*See 1.56, 1.58, 1.63*)

1.66 While perceiving, we know that the perceived is not the real object. (*See 1.65*)

1.67 An Actuality is adumbrated when and as an indicated and contemplated are united in a judgment. (*See 1.56, 1.64*)

1.68 The adumbrated conveys knowledge. (*See 1.65–67*)

1.69 Perceptual content grounds generalizations, specifications, and other inferences. (*See 1.59*)

1.70 An idea has an empirical meaning if there is a perceptual contemplated from which the idea can be derived. (*See 1.69*)

1.71 The meaning of an idea is any other, perceptual or not, as qualified by that conceivable transformation which would convert it into the former. (*See 1.69, 1.70*)

1.72 An idea of something nonempirical can be transformed into an idea of something empirical by subjecting it to the conditions of experience. (*See 1.71*)

1.73 An idea of the empirical is transformable into an idea of the nonempirical by freeing it from the conditions of experience. (*See 1.72*)

1.74 What is independent of experience can be understood in terms of the empirical, and conversely. (*See 1.72, 1.73*)

1.75 Different types of transformation provide supplementary ways of defining the meaning of a given idea. (*See 1.71, 1.74*)

1.76 Memory reverses transformations produced by the passage of time. (*See 1.75*)

1.77 Expectation is a waiting for determinations for some idea. (*See 1.41, 1.76*)

1.78 Ideas can be imagined. (*See 1.73*)

1.79 Thinking is the act of transforming an idea or judgment into another. (*See 1.69*)

1.80 A sound inference is a thinking which terminates in the warranted qualification of an idea. (*See 1.79*)

1.81 Inference is governed by rules, conformity to which determines the warrant of a transferred or transformed qualification. (*See 1.80*)

1.82 All thinking exemplifies rules and terminates in necessitated conclusions. (*See 1.44, 1.80, 1.81*)

1.83 A particular conclusion has content, meaning, implications beyond that expressed in a general rule. (*See 1.41, 1.81, 1.82*)

1.84 A process of moving to a conclusion ends with what is not wholly predictable. (*See 1.41, 1.83*)

1.85 Premiss and rule together define only a possible conclusion. (*See 1.43, 1.83, 1.84*)

1.86 All inference is logically necessitated and creatively free. (*See 1.44, 1.82, 1.83, 1.85*)

1.87 All making is rational as well as creative. (*See 1.42, 1.86*)

1.88 To produce well is to engage in an art; to produce for an enjoyment which awakens an awareness of an adumbrated is to engage in a fine art. (*See 1.67, 1.87*)

1.89 Inquiry is a chain of inferences designed to reach a source of desired judgments or their elements. (*See 1.69, 1.77, 1.86*)

1.90 A science is an inquiry well conducted. (*See 1.88, 1.89*)

1.91 Philosophy is at once a science and an art. (*See 1.88, 1.90*)

1.92 Philosophy's method is speculative; i.e., it infers to presuppositions. Its argument is primarily dialectic; i.e., it infers to what would complete the already known. And its attitude is at once sympathetic and critical. (*See 1.91*)

1.93 Philosophy is a circular enterprise. (*See 1.91, 1.92*)

1.94 The essentials of any cognition are expressed in a category or principle embodied in whatever is apprehended. (*See 1.64, 1.75*)

1.95 The primary category is inescapable. (*See 1.94*)

1.96 The category embodies the law of contradiction. (*See 1.94, 1.95*)

1.97 The primary category must be applicable to the contingent as well as to the necessary. (*See 1.94, 1.95*)

1.98 The primary category must be applicable to the false as well as to the true. (*See 1.94, 1.95*)

1.99 The primary category must have at least two parts. (*See 1.96*)

1.100 The primary category must inwardly make reference to the content which it organizes. (*See 1.94, 1.95, 1.97*)

1.101 The parts of the category and the content for it must already exemplify it. (*See 1.94, 1.95*)

1.102 The category is a unity, representing an external unity in which its parts are embodied. (*See 1.65, 1.94, 1.95, 1.101*)

1.103 The category has four facets. (*See 1.01, 1.11–13, 1.99, 1.100, 1.102*)

1.104 The relations of the various guises which the category assumes are themselves cases of the category. (*See 1.97, 1.98, 1.101*)

1.105 An Actuality seeks to realize possibilities, and the Actuality which is man seeks to realize an all-inclusive possibility. (*See 1.11, 1.21, 1.47–50, 1.51*)

1.106 The all-inclusive possibility which man seeks and ought to realize is The Good. (*See 1.105*)

1.107 The Good is specified in the form of limited objectives which men sometimes consciously acknowledge and bodily realize. (*See 1.21, 1.106*)

1.108 Men have a freedom of preference. (*See 1.107*)

1.109 Men have a freedom of choice. (*See 1.107*)

1.110 Desire for The Good is good. (*See 1.106*)

1.111 The Good needs more realization than it gets from preference, choice, or desire. (*See 1.108, 1.109, 1.110*)

1.112 Men have a free will. (*See 1.20, 1.50, 1.111*)

1.113 The values of all beings should be maximized. (*See 1.14, 1.106, 1.111*)

1.114 No one can do only what is right. (*See 1.109, 1.113*)

1.115 No one can do only what is wrong. (*See 1.114*)

1.116 Men are necessarily guilty. (*See 1.106, 1.114*)

1.117 All rewards are undeserved. (*See 1.116*)

1.118 Men can do all the good that ought to be done if they can ultilize other powers besides their own. (*See 1.106, 1.116, 2.14, 2.69*)

Ideality

2.01 Whatever is possible must be internally coherent. (*See 1.11*)

2.02 Some possibilities are ingredient in, i.e., are idealizations of Actualities, Existence, and God. (*See 1.21, 1.25*)

2.03 A real possibility is what in fact can be. (*See 2.01, 2.02*)

2.04 Real possibilities have a being exterior to Actualities and whatever else there be. (*See 2.03*)

2.05 Real possibilities are relevant to other realities. (*See 1.21, 1.26, 2.03, 2.04*)

2.06 Real possibilities change in the course of time. (*See 2.05*)

2.07 Real possibilities form linkages. (*See 2.05, 2.06*)

2.08 Real possibilities are systematically connected. (*See 1.14, 2.05, 2.07*)

2.09 Real possibilities are relevant and realizable. (*See 2.03–6*)

2.10 The Good is a possibility which ought to be realized. (*See 1.106, 1.118, 2.09, 2.14*)

2.11 Real possibilities are to some extent internally indeterminate. (*See 2.03, 2.06, 2.07*)

2.12 The difference between the possible and the Actual, or any other reality, is not merely possible. (*See 2.11, 4.109*)

2.13 Real possibilities must be realized somehow and somewhere. (*See 2.03, 2.05, 2.10, 3.44*)

2.14 Normative possibilities must be satisfied by a being outside both them and Actualities. (*See 1.118, 2.10, 2.13, 3.109, 4.93*)

2.15 The Good is an all-inclusive possibility, or Ideal, as relevant to Actualities. (*See 1.106, 1.107, 2.10*)

2.16 The Ideal is incomplete. (*See 1.14, 1.15, 2.15*)

2.17 The Ideal presupposes Actualities. (*See 1.14, 1.15, 2.15, 2.16*)

2.18 The Ideal presupposes Existence. (*See 2.16, 2.96, 3.07, 3.104*)

2.19 The Ideal presupposes God. (*See 2.16, 2.97, 4.18, 4.89, 4.90*)

2.20 The Good's attempt to encompass all Actualities is qualified by the Ideal's need to keep abreast of Existence. (*See 1.26, 2.17, 2.18*)

2.21 The Good's attempt to encompass all Actualities is qualified by the Ideal's need to accommodate a divine intent. (*See 1.28, 2.17, 2.19, 2.20*)

2.22 The Ideal's effort to keep abreast of Existence occurs together with its effort to accommodate the intent of God and its effort to encompass all Actualities. (*See 2.18, 2.20, 2.21*)

2.23 The Good encompasses Actualities to some degree by making them desirous. (*See 1.29, 1.45, 1.110*)

2.24 The Good encompasses more of a man when it makes him into a being who prefers than it does when it makes him merely desirous. (*See 1.108, 2.23*)

2.25 The Good encompasses more of a man when it makes him into a being who chooses than it does when it makes him into a a being who prefers. (*See 1.109, 2.24*)

2.26 The Good encompasses more when it makes a man into a being who creatively wills than it does when it makes him into one who chooses. (*See 1.112, 2.25*)

2.27 It is good for the Good to be fulfilled. (*See 2.10, 2.26*)

2.28 Men, as forming a community, can encompass a wider range of goods than is possible in a group. (*See 2.27*)

2.29 A class is a group in whom the common character controls the activities of the members. (*See 2.27*)

2.30 There ought to be classes functioning on behalf of the community. (*See 2.28, 2.29*)

2.31 The community should contain a number of classes. (*See 2.30*)

2.32 A class of reasonable men is one whose members' grasp of causal processes and whose adjustments are accepted as representative by the rest. (*See 1.17, 1.43, 2.31*)

2.33 A class of prestigious men is one whose members' behavior, values, or standards of what is important are models for the rest. (*See 1.49, 2.31*)

2.34 The members of a class of empowered men have control of the might of a community. (*See 2.31*)

2.35 A mature community contains at least three harmonized classes of men. (*See 2.28, 2.31, 2.32–34*)

2.36 A model community makes provision for the good of men outside it. (*See 2.28, 2.35*)

2.37 Men are justified in claiming to have their natures preserved or enchanced. (*See 1.113*)

2.38 Each man makes a number of essential claims to have his nature preserved or enchanced. (*See 2.37*)

2.39 A native right is an essential claim defined in terms of others as required to satisfy it. (*See 2.38*)

2.40 A right denied is a right alienated, and entails the insistence on some having a stronger case because better able to satisfy a superior claim. (*See 2.38, 2.39*)

2.41 Not all rights can be justifiably alienated at any one time. (*See 2.40*)

2.42 Men with the same type of right may be in conflict. (*See 2.39*)

2.43 Men have the privilege of ordering and interrelating their native rights. (*See 2.39, 2.42*)

2.44 Men have the privilege of exercising every one of their rights. (*See 2.39, 2.41, 2.43*)

2.45 There is no privilege to exercise all rights at any one time. (*See 2.42, 2.44*)

2.46 Men have the privilege of alienating any of their specific rights. (*See 2.40, 2.44, 2.45*)

2.47 Men have the privilege of alienating all their specific rights. (*See 2.46*)

2.48 Men have the privilege of constituting a single unitary right. (*See 2.41, 2.47*)

2.49 Man's unitary right cannot be justly alienated. (*See 2.48*)

2.50 Man's unitary unalienable right is the right to benefit from social existence. (*See 2.45, 2.49*)

2.51 Society dictates in part which specific rights are to be satisfied, when they are, and how. (*See 2.29, 2.50*)

2.52 Society should satisfy a man's unitary right to benefit from social existence. (*See 2.50, 2.51*)

2.53 Society is justified in denying satisfaction to some rights. (*See* (*See 2.48, 2.51, 2.52*)

2.54 Civil rights are correlate with duties in others to do or forbear. (*See 1.109, 2.39, 2.48, 2.51*)

2.55 Rights are satisfied with the aid of a might outside themselves. (*See 2.51, 2.54*)

2.56 Might has the right to be preserved or enhanced. (*See 1.113, 2.37, 2.55*)

2.57 The right of might can be alienated only by might. (*See 2.56*)

2.58 The right of might can be justly alienated. (*See 2.40, 2.56, 2.57*)

2.59 Might has rights and duties in relation to men. (*See 2.54, 2.55*)

2.60 It is the sovereign duty of might to help man achieve an eventual satisfaction of his alienated rights. (*See 2.47, 2.48, 2.50, 2.59*)

2.61   Might must alienate its right. (*See 2.48, 2.57, 2.58, 2.60*)

2.62   Might should be divided just so far as this promotes the satisfaction of man's rights. (*See 2.55, 2.61*)

2.63   Each of the classes of a mature community satisfies part of man's unitary right. (*See 2.35, 2.48*)

2.64   The divisions of might should answer to the needs of three classes of men. (*See 2.35, 2.62*)

2.65   A political whole correlates self-divided might and the classes of a community. (*See 2.35, 2.64*)

2.66   A political whole has three essential organs. (*See 2.65*)

2.67   A state is a persistent political whole forcing classes and institutions into harmony. (*See 2.65, 2.66*)

2.68   A man ought to acquire the habit of functioning as a man should. (*See 1.106, 1.111, 1.113*)

2.69   Men should be taught virtue and be forced to act virtuously. (*See 1.118, 2.68*)

2.70   There is a natural law. (*See 2.69*)

2.71   Natural law is germane to all societies. (*See 2.36, 2.70*)

2.72   There ought to be a common law. (*See 2.70*)

2.73   There ought to be positive laws, public delcarations of what is to be done or avoided in a given society. (*See 2.71, 2.72*)

2.74   Positive laws threaten realizable punishments for violations. (*See 2.55, 2.69, 2.73*)

2.75   Positive laws are backed by might. (*See 2.55, 2.74*)

2.76   Positive laws should be expressed in an official language. (*See 2.34, 2.73*)

2.77   Positive laws should be impartial. (*See 2.73, 2.76*)

2.78   Positive laws ought to define a man's civil rights and duties. (*See 2.39, 2.51, 2.54*)

2.79   Positive laws require interpretation in relation to social power, social expectations, and social values. (*See 2.32, 2.33, 2.34*)

2.80   Judges interpret the law in a threefold way. (*See 2.79*)

2.81   A wise, creative judge guides his interpretations by universal natural law. (*See 2.71, 2.80*)

2.82   In the ideal state citizens are law-abiding and law-controlled, and guided by the interpretations of wise, creative judges. (*See 2.81*)

2.83   The Good is most completely publicly fulfilled in a perfect state, a state where all are wise, creative judges. (*See 2.27, 2.81, 2.82*)

2.84   The good in a state fails to encompass the ethical man. (*See 2.26, 2.83*)

2.85   The good in a state fails to encompass the aesthetic man. (*See 1.88, 2.84, 3.54*)

2.86   The good in a state fails to encompass the religious man. (*See 1.28, 2.84, 3.80, 4.96*)

2.87   The good in a state fails to encompass the speculative man. (*See 1.92, 2.84*)

2.88   Education is the art of reconstituting individuals so that the Good can be maximally achieved in and by them. (*See 2.51, 2.69, 2.84–7*)

2.89   Education should include discipline, the subordination of the individual to the group. (*See 2.72, 2.84, 2.88*)

2.90   Education should include training, the mastery of techniques. (*See 1.88, 2.73, 2.88*)

2.91   Education should include the art of civilizing, the acquisition of professional competence. (*See 2.69, 2.70, 2.85, 2.88*)

2.92   Education should include a mastering of values. (*See 2.71, 2.86, 2.88*)

2.93   Education should teach men to engage in the creative, intellectual mastery of the total Good, social and nonsocial. (*See 2.83, 2.87, 2.88*)

2.94   Liberal education should terminate in an understanding of the Ideal. (*See 1.92, 2.15–19, 2.85–87, 2.88, 2.93*)

2.95   The Ideal provides testimony to the reality of Actualities. (*See 1.11, 1.21, 2.17*)

2.96   The Ideal provides testimony that there is a real Existence. (*See 2.18, 3.07*)

2.97   The Ideal provides testimony that there is a God. (*See 2.14, 2.19, 4.18*)

2.98   The Ideal partly satisfies the needs of Actuality. (*See 1.14, 2.17, 2.95*)

2.99   The Ideal partly satisfies the needs of Existence. (*See 2.18, 2.96, 3.13, 3.104*)

2.100   The Ideal partly satisfies the needs of God. (*See 2.19, 2.97, 4.85*)

2.101   The Ideal provides Actualities with a desirable permanence. (*See 1.18, 2.98*)

2.102   The Ideal provides Existence with a desirable intelligibility. (*See 2.99*)

2.103   The Ideal provides God with a desirable relevance to what else there be. (*See 2.100*)

2.104   The Ideal, while guaranteeing the satisfaction of some needs of the other modes, fails to do full justice to any mode. (*See 2.22, 2.101–3*)

Existence

3.01   Existence is being, as engaged in the act of self-division. (*See 1.12, 2.96*)

3.02   Existence perpetually divides. (*See 3.01*)

3.03   The endless expansion of energy, towards which Existence tends, is restrained by Actuality, Ideality, and God. (*See 1.27, 2.20, 3.02, 4.91*)

3.04   The endless expansion of time, towards which Existence tends, is restrained by Actuality, Ideality, and God. (*See 3.03, 3.103–5*)

3.05   The endless expansion of space, towards which Existence tends, is restrained by Actuality, Ideality, and God. (*See 1.09, 3.03, 3.04, 3.103–5*)

3.06   Existence as separated from Actualities is their spatial field. (*See 1.09, 1.12, 3.05*)

3.07 Existence as separated from the Ideal is its causal ground. (*See 1.39, 2.99, 3.04*)

3.08 Existence as separated from God is his cosmic vitality. (*See 3.05, 3.105, 4.86*)

3.09 From the perspective of Actualities, Existence is that which makes them contemporaries. (*See 1.27, 3.06*)

3.10 From the perspective of the Ideal, Existence is that which adds implications to those derivable from what is merely possible. (*See 2.96, 3.07*)

3.11 From the perspective of God, Existence is the power to make something become, by making others pass away, and conversely. (*See 3.08*)

3.12 From the perspective of Existence, Actualities are focal points, the Ideal is future, and God is essence. (*See 3.06, 3.07, 3.08*)

3.13 The failure of Actuality, Ideality, and God to do full justice to one another imposes a burden on Existence. (*See 1.14, 2.20, 2.98, 2.99, 2.104*)

3.14 Existence is unified by the other three modes. (*See 2.21, 3.09–11, 3.13*)

3.15 Existence is intelligible. (*See 2.102, 3.10*)

3.16 "Existence" is a predicate. (*See 1.67, 2.12, 3.15*)

3.17 "Existence" is predicable of every idea and predicate. (*See 1.67, 1.80, 3.16*)

3.18 To know an idea is not yet to know the career it has. (*See 3.10, 3.17*)

3.19 The features of beings are involved in careers not identical with those they have as part of a mind. (*See 1.63, 1.65, 3.16, 3.18*)

3.20 The passage from what is in mind to the object known goes through Existence. (*See 1.65, 1.67, 3.01, 3.19*)

3.21 Predication produces a change in the meaning of the predicate. (*See 1.70, 3.19, 3.20*)

3.22 Attributes are altered by being abstracted from objects. (*See 1.70, 3.21*)

3.23   The perceived is contemporary with the perceiver. (*See 1.57–60, 3.22*)

3.24   What is in the mind tests what is in the body, and conversely. (*See 1.70, 1.74, 3.21, 3.22*)

3.25   A claim to truth is vindicatable if a consequence in mind is abstractable from a consequence in nature in a predesignatable way. (*See 1.67, 3.22, 3.24*)

3.26   A vindicatable claim to know the Ideal, Existence, or God requires a capacity to repeat the methods by which we obtained our initial knowledge of them. (*See 1.73, 3.25*)

3.27   A unique characterization is not an attribute. (*See 3.19, 3.21, 3.22*)

3.28   A "collective" disjunction is distinct from a "distributive" disjunction. (*See 2.14, 3.18, 3.20*)

3.29   An "extensional" conjunction is distinct from an "intensional" conjunction. (*See 3.18, 3.20*)

3.30   A negation in thought is distinct from a rejection in fact. (*See 3.18, 3.20*)

3.31   Formal implications are distinct from material implications. (*See 3.10, 3.18, 3.20*)

3.32   Inferences and processes are distinct. (*See 1.43, 1.86, 1.87, 3.31*)

3.33   Inference makes a difference to what is formally implied. (*See 1.83, 1.84, 1.86*)

3.34   Inference is an art in which one risks replacing a satisfactory premiss by an unsatisfactory conclusion. (*See 1.82, 3.33*)

3.35   Processes add to what is materially implied. (*See 1.87, 3.31–33*)

3.36   Formal implications and processes are not necessarily in accord. (*See 3.31–35*)

3.37   Each Actuality has its own Existence. (*See 1.22, 3.08, 3.09*)

3.38   Existence makes Actualities concordantly effective. (*See 1.27, 3.09, 3.37*)

3.39   Existence makes Actualities determinate. (*See 1.08, 3.09, 3.38*)

3.40   Actualities can lose their Existence. (*See 3.37*)

3.41   Facts are realities de-existentialized. (*See 1.10, 3.39, 3.40*)

3.42   Passing away is the conversion of an Actuality into a fact. (*See 3.41*)

3.43   The past is a tissue of facts. (*See 2.13, 3.41, 3.42*)

3.44   Nothing occurs in the past. (*See 3.38, 3.41, 3.43*)

3.45   Remembering is a present act. (*See 1.76, 3.44*)

3.46   Subsequent occurrences provide the past with new settings. (*See 3.44*)

3.47   The past is necessarily related to the present. (*See 3.42, 3.46, 4.17*)

3.48   To say "x existed" is to say that the Existence which x's fact had co-ordinate with it is co-ordinate with a present fact. (*See 3.37, 3.47*)

3.49   To reach Actualities as they are in themselves, they must be freed from the qualifications produced by Existence and other modes of being. (*See 1.19, 1.25, 2.02, 3.10, 3.38*)

3.50   The prescinding of qualities is a desirable dislocation. (*See 3.10, 3.22, 3.49*)

3.51   A dislocation of the natures of Actualities is desirable. (*See 1.07, 3.49, 3.50*)

3.52   The Ideal component in an Actuality should be dislocated, and conversely. (*See 1.21, 2.95, 3.49, 3.50*)

3.53   The divine component in an Actuality should be dislocated, and conversely. (*See 1.23, 3.49, 3.50, 4.95*)

3.54   Knowledge and art provide new carriers for freed Actualities, their qualities and natures. (*See 1.64, 1.88, 1.94, 3.49–51*)

3.55   Myth provides a new carrier for freed Ideals. (*See 3.50, 3.52, 3.54*)

3.56   Sacraments provide new carriers for a freed divine component. (*See 3.53, 3.54*)

3.57   Criticism is the establishment of the import of freed items as carried by new media. (*See 3.54–56*)

3.58   Maximal freedom from nonessential qualifications by Existence, objective and human, is achieved through epitomization. (*See 3.49, 3.54–57*)

3.59 Existence is made integral to and thus specified by Actualities when and as they change in state and position. (*See 1.31, 1.32, 3.37, 3.39, 3.48*)

3.60 Existence imposes a limit on what Actualities and other realities can do, and do with it. (*See 1.06, 3.01, 3.06–8, 3.59*)

3.61 At any moment beings are at different stages of typical careers. (*See 3.59*)

3.62 Attention has a temporal span. (*See 3.59*)

3.63 No evidence can be provided to show that nothing endures. (*See 3.59, 3.62*)

3.64 Evidence that beings are of different ages can be judged untrustworthy only if there is a truth more basic than that some beings are older than others. (*See 3.61, 3.63*)

3.65 Knowledge of the past is inferentially derived from present evidence that some Actualities have different ages, and thus had origins at different dates. (*See 1.76, 3.44, 3.46, 3.64*)

3.66 A history is reconstructive. (*See 3.65*)

3.67 Historic occurrences have significant beginnings and endings. (*See 1.43, 3.04*)

3.68 The beginning of an historic occurrence is relevant to its end. (*See 1.37, 3.67*)

3.69 History provides explanations of facts in terms of transformations produced by Existence. (*See 1.76, 3.65, 3.66, 3.68*)

3.70 Historic occurrences have different temporal spans. (*See 3.67, 3.68*)

3.71 There are unit measures for the historic past. (*See 3.43, 3.70*)

3.72 There are no determinate historic occurrences in the present. (*See 3.70, 3.71*)

3.73 Incompleted historic occurrences are grounded in the present. (*See 3.72*)

3.74 Every historic occurrence must be at least two moments long. (*See 3.67, 3.71, 3.72*)

3.75 An historic field contains a number of occurrences not related in sequence. (*See 3.74*)

3.76 An epoch is a field of works of art, structured by myth, and sacramentally unified. (*See 3.54–56*)

3.77 A civilization is a field containing great men, given direction by an ethical norm, and unified by a religion. (*See 3.58, 3.76*)

3.78 The men of a given civilization constitute a people. (*See 3.77*)

3.79 A guided people make up the body of a civilization whose nature is defined primarily by great men. (*See 3.77*)

3.80 A religious people make up the body of a civilization whose nature is defined primarily by a religion. (*See 2.86, 3.77*)

3.81 An ethical people make up the body of a civilization whose nature is defined primarily by an ethical ideal. (*See 3.55, 3.77*)

3.82 There are three types of civilization. (*See 3.79–81*)

3.83 A people exhausts its being and meaning in a civilization. (*See 3.78*)

3.84 A people's potentialities are not exhausted in a civilization. (*See 3.43, 3.78, 3.83*)

3.85 A people has a nature not exhausted in a civilization. (*See 3.73, 3.83, 3.84*)

3.86 A people has an organic unity not exhausted in a civilization. (*See 3.83, 3.84, 3.85*)

3.87 A people faces a standard not exhausted in a civilization. (*See 3.81, 3.83*)

3.88 Civilizations are comparable because there are principles which apply to all. (*See 3.84–87*)

3.89 Great men provide universal principles measuring the creative energies of a people and a civilization. (*See 3.58, 3.76, 3.79, 3.88*)

3.90 A religion provides a measure of the purity of a people and a civilization. (*See 3.80, 3.88*)

3.91 Ethical ideals provide a measure of the moral worth of a people and a civilization. (*See 3.81, 3.88*)

3.92 Peoples and civilizations have hovering natures, unities, and values exhausted only in a longer history. (*See 3.46, 3.73, 3.85–87, 3.89–91*)

3.93 The whole of history, and derivatively any people, may be unfulfilled, fail to be actualized maximally. (*See 1.47, 3.85, 3.88*)

3.94 The whole of history, and derivatively any people, may be incoherent, fail to be unified maximally. (*See 2.14, 3.86, 3.90, 3.93*)

3.95 The whole of history, and derivatively any people, may not be wholly good, because it fails to be idealized maximally. (*See 2.15, 3.87, 3.91*)

3.96 From the perspective of Actuality, the whole of Existence is only potentially excellent. (*See 3.09, 3.93*)

3.97 From the perspective of the Ideal, the whole of Existence is not wholly rational. (*See 3.10, 3.95*)

3.98 From the perspective of God, the whole of Existence is incoherent. (*See 3.11, 3.94*)

3.99 Actuality, the Ideal, and God are deficient from the perspective of Existence. (*See 3.12*)

3.100 Existence provides testimony to the reality of Actualities. (*See 1.27, 3.06, 3.12*)

3.101 Existence provides testimony to the reality of the Ideal. (*See 2.96, 3.12*)

3.102 Existence provides testimony to the reality of God. (*See 3.01, 3.14, 4.21, 4.86*)

3.103 Existence partly satisfies the needs of Actualities. (*See 1.14, 3.12, 3.40, 3.41, 3.100*)

3.104 Existence partly satisfies the needs of the Ideal. (*See 2.99, 3.07, 3.12, 3.101*)

3.105 Existence partly satisfies the needs of God. (*See 1.15, 3.04, 3.102, 4.86*)

3.106 Existence supplements the contributions other modes make to one another. (*See 1.14, 1.25, 2.20, 2.104, 3.13, 3.103–5*)

3.107 The Ideal relates Existence and Actuality. (*See 2.101, 2.102, 3.40*)

3.108 Actuality relates Existence and the Ideal. (*See 3.40, 3.107*)

3.109 Existence relates the Ideal and Actualities. (*See 3.01, 3.107–8*)

3.110 A "proof" of a mode of being involves the use of the other three modes. (*See 3.100–102, 3.107–9, 4.12, 4.56*)

God

4.01 Each mode of being is ingredient in the others. (*See 1.15, 1.25, 2.98–100, 3.60, 3.100–102*)

4.02 Each mode of being needs the others. (*See 1.14, 4.01*)

4.03 Each mode of being seeks to adjust itself to others. (*See 1.24, 1.25, 2.98–100, 3.103–5*)

4.04 Each mode of being partly satisfies the others. (*See 1.118, 2.98–100, 3.103–5, 4.02, 4.03*)

4.05 Each mode of being imposes a burden on every other. (*See 1.14, 2.21, 2.104, 3.13, 3.106*)

4.06 Each mode of being provides testimony to the reality of the others. (*See 1.11–13, 2.95–97, 3.100–102*)

4.07 Each mode of being provides both direct and indirect testimony to the reality of others. (*See 4.06*)

4.08 Each mode of being relates two other modes of being. (*See 3.107–9*)

4.09 A being is related to another by a third in a primary and a secondary way. (*See 4.07, 4.08*)

4.10 Each mode of being enables one to hold any other apart from the rest. (*See 1.82, 4.08, 4.09*)

4.11 Each mode of being permits of the detachment of a directly or indirectly originative being. (*See 4.10*)

4.12 A "proof" of a mode of being begins with testimony, acknowledges a relation, and terminates in the being. (*See 1.80–86, 3.110, 4.06–11*)

4.13 There are three basic and six subordinate testimonies for, relations to, and terminations in God. (*See 4.07–12*)

4.14 Teleological testimony offers evidence requiring God for its explanation. (*See 4.06, 4.07*)

4.15 A substantival teleology begins with primary Actualities offering direct testimony to the reality of God as their Absolute Other. (*See 1.08, 1.14, 1.16, 1.23*)

4.16 A rationalistic teleology begins with universals offering indirect testimony to a God concerned with the Ideal. (*See 1.16, 1.26, 2.19, 4.07, 4.15*)

4.17 An historical teleology begins with facts offering indirect testimony to a God concerned with Existence. (*See 3.41, 3.47, 3.102*)

4.18 A moralistic teleology begins with normative possibilities, directly testifying to an evaluating God. (*See 2.13, 2.14*)

4.19 A directional teleology begins with realizable possibilities which indirectly testify to a temporally oriented God. (*See 2.09, 2.13, 3.94, 4.18*)

4.20 A providential teleology begins with a cosmic possibility which indirectly testifies to a purposing God. (*See 2.18, 3.07*)

4.21 An architectural teleology begins with unified Existence as providing direct testimony to the reality of an effective God. (*See 3.01, 3.03, 3.102*)

4.22 A mathematical teleology begins with phenomenalized Existence as offering indirect testimony to the reality of a cosmic God. (*See 1.09, 1.12, 1.22, 3.102, 4.17*)

4.23 A structuralized teleology begins with idealized Existence as providing indirect testimony to an ordering God. (*See 2.99, 4.20*)

4.24 There can be no teleological proofs of God. (*See 1.81, 4.12*)

4.25 There are three primary and six cosmological approaches to God. (*See 1.81, 4.09*)

4.26 A formal cosmological approach to God relates some mode of being to him by means of the formal structure of possibility. (*See 4.12, 4.25*)

4.27 A devotional cosmological approach to God relates some mode of being to him by means of an individualized structure of possibility. (*See 4.25, 4.26*)

4.28   A naturalistic cosmological approach to God relates some mode of being to him by means of an existentialized structure of possibility. (*See 2.18, 3.03, 3.104, 4.25, 4.26*)

4.29   An individualized cosmological approach to God relates some mode of being to him by means of the structure of Actuality. (*See 4.12, 4.16, 4.25*)

4.30   An institutionalized cosmological approach to God relates some mode of being to him by means of the structure of Actuality when qualified by Ideality. (*See 2.16, 2.17, 4.25, 4.29*)

4.31   A worshipful cosmological approach to God relates some mode of being to him by means of the structure of Actuality when qualified by Existence. (*See 3.38, 4.25, 4.30*)

4.32   A materialistic cosmological approach to God relates some mode of being to him by means of the structure of Existence. (*See 3.02, 3.03–5, 3.15, 4.25, 4.30*)

4.33   An idealized cosmological approach to God relates some mode of being to him by means of the structure of Existence when qualified by Ideality. (*See 3.104, 4.23, 4.28, 4.32*)

4.34   An historical cosmological approach to God relates some mode of being to him by means of the structure of Existence when qualified by Actualities. (*See 4.22, 4.31, 4.32*)

4.35   There can be no cosmological proofs of God. (*See 1.81, 4.12, 4.24*)

4.36   Teleological and cosmological approaches to God are supplementary. (*See 4.24, 4.35*)

4.37   A conjunction of teleological and cosmological approaches cannot provide a proof of God. (*See 4.12, 4.36*)

4.38   A proof of God requires an act of ontological detachment of him from the structure of the proof. (*See 1.86, 1.87, 4.10–12, 4.37*)

4.39   There can be no ontological proofs of God. (*See 1.14, 4.12, 4.36, 4.38*)

4.40   There are three pure and six qualified modes of detaching God from a cosmological rule which begins with testimony to his existence. (*See 4.11, 4.38*)

4.41 The existence of God can be logically inferred. (*See 1.80–86, 4.40*)

4.42 The existence of God can be accepted through an intellectual assent qualified by the self. (*See 4.40, 4.41*)

4.43 The existence of God can be acknowledged through an intellectual assent qualified by Existence. (*See 3.104, 4.40, 4.41*)

4.44 God can be reached through faith. (*See 4.40*)

4.45 God can be reached through prayer, a faith qualified by possibility. (*See 2.103, 4.27, 4.40, 4.44*)

4.46 God can be reached through humility, a faith qualified by Exitence. (*See 3.103, 4.31, 4.40, 4.44*)

4.47 God can be reached through work. (*See 4.40*)

4.48 God can be reached through good works. (*See 2.86, 2.99, 4.47*)

4.49 God can be reached through dedicated work. (*See 2.102, 4.47*)

4.50 Teleological and ontological approaches to God are supplementary. (*See 4.24, 4.38, 4.39*)

4.51 Cosmological and ontological approaches to God are supplementary. (*See 4.35, 4.38, 4.39*)

4.52 A proof of God begins teleologically, is validated cosmologically, and terminates ontologically. (*See 4.12, 4.50, 4.51*)

4.53 There are nine basic ways of proving God's existence through faith. (*See 4.15, 4.18, 4.21, 4.26, 4.29, 4.32, 4.44*)

4.54 There are nine basic ways of proving God's existence through a logical inference. (*See 4.15, 4.18, 4.21, 4.26, 4.29, 4.32, 4.41*)

4.55 There are nine basic ways of proving God's existence through work. (*See 4.15, 4.18, 4.21, 4.26, 4.29, 4.32, 4.47*)

4.56 All proofs of God are circular and question-begging. (*See 4.41, 4.52, 4.53–55*)

4.57 A proof of God is satisfying only so far as God is encountered in other ways as well. (*See 1.84, 1.87, 3.34, 3.54, 4.56*)

4.58 God's nature, as apart from proof, includes all that has been truly testified regarding him. (*See 4.15–23, 4.24, 4.57*)

4.59 God's nature, as apart from proof, includes whatever is known of him through the agency of a systematic dialectic. (*See 1.14, 1.23, 1.92, 2.19, 3.99*)

4.60   Our most adequate idea of God is self-engendered. (*See 1.52, 1.74, 4.15, 4.57, 4.58, 4.59*)

4.61   Theoanalysis is the art of dealing with other realities in theological terms. (*See 1.13, 1.73, 2.14, 2.19, 2.97*)

4.62   In theoanalytic terms, Actualities are God's self-identity endlessly multiplied and combined. (*See 1.47, 1.96, 4.61*)

4.63   In theoanalytic terms, the Ideal is all-encompassing. (*See 2.100, 4.61*)

4.64   In theoanalytic terms, Existence is creativity. (*See 3.11, 4.61*)

4.65   God's nature, mind, and expression are one with the being, knowledge, and creation of all there is. (*See 4.62–64*)

4.66   God internally reproduces other modes of being. (*See 4.62, 4.65*)

4.67   God has a direct awareness of exterior Actualities. (*See 4.15, 4.66*)

4.68   God has an indirect awareness of Actualities in relation to the Ideal. (*See 1.118, 2.21, 4.16, 4.63*)

4.69   God has an indirect awareness of Actualities in relation to Existence. (*See 3.41, 4.17, 4.67–68*)

4.70   God has a direct awareness of a normative Ideal. (*See 2.09, 2.14, 2.100, 4.18*)

4.71   God has an indirect awareness of the Ideal in relation to Actualities. (*See 2.13, 3.92, 4.19, 4.70*)

4.72   God has an indirect awareness of the Ideal in relation to Existence. (*See 2.13, 4.20, 4.28, 4.70*)

4.73   God has a direct awareness of an extensive Existence. (*See 4.21, 4.65, 4.66*)

4.74   God has an indirect awareness of Existence in relation to Actualities. (*See 3.100, 4.22, 4.73*)

4.75   God has an indirect awareness of Existence in relation to the Ideal. (*See 4.23, 4.73, 4.74*)

4.76   God is omnipotently omniscient, providential, and self-expressive. (*See 4.66, 4.67, 4.70, 4.73*)

4.77   Actualities relate God's reproductions to the objects of his awareness. (*See 1.67, 4.29, 4.66, 4.67–75, 4.76*)

4.78   The Ideal relates God's reproductions to the objects of his awareness. (*See 4.26, 4.67–75, 4.76*)

4.79   Existence relates God's reproductions to the objects of his awareness. (*See 3.37, 4.32, 4.67–75, 4.76*)

4.80   God arrives at the other three modes of being through the agency of love. (*See 4.10, 4.44*)

4.81   God arrives at the other three modes of being through the agency of divine understanding. (*See 4.10, 4.41*)

4.82   God arrives at the other three modes of being through the agency of grace. (*See 4.10, 4.47*)

4.83   Beginning with God, there are nine primary ways of proving the existence of each mode of being. (*See 4.08, 4.53–56, 4.67, 4.70, 4.73, 4.77–82*)

4.84   God needs and makes use of Actualities. (*See 1.14, 2.86, 4.15, 4.60*)

4.85   God needs and makes use of the Ideal. (*See 2.100, 2.103, 3.106, 4.18, 4.60*)

4.86   God needs and makes use of Existence. (*See 3.08, 3.102, 3.105, 4.21, 4.60*)

4.87   God preserves Actualities (*See 4.17, 4.62, 4.66, 4.84*)

4.88   God preserves whatever excellencies can be obtained from Actualities. (*See 4.69, 4.87*)

4.89   God establishes the Ideal as a perpetual standard of value. (*See 2.19, 2.21, 2.100, 3.92, 4.70, 4.85*)

4.90   God provides the Ideal with satisfying Actualities and Existence. (*See 1.118, 2.14, 2.21, 2.22, 2.99, 2.104, 3.104, 4.85, 4.89*)

4.91   God unifies Existence. (*See 3.01, 3.08, 4.73, 4.86*)

4.92   God eternalizes Existence as his private extensionality. (*See 3.03–5, 4.66, 4.91*)

4.93 God supplements the work performed by any pair of modes on behalf of a third. (*See 2.14, 2.21, 2.104, 3.12–14, 3.106, 4.84–92*)

4.94 Each mode completes work God should do on behalf of the other modes. (*See 3.14, 3.106, 4.05, 4.93*)

4.95 All the modes of being merge with the being which is God. (*See 4.01, 4.60*)

4.96 A religious man seeks God as apart from him, convinced that the search will be successful. (*See 1.28, 2.86, 4.15, 4.40, 4.53, 4.55, 4.95*)

4.97 The search for God is provoked by evil, tragedy, sorrow, pain. (*See 4.88, 4.96*)

4.98 God can be sought and found anywhere. (*See 4.14, 4.95, 4.96*)

4.99 The search for God can never come to an absolute end. (*See 4.53–55, 4.58, 4.59, 4.95, 4.97*)

4.100 God reaches to and finds every other being. (*See 4.67–75, 4.80–83, 4.95*)

4.101 God and men are related in a common field. (*See 4.15, 4.67, 4.95, 4.99–100*)

4.102 The mystic traverses the field he constitutes with God. (*See 4.98, 4.101*)

4.103 God completes the work of man. (*See 1.118, 2.13, 2.14, 3.92, 3.94, 4.93*)

4.104 Trust is the belief that what man takes to be good is good in God's sight. (*See 4.90, 4.97, 4.103*)

4.105 Ethics and peremptory religion make independent demands. (*See 1.118, 4.104*)

4.106 Scientific and religious claims are independent. (*See 1.90, 4.97, 4.105*)

4.107 Psychology and religion are grounded in independent attitudes. (*See 1.50, 4.99, 4.105*)

4.108 A proper adjudication requires neutrality. (*See 4.105–7*)

4.109 A genuinely neutral treatment of what is the case is at once prescriptive and descriptive of all the modes. (*See 4.56, 4.108*)

Index

achievements of, 458; action of, 16, 123, 186, 225, 290, 336; affected by Actuality, 270, 296, 304, 342, 356, 357, 377, 533, 537, 538; affected by future, 125, 297; affected by God, 296, 356, 537; affected by Ideal, 304, 356, 357, 537, 538; analytic components of, 199; and Actualities, 16, 18, 128, 186, 223, 234, 284, 340, 367, 444, 445, 452, 453, 457, 467, 468, 477, 487, 529, 533, 534, 537; and art, 236; and category, 93, 193, 198; and essence, 114; and facts, 225, 230; and field, 33; and future, 122–25 *passim*, 297, 328, 475; and God, 16, 180, 291, 326, 350, 474; and history, 252, 263, 268; and Ideal, 16, 120, 121, 122, 180, 182, 221, 270, 369, 420, 421, 444, 467, 469, 488; and individual, 52, 180, 290; and knowledge, 205; and logic, 194, 325; and man, 16; and mind, 205; and motion, 38; and other modes, 187, 374; and past, 226; and perception, 200; and possibility, 200; and self, 52; and space, 119; and The Good, 14, 335, 445, 467, 468, 478; and time, 119; effect of, 197, 230; effect on Actuality, 178, 184, 192, 232, 241, 273, 534; effect on God, 184, 235, 539, 540; effect on Ideal, 184, 191, 194, 273, 535, 536; effect on men, 96
— a perfection, 308; as carrier, 234, 546; as destructive, 183; as detaching, 309; as energizing, 343; as field, 33, 123, 296, 343, 351; as medium, 208, 546; as a mode of being, 190; as norm, 540; as phenomenon, 296, 304; as relation, 283, 345, 489; as supplementary, 273, 468; as temporal, 343; as terminus, 284; being of, 185, 191, 296, 336; boundaries of, 185, 196, 356, 537; burdens of, 123, 124, 181, 182, 184, 196, 273, 280; career of, 231, 268; category of, 93, 193, 198, 530; changing, 231, 350; continuity of, 189, 192, 224, 274, 303, 537; con-

trol by, 125, 193, 197; control of, 122, 183, 188, 194, 202, 357; correlative of, 441; cosmic, 295, 303; creativity of, 335, 486; curvature of, 189; defects of, 268, 269, 289, 353, 419; derivatives from, 27, 262; direction of, 122, 181, 184, 186, 191, 197, 271, 272, 297, 535, 537, 538; disjunction in, 214; distortion of, 189, 190; division of, 119, 182, 186, 187, 188, 192, 196, 198, 241, 270, 274, 295, 332, 343, 344; energy of, 121, 269, 481; epitomized, 254, 257, 263, 463; essence of, 14, 184, 186, 187, 197, 198, 199, 271, 295, 355, 357, 468, 475, 492, 537; eternalized, 186, 192, 355, 493; evaluated, 341, 466; extended, 189, 217, 270, 351, 488, 538; existence of, 190, 241; expansion of, 303, 350, 537, 538; failures of, 196, 357, 363; force of, 534; freed, 253, 545; from other perspectives, 172, 193, 268, 335, 336; fulfillment of, 343, 466; geometry of, 33, 296, 328, 342, 475; Ideal in, 126, 253, 264, 268, 274, 377, 467; idealized, 105, 297, 416, 475; idea of, 194, 241; identity of, 231, 241, 537; implications of, 195, 250, 268; in Actuality, 52, 190, 192, 195, 223, 224, 231, 242; incoherence of, 269, 467; in God, 189, 192, 195, 205, 223, 242, 254, 350, 378; in Ideal, 191, 223, 242; in ideas, 241; in itself, 198; in other modes, 188, 197, 202, 270; in present, 11, 297; in proof, 286, 308; in relation to Actuality, 119, 123, 182, 186, 190, 193, 274, 342; in relation to God, 182, 183, 191, 196, 197, 274, 342; in relation to Ideal, 119, 194, 274, 342; in relation to other modes, 443, 444; intelligibility of, 182, 185, 191, 198, 199, 297, 346, 357, 441, 446; in others, 33, 189, 191, 218; irreducibility of, 180, 185, 446; irregularity of, 270; knowledge of, 185, 194, 198, 199, 211, 446; language appropriate to, 278; laws of, 188, 194, 195, 217, 242, 245, 301, 537;

200; facts in, 227; historic, 250, 461; magnitude of, 460; moving, 230, 536; sequence of, 220; "specious," 458; units in, 250

Prescinding, act of, 455

Preservation, 36, 136, 137, 146, 182, 314, 359, 491

Pressure: social, 159, 161

Presuppositions: 23, 85, 511; daily, 82; inference to, 82, 409; knowledge of, 81; minimum, 9; of Actuality, 327; of Existence, 326, 327; of God, 325, 326; of good, 172; of inference, 325; of modes, 15; of possibility, 327; of proof, 275, 276, 325, 327, 349; of thought, 81; search for, 81

Priests, 133, 317

Principles: 5, 82, 85, 158, 265, 464; of Perfection, 122, 124, 126; universal, 262, 264, 373, 410, 476

Principia Mathematica, 201, 212

Privacy, 10, 30, 37, 46, 49, 52, 62, 145, 146, 172, 330, 452, 462

Privilege, 140–52 *passim*, 426, 427

Probability, 5, 61, 83, 221, 396, 520

Process: 197, 218; and cause, 44; and implication, 220, 221; and rules, 76, 77, 78; awareness of, 69; causal, 188, 423, 452; dialectical, 84; freedom of, 45, 408; intelligibility of, 451; of inference, 300; philosophy, 121; rationale of, 89; regular, 296; structure of, 451; time in, 220, 221; types of, 541

Procreation: human, 47

Production: 22, 41, 218, 396, 397, 408, 456; and desire, 100; and laws, 43, 44; and universals, 43; of consequences, 194; creative, 457; deductibility of, 43, 44; evaluation, 457; free, 44, 45; good, 78; human, 238; immediacy of, 44; intelligibility of, 43; limits of, 45; of facts, 226; types of, 541

Productivity, 197, 331, 397

Professions, 175, 439

Progress, 261, 294

Prohibition amendment, 162

Projection, 207

Prometheus: myth of, 235

Promise, 57, 96, 136

Proof: 240, 284, 358; and longing, 359; as introduction, 327; beginning of, 179, 275, 276, 285, 311, 318, 473, 479, 482; by faith, 319, 320, 321, 483; by fire, 309; by God, 344, 347, 351, 361; by inference, 483; by work, 323, 483; circularity of, 324, 329, 349, 484; confessional, 320; cosmological, 305, 478; daily, 324; data for, 319; detachment in, 285, 316; ending of, 275, 276, 285, 311, 328, 482; existential, 323; humanistic, 322; incompleteness of, 348; intellectual, 285, 312; legitimacy of, 310; locus of, 312; logical, 286, 309, 321, 476; modes in, 285, 327, 348, 349, 469; nature of, 179, 285, 299; need for, 179, 306; number of, 348; of God, 202, 271, 287, 289, 305, 319, 358; of modes, 179, 275, 276, 282, 298, 326, 347, 348, 469, 473, 490, 517, 518; ontological, 308, 479; parts of, 319; personalized, 476; philosophical, 321, 322; plurality of, 476; practical, 324; presuppositions of, 275, 276, 325, 327, 349; question-begging, 484; rational, 322; religious, 320, 323; routes of, 285, 311; sacramental, 324; satisfactory, 327, 476; structure of, 305, 306, 319, 320, 327, 473, 479; subordinate, 222; teleological, 288, 297, 476; terminus of, 179, 284, 319, 473, 482; theological, 321; traversal in, 285; utility of, 329, 349; valid, 473, 480, 482; value of, 328

Property: right to, 139

Prophecy, 291

Prophets, 133, 253, 255, 257, 274, 344

Propositions, 85, 201, 203, 216, 285, 307, 310, 450, 451

Prospects, 11, 109, 114, 126, 191, 341

Prosperity, 168, 169

Providence, 107, 125, 197, 295, 311, 328, 343, 344, 345, 350, 377, 489